1993

Canada's Health Care System: Bordering on the Possible

Canada's Health Care System:
Bordering on the Possible

by Jane Fulton, PhD

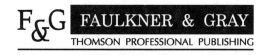

Faulkner & Gray, Inc., New York
Healthcare Information Center, Washington DC

ISBN 1-881393-08-9

The sponsoring editor was Luci S. Koizumi; production
director was Susan Namovicz-Peat; project editor was
Amy Kilgallon Lee; indexed by L. Pilar Wyman.

Published by Faulkner & Gray's
Healthcare Information Center

1133 Fifteenth Street, NW
Washington DC 20005

PRINTED IN THE UNITED STATES OF AMERICA

DEDICATION

This book is dedicated to my parents, Margaret and Blair Fulton, who demonstrate in their lives the true meaning of health and who continue to share the joy of living with their friends and our family across Canada.

ACKNOWLEDGEMENTS

I would like to acknowledge the energy of my research assistant, Amy Fraser, who devoted herself to the development of the book and its readability. Dr. Ralph Sutherland agreed to the use of portions of the jointly authored text *Health Care in Canada* and offered valuable information and criticism. Diane Fontaine managed the word processing while the editors at Faulkner & Gray polished the text. I would especially like to acknowledge the enthusiasm of my editor, Luci Koizumi, for making this book a reality. Any remaining errors or omissions are mine.

I live on a small farm in the Ottawa Valley. I would like to thank my four daughters Jean, Amy, Sarah, and Lila for managing the farm — haying, shearing sheep, spraying for potato beetles, feeding pigs, canning and freezing, and cutting firewood for the winter — during the months I needed to prepare this book. They were cheerful throughout. I would also like to thank my parents for taking us all on a hiking holiday in the Assiniboine when the book was done.

PROLOGUE

Americans' interest toward the Canadian health care system has become more and more evident during the last ten years. This is no surprise. Many authors have recently described how universal access on equal terms and conditions, has kept overall costs in Canada more or less in line with the growth of national income, rather than eating up a steadily increasing share of it as in the United States.

Before 1971, health care costs consumed a virtually identical share of national income, roughly 7.5 percent, in both the United States and Canada. This share rose steadily, stabilizing at 8.6 percent in Canada for 1987, compared with an estimate of 11 percent in the United States for that same year. By 1992, Canadian consumption of GNP had risen to 9 percent for health care, while U.S. estimates exceeded 12 percent.

As Evans and his co-authors state in *The New England Journal of Medicine* (March, 1990): "The large and growing gap between the United States and Canada drives home the point that, for good or ill, the form of funding adopted by Canada does permit a society to control its overall outlays on health care. Furthermore, it is unnecessary to impose financial barriers to access in the process."

The authors recognize, on the other hand, that such a system, although successful in general, can be a "bruising political process, producing much sound and fury."

Health care is a complex process, with less than full agreement about causes of illness, treatment choices, and expected outcomes. The organization of systems to support health through health care is also plagued by lack of consensus. Throughout this book, efforts are made to offer current data from OECD, Canadian, and American sources that compare apples with apples. The analysis of the data and the conclusions drawn represent current literature about the Canadian system.

This is by no means the definitive text on Canada's health care system, but an effort to present useful information that will add to the informed debate about health care reform in America.

The greatest attributes of universal insurance are, first, the opportunity to provide care quickly to those who need it, regardless of wealth or employer, and second, the almost complete absence of fear of the cost burden of illness, aging, or childbirth that is prevalent in America. The common problems of the Canadian system are detailed throughout the chapters and current thinking about solutions to those problems is explored. The reason for clearly identifying these issues is to, again, assist in an informed debate in America. Every public policy choice brings with it benefits and burdens. Canada has chosen universal insurance, federal principles and legislation, provincial planning, reasonable implementation of technology, and modest public support of medical research. The product of these choices is a system that looks like America in its hospital sector but more like European nations in its community health and social support.

The provinces are now moving towards regional planning and envelope funding. Hospitals are using population data to make decisions about programs and physicians are advising patients about the probabilities of treatment outcomes to achieve fully informed consent. Many of these management strategies were developed in America and we have adapted them to our needs. Perhaps it is now our turn to offer some knowledge and experience about structure and funding to America.

TABLE OF CONTENTS

Chapter 1
The Structure of Canada's Health Care System ———————————— 1

Chapter 2
Costs and Financing ———————————————————— 25

Chapter 3
Social, Political, and Structural Factors in
Canadian Health Services ————————————————— 45

Chapter 4
The Role of Physicians ————————————————————— 65

Chapter 5
Short Term Acute Treatment Hospitals ———————————————— 89

Chapter 6
Community Health Services ————————————————— 119

Chapter 7
Technology, Pharmaceuticals, and Research———————————— 137

Chapter 8
Mental Health Services——————————————————— 153

Chapter 9
Long Term Care Services ——————————————————— 171

Chapter 10
Emerging Health Professions, Dental Services,
and Emergency Services ——————————————————— 195

Chapter 11
The Health of Canadians ——————————————————— 211

Chapter 12
Ethical Issues, Cost Control, and Evaluation ——————————— 229

Chapter 13
What Can the United States and Canada
Learn From Each Other? ——————————————————— 253

Glossary ——————————————————————————— 269

Index———————————————————————————— 285

CHAPTER 1

The Structure of Canada's Health Care System

Introduction

T
he *Constitution Act*, of 1867, which created Canada, established two levels of government, one central or federal, the other provincial. Each province has its own legislative assembly and adopts legislation in areas falling under its jurisdiction. The Premier and Cabinet exercise executive power; they are responsible for administering legislation and adopting related regulations. They also define government policy.

Canada's health system has opted for more public administration, more universality, less competition, and a smaller private sector role than the United States. Canada also has chosen a smaller government role in the administration and delivery of care than Great Britain. Like the United States, Canada has a mixture of government, nonprofit agencies and institutions, and for-profit agencies involved in the delivery of health care.

Universal insurance was made possible by an environment of voluntary efforts to protect citizens against the cost of unpredictable hospital and medical care through pre-payment. These groups included churches, community groups, and employees covered by contracts such as the Canadian railway workers.

Public financing of health care insurance became a growing political issue during the depression of the 1930s and the hardships imposed by World War II. By 1945, the federal government attempted to initiate sponsorships of provincial insurance plans but provinces would not agree. Blue Cross and Blue Shield pre-payment plans, sponsored by hospitals and doctors, took on a major role in the industry. They offered first dollar coverage and no extra billing.

Only in 1957 did the federal government get enough agreement from the provinces that it could initiate a national program to fund hospital care costs. Until this time some provinces would not agree to the cost-sharing formula. The *Hospital Insurance and Diagnostic Services Act* sent funds to provinces to ensure comprehensive coverage for inpatient services. The benefits were portable across provinces and available to all residents on equal terms. The more per-capita a province spent on hospitals, the more money the federal government transferred to the program. By 1958 the provinces were all members of the plan.

Insurance for medical care gained a national prominence in November, 1961, when Tommy Douglas, Premier of Saskatchewan, used some hospital insurance funds to support the province's medical insurance program, already 15 years old. The doctors in Saskatchewan went on strike in 1962, but the program was implemented and became the trigger for the Hall Commission in 1964.

The Hall Commission recommended a comprehensive, universal health services program for all Canadians. This system was based upon freedom of choice, it was publicly funded and directed toward the effective use of the nation's health resources to attain the highest possible levels of physical and mental well-being.

This program, called "Medicare" in Canada, has made a major contribution to equalizing the health care opportunities for Canadians. In typical Canadian fashion, health care is based on Constitutional division of legislative powers, so that the federal and provincial governments each play specific roles. Medicare was accepted and implemented in every Canadian Province, including Quebec, by 1971.

In 1977, the Established Program Financing (EPF) arrangements replaced the earlier hospital and medical care insurance acts. Under EPF the federal contribution to health care became tied to population size and economic growth. Changes are based on increases in GNP and the rate of inflation.

Our Canadian health services network is dominated and characterized by a number of features, trends, and problems or issues. They are summarized briefly here and discussed in greater detail throughout the text.

Philosophies and priorities:
- ☐ Health services are primarily nonprofit.
- ☐ There is equal and unlimited patient access to health care services that are under the public umbrella.
- ☐ There is increasing willingness to decrease the previous degree of physician autonomy, which was almost absolute.
- ☐ There is freedom of choice of providers by users, and of users by providers.
- ☐ There is increasing discussion of the importance of quality of life.
- ☐ There is public rejection of cost at the time of service.
- ☐ There is an emphasis on expensive types and sources of care; for example, acute hospital care is usually the first point of access.
- ☐ There is increased attention to health promotion and health maintenance including an attempt to acquaint Canadians with the extent to which their health is the product of their own individual actions and, therefore, is their own responsibility.
- ☐ Physical health problems have a higher priority than mental health problems.

Organization and Administration. Canada is an example of the public insurance model. There are ten independent provincial health care networks, plus the federally determined arrangements in the Yukon and Northwest Territories and areas of federal jurisdiction such as native health. The administration of health services takes place, predominantly, at the local level, through nonprofit, independent boards who govern privately held corporations. Private practitioners remain uncoordinated and highly independent. In fact, urban physicians increasingly have no hospital affiliation. Provincial approaches to public health and mental health are quite variable. Because of this provincial independence, progress toward coordination, or integration, of health services and other social services is variable. Finally, for better or worse, the medical model of care is dominant.

Policy and Planning. Planning decisions are usually centralized at the provincial level. The use of quasi-public agencies for policy development and advice varies among the provinces. The presence of these agencies, however, is often significant in the decision-making process. Regional planning agencies are increasingly responsible for agency functions and coordination; and there is no private insurance of services under the public umbrella. In other words, a monopsony exists. Federal influence through financial leverage is less evident since the Established Program Financing (EPF) legislation in 1977.

Financing and Costs. The percentage of each Canadian health dollar that is spent on institutional care increased until 1992 where it has been stabilized by a "no growth" policy in most provinces. Ontario, for example, held hospital global budgets to a 1 percent growth — currently below inflation. Public programs are financed primarily through general revenues, with premiums or employer health tax still being charged (1992) in Ontario, Alberta, British Columbia, and the Yukon.

Resources. There has been a rapid increase in physician supply with the first ever 10 percent cutback in medical school enrollment scheduled for September, 1993. The acute treatment hospital bed supply per 1,000 residents appears to have stabilized after 15 years of decline. To date, the family physician has been successfully preserved. One-third of new physicians choose to go into family practice. There is, however, a major shortage of nonclinical health services research and researchers and a perception, probably overstated, of slow acquisition of new technology in major hospitals.

Utilization. The number of physician contacts per person, per year, by fee-for-service physicians continues to climb; however, hospital utilization (days of inpatient care per 1,000 per year) has stabilized. The number of surgical procedures per year per 1,000 residents continues to rise with the growth of outpatient and ambulatory care while the volume of laboratory investigations and diagnostic radiology services continues to rise as well.

Problems and Issues. Two big problems are a system still dominated by the concept of cure and a patient group increasingly dominated by degenerative diseases that cannot be cured. It promotes an emphasis on physical perfection and quantity of life, with death as the enemy. There is also a continuing, although perhaps slightly reduced, neglect of emotional distress, environmental stress, and the quality of life. The undisciplinary medical model of care dominates the system. This model is promoted by fee-for-service and characterized by episodic and fragmented care. The health services provided are primarily reactive rather than proactive. Services are regularly provided, often in large volume, because some individual, group or public policy failed to prevent easily preventable disease or injury.

Information systems and payment arrangements that are inappropriate for health care networks are increasingly delivering multidisciplinary and long term care. Canadians have also found that the modern trend towards user decision-making based on complete information is incompatible with paternalistic providers who tend to decide what kind of care the user gets as well as from whom, where and at what cost.

There is a conflict between individual needs or benefits and collective needs or benefits. The public has, in the past, been told, and providers still often believe, that the objective is "the best health care for everyone." Meeting this objective is now impossible and not socially desirable because of the massive trade-offs required. Perfect care for anyone usually means a decreased amount of care for someone else.

A major gap exists between what the system is capable of (with the resources available) and what is delivered. There is great uncertainty and ambiguity about consumer and community roles, including confusion with respect to technocracy versus democracy. Canadians want an integrated system with privately controlled segments of the system the plan and operate independently but the system just can't quite do it.

An increasing governmental interest in the quality of health care has developed but that interest has been met with professional objection to quality review by anyone but practicing peers. No one seems sure which things are worth doing or which are most useful. This makes it difficult to reduce resource consumption rationally.

The main principles of our health system were enshrined in *The Canada Health Act* in 1984. They are universality, non-profit administration, portability, no extra billing, and equity of access. These principles have been jeopardized by the 1991 *Federal Restraint Law* which reduces the obligation of the federal government to maintain financial contributions to the provinces for health care.

The Political Nature of Health Care

In Canada's health care network, decision-making power is widely dispersed among caregivers, other workers, institutions, consumers, communities, taxpayers, for-profit and not-for-profit private corporations, and all levels of government. The recent increase in grass roots power and in the power of providers other than physicians is changing all that.

Power does not flow only from constitutions, statutes, and elections. The highly personal and often frightening nature of illness or injury, the miracles of modern medicine, and the high (often unreasonable) levels of expectation in the public have created an environment in which logic and mandate may be no match for a charismatic politician or professional. Those who wish to have influence must often understand the political and behavioral elements of decision making better than they know how to handle data, conduct research or scientifically evaluate the options.

Individual caregivers have power based on their expertise, their ability to withhold or supply needed care, the information they control and statutes or regulations. They also derive power from a culture in which the client/patient and/or the family believes the caregiver should be in charge and make decisions. Any **individual** can have power through oratorical or other charismatic skills. **Canadian government** derives its power from the public acceptance of democratic traditions in which government may, within areas of jurisdiction, pass laws and see that they are enforced. By virtue of their policy-writing mandate **government**, **boards** and **administrators** can, in their respective areas of control, start, reduce, expand, or stop programs. **All parties** can exert influence beyond their areas of jurisdiction through activities such as lobbying, harassment, passing resolutions, sending letters to the editor, or complaining, but these extra-parliamentary processes are particularly important to individuals and communities who lack formal power. **Courts** have power because governments, culture and tradition have given it to them. **Bureaucrats** have power through their expertise, their direct access to political policy makers and their capacity to obstruct, sabotage, or ignore policies with which they do not agree. Throughout health services there are innumerable networks with power based on internal loyalty. These might include the "old boys network" that is, the graduates of a particular university or school or members of the same occupational, religious, ethnic, or political group. Any group can also be powerful if they are able to offer money or withhold it, and people can have power because of the information they control.

In Canada, whether one is a politician, an administrator, a caregiver, or a consumer, one's capacity to change health services or health policy is routinely dependant on the support of others. An understanding of networking, group dynamics, and participatory leadership are routinely useful, if not essential. Changes being proposed must, in principle, be acceptable to, and preferably attractive to, a variety of social or bureaucratic entities, and the details of the proposal should be hammered out in a mood of compromise so that the necessary range of allies can be retained.

The amount of change that can be caused or prevented by a person, group, institution, or government depends, not only on the amount of formal or informal power held, but also on the skill with which it is used and the skill with which the power of opposing forces is neutralized. The governments of Saskatchewan in 1962 and Ontario in 1986 could have averted or emasculated their doctor strikes by showing early sensitivity to minor issues that eventually led large numbers of physicians to support the militant minority. The governments failed to neutralize the power of their opponents. Physicians, as a group, routinely demonstrate poor tactics, insufferable self-righteousness, and a lack of acceptance of social change. Their lack of understanding of issues and their lack of tactical skills has regularly resulted in physicians having minimal influence in situations in which they have major interest — even when their sensible participation would be helpful to all parties. A poor understanding of process reduces their power.

Competition for territory and power within the health services network is intense. Hospitals see themselves as the hub and routinely wish for more and more of the system to be within their circle. Within the hospital family, the tertiary care (university teaching) hospitals constitute a form of royalty. These hospitals and their super specialists see themselves as the elite whose services deserve limitless access to funds and growth, a position put forward in 1984 in a Medical Research Council submission to Health and Welfare Canada. Nursing homes see themselves as the "keystone" in long-term care (LTC), a position vigorously rejected by almost (if not all) other parts of the LTC network. Community health centers (by many names) remain an optimistic group who see themselves as the logical entry point and gatekeeper to medical treatment.

A few examples may show how difficult it is to predict who, or what, will be most powerful in a given situation or at a particular moment in time.

Physicians tried to stop chiropractors from being given statutory recognition, but they could not. Nurses, through their associations, their clinical importance, and their large numbers should dominate in matters of nursing policy, but their objections to formally trained nursing assistants were ignored by both governments and educators.

In 1987, hospitals, provincial governments, consumer groups and most of the public opposed patent law changes that would raise the price of drugs in Canada but the political clout of the pharmaceutical industry was greater and new legislation was approved by the House of Commons. A new and unexpected player, the Senate, complicated the process but the outcome was only delayed, not changed. When the Ottawa Civic Hospital planned a major building program in 1978-79 but neglected to discuss traffic, parking and other such issues with the neighborhood, the hospital found it could not get a building permit. The entire project had to be redrawn. The community association and a sympathetic city hall were more powerful than the hospital.

The unanimous passage of the *Canada Health Act* in 1985 demonstrated the power of the extraparliamentary processes. Opinion polls, petitions, and public discussion convinced even traditionally conservative physicians, who personally approved of extra-billing, that extra-billing must go. These examples are not meant to have anything in common; they merely demonstrate the existence of a wide range of players in situations of conflict and the unpredictability of the outcomes.

Of all the players who wield power, the provincial governments are probably the most important, but because there are so many players, victory, or partial victory, usually goes to those who have most carefully done their lobbying, built their networks, and neutralized major opponents. Good tactics, the art of compromise, the talents of good leadership, and the ability to offer or withhold money are often more important to success than good data or legal/administrative control.

Policy and Planning

Policies represent intent and may represent practice. They are not recommendations. They are statements of what is to be done. They infer a capacity to implement. In Canada, the provinces are the *major* planners and paymasters.

The processes of policy creation and of planning are often difficult to separate. They both occur at many levels and places in the health system. A policy is a decision that has been made whereas "planning" refers more to either the process through which the decision was selected or the process by which it is implemented.

Statutes (laws) relevant to health are enacted only by federal and provincial governments but the list of bodies which write health policy includes

□ institutional boards of trustees,
□ children's aid societies,
□ boards of health,
□ boards of education,
□ municipal governments,
□ some regional planning agencies, and
□ all those other boards, councils, and executives of profit and nonprofit agencies which establish rules about financing and resource allocation.

The legislative stages of public policy adoption are highly visible but policy often passes through a complicated, tortuous, and time consuming multistage process before ending in a legislature or other forum able to approve policy. A policy proposal can originate within government or from outside. It can come from special interests, from special studies or inquiries, from the example of other jurisdictions, from a coroner's inquest or a court, from citizens or civil servants. Proposals tend to be examined, initially, in one department and reviewed by one minister. If supported at this level, they may then go to a cabinet committee (or more than one) and to various departments, for financial, social, political, or organizational evaluation.

After passage of an act in a legislature, it becomes law when proclaimed. There may be a considerable delay between final debate and approval in the legislature and actual proclamation, sometimes so that the regulations under the act can be written. Statutes may set out only the general principles, with the details being written into the regulations. Statutes are difficult to amend but regulations can be easily altered. Statutes can only be amended by a legislature whereas regulations can be changed by Order in Council or a minister.

Advisory groups, regardless of their permanence or reputation, do not write policy. The Economic Council of Canada, for example, may make recommendations and be quoted often, but these recommendations are not policy and most of them do not become policy. In 1980, an Ontario Royal Commission into the Confidentiality of Health Information brought forth 179 recommendations. By 1987, only one of these had become law. Task forces, commissions and other such bodies have the habit of producing reports which include very long lists of impractical and unpriorized recommendations — a habit which may help explain why so few recommendations become policy.

The role of the informal caregiver and the voluntary agencies as creators and shapers of programs that later become universally accepted is impressive. Palliative care, programs for persons with Alzheimer's disease, sheltered housing for the disabled and home-support services of various kinds exist because someone in the community saw a need and responded to it.

The Regulation of Institutions and Providers

Health services statutes and their related regulations tend to affect one or more of the following.

1. **Quality and safety**. These are affected by legislation (and their regulations) governing such things as the running of hospitals and nursing homes, the handling of radioactive substances, and the disposal of toxic wastes.

2. **Professional entry or function**. Licensing regulations limit the entry of individuals to specified professional groups and, to varying extents, prevent other persons from performing certain of the acts that are performed by the licensed group. For example, physicians and dentists have exclusive practice arenas. Certification is associated with entry restriction but does not convey exclusive functional domain, for example, nurses and physiotherapists. Others who do not qualify for certification can legally perform these duties.

3. **Rate or price regulation**. Rates of payment — fees, sessional payments and salaries — can be determined by the government. Governments can vary rates of pay on the basis of location or other factors.
4. **Income regulation**. Governments can place ceilings on incomes per year or month, from a particular paying agency.
5. **Authority to deliver services**. Hospital legislation, for example, can enable the building of a new hospital and provide capital funds for this purpose.
6. **Matters of ethics or human rights**. The 1985 *Canadian Charter of Rights*, for example, outlaws discrimination while establishing some grounds for exemption.

Policy Examples

Policies are a reflection of the values and priorities of those who influenced and authored them. In 1984, the government of Ontario found $45 million to bail out a financially sinking, luxury resort in northern Ontario. At the same time, it could not find $45 thousand to bail out the Kenora (Ontario) Children's Aid Society, overwhelmed with the products of family breakdown in that northern community. Also at the same time, there was almost no help available for hundreds of ex-psychiatric patients recently discharged from Toronto psychiatric institutions. The values and priorities of policy makers have a direct effect on the services available to people. Several provinces are actively attempting to set out overall goals which will provide a framework within which policies and plans can be created. Ontario and Alberta are examples.

The policy creation process in Canada is influenced by the concepts of democracy, pluralism and federalism, each of which reduce the ease with which leaders can do as they please. In our society, there are well-defined "limits to governing," especially when all interested players understand the process and play the game in the way that is their right.

Health Planning

Health planning, at one time, often consisted merely of selecting resource-to-population ratios such as one public health nurse per 5000 population or 6 acute treatment beds per 1000 population. This arbitrary selecting is still done but is now partly replaced by needs planning. Through this planning, the needs of a population are documented and plans are then developed to meet those needs. As with all change, however, the conversion to needs based planning has not been without its pitfalls.

Other factors also reduce the quality of Canadian health planning. Responses are too often reactive rather than proactive — of the firefighting variety. We also do not know enough about the effects of various services and expenditures on the health of communities. Health planning has, to a large extent, assumed that if *physicians* think an action is useful then it is, in fact, useful, an assumption that has lead us into many high costs, high volume activities that probably have modest if any effect on either the quantity or quality of the life or health of a community.

Municipal and regional governments are usually seen as very minor players in health planning but their areas of jurisdiction include land use (zoning), providing and routing general and special public transportation, planning traffic patterns, handling and disposing of toxic wastes, adapting facilities to the physically handicapped, establishing parking requirements, assigning heritage designations and appointing some trustees. Local governments also usually influence or control the degree to which the community is served by a broad range of health-related social services and institutions such as public housing, day care, recreation, halfway houses, and group homes. These decisions have an impact on health planning. Local governments can also finance health services, especially capital costs. This role was largely abandoned to provincial governments for many years but is, again, emerging.

Labor-Management Relations

Prior to the appearance of public insurance programs, very few Canadian health care workers were unionized and the majority were poorly paid compared to similar workers outside the health sector. With unionization of most health sector workers, pay scales have risen rapidly. Nurses, for example, achieved 40-75 percent pay increases in several provinces with the signing of their first negotiated contract. A number of other worker groups had similar successes. Salaries and wages throughout the health care industry are now comparable to those paid elsewhere.

In most provinces, collective bargaining occurs only between the ministry and provincial unions. In Ontario, bargaining is not a provincial function but hospitals voluntarily act collectively to establish master contracts. In most provinces, strikes by hospital workers are illegal. British Columbia is an exception, and a rotating strike of hospital workers occurred in the spring of 1992.

Physicians in several provinces are now officially unionized with the provincial medical associations (or the two separate specialist and family practitioner "syndicates" in Quebec) as the bargaining units. The Quebec Medical Association, with both specialist and nonspecialist members, has tried, unsuccessfully, to replace the two separate syndicates as the bargaining agent for all physicians.

Physicians negotiate fees or incomes through a variety of mechanisms. Nova Scotia, Manitoba, and British Columbia have tried to settle disputes through binding arbitration but are now wary of this process. The arbitration awards were unacceptably generous. In most provinces, the final fee increases are determined by government after discussions with the physician representatives. There may or may not be a mutually accepted fee increase; usually physician demands are not met. Ontario is attempting to reduce acrimony between physicians and government with the development of a Joint Medical Commission to deal practically with fees and other issues.

Coordination and Integration

Both integration and coordination can occur at the point of delivery of service or at any higher level in the administrative hierarchy. These are important strategies in the evolution of efficient organization of health care in

Canada. Coordination helps separated (discrete) administrative units or care delivery teams to work together. Integration is defined as a fusion of either two or more administrative units or two or more information systems, inventories, or other such services. "Coordinated" units may be in the same organization, as is the case with departments in a hospital, or they may be in quite different organizations as is the case with a public health unit and a community health center.

Integration is routinely a centralizing phenomenon. Successful coordination, on the other hand, is frequently a prerequisite to the preservation of a decentralized arrangement in which functionally related but organizationally separate units must work together. The health services network exists to serve individuals and groups of individuals whose problems do not fit within convenient bureaucratic and professional boundaries. The problems are emotional, physical, functional, social, spiritual, financial, or all of these in the same person at the same time. It would be organizationally convenient if the problems of the person could be separated into parts and each part handed out to a particular system — a bit to a priest, a bit to a lawyer, a bit to a welfare office, a bit to a marriage counsellor, a bit to an ambulance, and so on. Unfortunately, bureaucracies and professionals are trained to cope only with specific problems and, therefore, they sometimes chop people into a set of discrete problems, each one the property of a particular agency or worker or statute. This dissociation is a major hazard to quality and convenience when the problems are interacting, as they usually are, and the hazard is reduced only by the coordination of agencies and professionals.

The purposes of coordination and integration include:

1. Providing improved service delivery, especially to multiproblem patients or families. These clients with complex problems, such as alcoholics and the severely disabled or chronically ill, require a variable and often sophisticated mix of health services and often other social services.
2. Providing improved productivity through job sharing, information sharing, or simplified transfer of tasks or patients.
3. Decreasing opportunities for client manipulation of the system. This objective has, to date, been limited primarily to situations in which a client could obtain similar social support services from multiple sources.
4. Achieving better planning through a capacity to affect a greater number of components of a network, and a greater capacity to standardize data and procedures.
5. Achieving greater likelihood of conflict resolution within the service network or bureaucracy.

Integration has the added advantage of reducing or eliminating legal barriers to information transfer.

Prerequisites to successful coordination include the official and personal support of highest level bureaucrats. There must be a willingness by all parties to become acquainted with the goals, fears, culture, and operations of other parties and an absence of serious levels of mistrust or competition. A willingness to develop new skills including those of consensus seeking, conflict resolution, and negotiation must be present, as well as a willingness to accept delays and failures so that common goals may eventually be better served. Another desirable prerequisite is the availability of successful role models or examples from which to learn.

Although coordination and integration often seek the same ends they must, because of their inherent differences, use quite different techniques. They are also used in quite different circumstances. Integration is used when merging or fusion is practical, whereas coordination can be useful and can be carried out almost anywhere at almost any time.

Techniques which promote coordination include:

☐ **Multiagency committees or boards**. These organizations include federal-provincial committees of ministers of health or of deputy ministers of health, special federal-provincial technical advisory committees dealing with such subjects as manpower, laboratory services or health insurance, and committees of regional planning bodies. The old voluntary hospital planning councils, the Halifax-Dartmouth Mental Health Planning Board and social planning councils are other examples. These multiagency committees may be standing or ad-hoc and may be highly formal or quite informal. They may exist at all levels of bureaucracy or community and may be voluntary or mandatory.

☐ **The case conference**. This forum is quite analogous to the multiagency committee but it operates at the point of delivery of care. It brings together a number of providers with different skills and points of view that are important in solving a problem or in providing care to a patient. It improves the coordination of the many disciplines involved in the care of the patient.

☐ **Secondment of staff**. There have been many examples of public health nurses playing a liaison and referral function in hospitals, physicians' offices, and community health centers. Some multiservice centers will have on-site staff who are employees of provincial welfare programs, mental health agencies, or children's aid societies. This arrangement, which encourages coordination, allows staff from several agencies to work together in a single office without unduly disturbing established and, perhaps, parochial agencies.

☐ **Interlocking board memberships**. In Quebec, board member exchange is mandatory for hospitals, regional planning councils, CLSCs and other components of the regional health and social services network.

☐ **Devices for information exchange**. Information availability and transfer is improved by, for example, having a central community information service, adhering to a standard set of definitions and to a standard format for data collection, producing of simple but informative annual reports and holding regular regional or local conferences and seminars.

☐ **Formal agreements**. Coordination is easier and better when the rules are produced by, acceptable to, and accepted by all parties. An example of this is the agreements between educational and service units which assure field based training for professional and technical students.

Examples of integration are also common and include:

- ☐ **Long-term care patient placement services with the authority to control placement**. These organizations centralize functions formerly served by independent admissions offices.
- ☐ **Multi-institutional organizations**. These usually consist of two or more hospitals but also often include LTC facilities, ambulatory care units, and public health programs. These are now common throughout Canada with the western provinces leading the way. Health Science Centers were an early phase of institutional amalgamation.
- ☐ The **merging of the departments of health and of social services** into one department.
- ☐ The **merging of small public health units** in Ontario into county or multicounty units.

All large institutions and other bureaucracies are examples of integration although they are not always thought of as such. They represent the integration of such diverse functions as emergency services, hotel services, business services, education, psychiatric services, and diagnostic services. When cared for in the community, patients who are quite similar to many institutional inpatients receive their care from multiple sources that are not integrated, or even coordinated.

The concepts of coordination and integration are inherent in such terms as "one-stop shopping" and "single-point-of-entry." The general hospital is an example of an institution bringing many types of services together rather than having different types of workers deliver care from organizationally separate units. In hospitals, the unification (integration, centralization) was primarily for technological and administrative reasons rather than for client convenience, but inpatient hospital care certainly illustrates the one-stop shopping principle.

Community health centers and a variety of multiservice centers are also designed to bring a mix of health and social service professionals to one spot under one management. Group medical practices bring convenience to the client through the proximity of a mix of medical specialties and easy internal referral.

The "single point of entry" concept commonly refers to an arrangement in which persons in need of continuing care are referred to, and assessed by, a standardized process based in a single agency. After review, the person is referred to the appropriate community based or institutional program for ongoing care. This arrangement is a great improvement over unintegrated options in which many agencies, programs and institutions use their own, often unique, referral and assessment practices.

Despite the acknowledged importance of coordination it is often inadequate. It is often impeded by the following:

1. **Geographic dispersion**. Often, offices are nowhere near the laboratories that provide services.
2. **Obvious or latent competition between agencies or individuals** whose cooperation is important to the client. There can, for example, be competition between hospitals, between physicians or between agencies providing similar services such as pre-natal classes or home support services. Client or community interest becomes secondary to institutional or worker self interest.
3. **Unwillingness to share information**.

4. **Unwillingness to change**. Coordination may require adaptation, sometimes with a sharing of functions or even the loss of specific functions. Counselling, for example, may move from physicians to social workers and psychologists. Coordination may also require a modification of currently used vocabulary and reporting. All of these changes may be resisted.

5. **Interprofessional hostility or disdain**, such as that which exists between physicians and chiropractors, physiotherapists and athletic therapists, or chiropodists and podiatrists.

6. **Different priorities and objectives**. Highly technological workers may rank client needs much differently than someone whose service area is housing, advocacy, spiritual health, employment, or long term care.

7. **Differences in self-image and external image**. Health care workers, especially acute care workers, often have a higher social profile and status than social service or long term care workers.

8. **The fee-for-service payment system**. Practitioners on fee-for-service find it difficult to coordinate or cooperate with other workers and agencies because their income is tied entirely to what they do and who they see. Shared services or transferred services may result in lower income or to difficulties with a paying agency.

9. **Legal obstruction to easy exchange of information or delegation of functions**.

Almost all of the factors that impede coordination also impede integration, but the list of impediments to integration also includes objections to an integrated patient record (such as is able to be used in a hospital), objections to loss of provider "freedom" and a desire for corporate survival.

People and agencies may be reluctant to put the public interest ahead of their own. Personal freedom, personal income, agency survival, and both agency and professional jurisdiction are not usually surrendered easily even if the change will improve the access, convenience, quality and/or cost-effectiveness of some service needed by some client or groups of clients.

The Evolution of Regionalization in Canada

Health programs and facilities in Canada were once quite independent. To varying degrees, they raised their own money and did their own planning. This autonomy has now been largely replaced by multiagency or regional arrangements that fall within the concept of regionalization.

Alberta has, for some time, been regionalizing its hospital boards. Instead of each hospital having its own board, one board administers a number of institutions. One budget has replaced a number of budgets and one executive director/ president replaces several. In this example there is no significant change in hospital financing, planning, or evaluation, but legal responsibility is centralized with probable changes in personnel management, resource allocation, and other functions.

In many urban areas there has been regionalization of a number of clinical specialty services such as cardiac surgery, hemodialysis, pediatrics, and obstetrics. There is no change in the number of organizationally separate institutions but a particular service which was formerly provided from several sites is now provided at only one.

When a number of institutions lose their in-house laundries and a new and quite separate organization is formed to provide this service to all, this change is also called regionalization. Not only is an activity centralized but a new regional financing and management arrangement is put in place.

When a provincial or federal ministry of health, or some part of a ministry, creates regional offices, this creation is again called regionalization. There may have been little or no change in policy, organization, or function.

In Quebec in the 1970s, both institutional and noninstitutional services were affected by regionalization. Functions were changed, a number of traditional programs disappeared, many new boards and agencies came into being and planning, financing, and administration processes were significantly revised.

In Ontario, the old Regional Hospital Planning Councils have been replaced by another type of purely advisory body, the District Health Councils. The Councils have no executive authority over any health services but they give advice on the planning of a broad range of health services. They are only advisory and are concerned only with planning, but they also are an example of regionalization.

In Prince Edward Island public health services were decentralized to four regions, each with a population of 30-40,000. Some of the units created were similar in size to those that were abolished through centralization of public health services in Ontario two decades ago. In both Prince Edward Island and Ontario the change was referred to as regionalization.

Ontario is currently regionalizing emergency services through the categorization of emergency rooms. Some emergency departments will provide the most complex kinds of care and some will remain open only 14-18 hours per day. In this example of regionalization, it is probable that no organization charts will be altered although functions will change and some global budgets will be adjusted.

The examples reveal little if any pattern. Regionalization can deal with populations of 30,000 to 2,000,000. It can affect one health service or program or many. It can affect the delivery, planning, financing, administration, or evaluation of care. Any number of specialized administrative functions can be affected such as management information systems (MIS), quality control and education. One type of patient (renal failure patients, hemophiliacs) or one specific activity (computers or collective bargaining), may be affected or a broad range of both care and management functions (Quebec Regional Health and Social Services Council, or CRSSS; Manitoba rural health and social service boards) may change. It can involve major authority transfer (regional public health units, multihospital boards) or none at all (District Health Councils in Ontario). It can lead to smaller units being amalgamated (the food commissariat in Ottawa), or to completely new units being created (the Greater Vancouver Mental Health Service), or, very rarely, to new and smaller units being created to replace a larger one (the creation of community based public health and social service centers). Sometimes decision making or some other activity moves to another community but stays in the same organization (for example the creation of the regional offices of the Department of Indian and Northern Affairs), and sometimes it stays in the same community but moves to another organization, as with a regional laundry. There appears to be no limit to the variations possible within the theme of regionalization.

Institutions, agencies, and communities often believe that, with regionalization, there will be decentralization of provincial powers. This seldom happens. Regionalization is much more likely to lead to increased centralization, as is the case when enlarged hospital boards or public health units are created or when laundries are amalgamated.

The Variability of the Characteristics of Regional Authorities, Agencies, Commissions, Boards, Councils, Departments, Committees, or Programs

Objectives and Philosophy. The motivation for regionalization can be social, technological, managerial, political or some combination of these. The objectives and philosophies of different examples of regionalization may be overlapping or in conflict. Most examples can meet only some of the objectives in the following list because the list is generic and not broadly applicable in its entirety.

1. Develop policies and programs which reflect the character and priorities of the region.
2. Reduce intraregional disparities in such areas as access, cost, availability, and quality.
3. Provide greater opportunity for and degree of consumer and community influence and control. (Sometimes stated much more strongly as local control rather than central control.)
4. Reduce the parochialism found in individual programs and facilities.
5. Attain financial savings through economies of scale, reduce undesirable duplication, and reduce undesirable competition.
6. Make movement and referral of patients easier.
7. Increase standardization.
8. Create better information flow.
9. Integrate/coordinate related services.
10. Distribute personnel and facilities more efficiently.
11. Develop better quality control techniques.
12. Train staff better.
13. Attain the "critical mass" of cases (or services) necessary if quality and efficiency are to be satisfactory. This critical mass attracts competent staff, allows this staff to remain competent, makes it more likely that equipment will be up-to-date, promotes research, and encourages a motivating professional atmosphere.
14. Reduce the power of some central agencies by creating a smaller jurisdiction and delegating to that jurisdiction some of the powers that were formerly exercised centrally.
15. Develop a regional approach to such functions as priority setting, planning, delivery and administration by bringing a broad range of services and administrative functions under one regional jurisdiction.
16. Rationalize services.
17. Provide greater career opportunities for staff.

18. Create one agency responsible for servicing a specified population with a broad range of services.
19. Create a system whereby consumers may more easily interact with administrators and planners.

Optional sources of authority for regionalization.

☐ **A statute**, such as the ones which established the consolidated Boards of Health in Ontario or the CRSSS in Quebec.

☐ **An Order in Council**, such as was used to establish each District Health Council in Ontario.

☐ **A decision of a minister or a bureaucrat**, such as that which centralizes the intern and resident payroll function in one regional hospital or which gives a particular laboratory responsibility for certain tests.

☐ **Letters patent**, which might establish a separate corporation such as a regional laundry.

☐ **A decision by another regional body**.

Degree of influence or authority of the regional body. It can be purely advisory, perhaps with an advocacy function, as is the case with the Ottawa-Carleton Council on Aging and the Social Planning Council. The authority, while purely advisory can have major influence assured by government policy, as with an Ontario District Health Council. There can be limited decision-making authority, such as the Quebec CRSSS, or major decision-making authority, such as the Ontario Boards of Education and the Ontario Boards of Health.

Methods of selection of members of a regional board, commission, council, or committee. New members may be elected by a total regional constituency, as occurs with a regional and municipal government and with most boards of education, or by a membership, as occurs with the Ottawa-Carleton Placement Coordination Service. Members could be appointed by a minister (as with appointments to a District Health Council in Ontario), by designated agencies (as is the case with the Ottawa-Carleton regional food services and regional laundry) or by someone else designated in law. The agencies which are to be represented on a board or council may be named in a charter, a statute or the regulations under a statute. Selections may also be made by any combination of the above.

Methods of financing.
☐ Budget from one or more levels of government (as is the case with Boards of Health, District Health Council or DHC, CRSSS).
☐ Fees from users (as with regional food services or regional laundries).
☐ Government grants.
☐ Philanthropy.
☐ By direct taxation, as is the case with Union Hospital Districts in Saskatchewan or boards of education in several provinces.

In some cases of regionalization no new financing is required, merely redistribution.

Devices for intraregional liaison and consensus seeking.

☐ **Interlocking board memberships.** Quebec offers the only formalized and province-wide example.

☐ **Regional committees with multiagency representation.** Once again Quebec offers the only example which is province-wide and proscribed by law, but other examples are common. The DHCs in Ontario usually have a number of such committees which advise with respect to types of service such as long term care or categories of consumers such as children.

☐ **The extraparliamentary and less formal processes,** which include lobbying, submitting briefs and writing letters.

Techniques for Institutional or Program Obstruction of Regional Approaches

Regionalization is not always welcomed, nor is it always passively received. There are techniques by which agencies or groups show their displeasure. Groups may make "end runs" to the province. This term is applied to instances in which agencies who do not get what they want at the regional level go directly to the ministry for approval. Other groups may simply refuse to cooperate. Institutions may fail to participate on committees and boards, fail to provide information or fail to perform assigned functions, or proceed with institutional initiatives that are inconsistent with regional plans or with assigned functions.

Groups may also use of the media to show their displeasure. Common approaches include scare tactics such as releasing misleading descriptions of waiting times or the length of waiting lists, dramatizing deaths that might have been avoided, distorting facts through the exploitation of anecdotal events that are inconsistent with norms, or making appeals which imply that institutions are the only defender of some patient group. When such strategies are used the provincial, regional, or municipal governments are often portrayed as callous and disinterested.

Prerequisites or Devices for Strengthening Regional Approaches

Provincial support is the most important prerequisite. Advisory regional planning bodies, such as DHCs in Ontario, can only be successful if the ministry refuses to recognize attempts at end runs, and if the ministry provides adequate operating funds and start up funds. Support among local health administrators is equally important. The process also works better if leaders have good consensus seeking skills, can maintain broad local involvement, and know how to find solutions that bring rewards to at least most of the major players.

Area-Wide (Regional) Health Planning Agencies

Planning is one of the functions with which regionalization is closely associated. The desirability of comprehensive area-wide (regional) health planning is no longer questioned, but because major tertiary care services require a population base of one million or close to it (some countries use a minimum base of two to three million), many provinces cannot regionalize tertiary care planning. Regions with populations of less than one million or thereabouts can play a role in planning certain kinds of services such as those which provide less sophisticated long term care or primary care, but they find it difficult to plan a total health services network except in cooperation with other geographic units.

From 1945-65 area-wide comprehensive health planning was largely carried out by voluntary hospital planning councils. Though they were a useful evolutionary phase they could not handle situations in which decisions were unacceptable to one or more of their members. These voluntary models were gradually replaced by government sponsored regional planning arrangements with the province often quite unavoidably being the planning region.

District Health Councils (DHCs) in Ontario. The first DHCs were established in 1973. By 1986 there were 26 of them serving almost all of the province. The establishment of DHCs was promoted by the province but they were not set up until there was a request from the region. They are established by Order in Council, that is, at the request of the Minister of Health, with the support of the cabinet, and with the approval of the Lieutenant Governor. They report directly to the Minister. DHCs have 15 to 20 members usually appointed for 3 year terms. Members are appointed by the Minister of Health and include representatives of consumers, providers, and the regional municipality. The DHCs serve regions with populations ranging from 150,000 to 2,000,000. Annual basic budgets, as provided by the Ontario Ministry of Health, are at one of two levels. Depending on whether the population served is under or over 200,000, the budget is sufficient to hire approximately 4 or 6 professional staff. Additional funds are granted on a project basis.

The mandate of DHCs is to advise the Minister of Health on the planning and coordination of health services. They are expected to identify needs, set priorities, plan a comprehensive health care program, coordinate health services, and evaluate and promote cooperation within the regional network. They must also make specific recommendations regarding all of these. The councils may initiate studies themselves or may respond to proposals made by agencies or institutions.

Proposals considered by the DHCs tend to come from one or more of a series of task forces or committees usually representing a major user group or service type. These groups include primary (ambulatory) care, mental health, hospitals, long term (continuing) care, pediatric services, and health promotion/disease prevention. Ad-hoc subcommittees are created as needed.

In some Ontario communities, the DHCs replaced Regional Hospital Planning Councils but, in Toronto, the Metropolitan Toronto Hospital Planning Council continues to operate. Duplication and competition seem inevitable. Overlap is probably further increased by the presence of OCATH (Ontario Council of Administrators of Teaching Hospitals).

District Health Councils should be considered at least a qualified success. They have led to major discussion between regional sources of care and have produced many fine studies. All DHCs undertake priority review exercises, usually annually, and may review hundreds of submissions (140 to 160 in Ottawa-Carleton). In the priority-setting exercise, each proposal is assessed with respect to such features as need, value for money, ease of implementation and extent of fit with council and ministry priorities.

With the maturing of DHCs, there appears to be a tendency towards increased provider domination. This trend is quite contrary to the concept within which DHCs were created. Perhaps provider representatives stay in the network whereas the community representatives come and go. Perhaps the more permanent members have co-opted the system. If a reasonable balance of power is to be maintained providers must become less dominant on DHCs and their committees, and perhaps provider representatives should be excluded from Council membership. In the early years, hospitals were unhappy with the appearance of DHCs and fought or ignored them; now they have decided to gain control. Providers, especially hospitals, have no difficulty exerting major influence when they wish.

The Quebec Health and Social Services System

Starting in 1961, the Quebec government gradually developed an original health care and social security system. Quebec has a population of more than 6.5 million people, of whom 5.3 million speak French. The population, of which half is centered in Greater Montreal, is distributed over about 10 percent of an area of 650,000 square miles. Its origins and culture are French, and its parliamentary system is British. Civil law is practiced, rather than common law.

Government structure. All Quebecers, regardless of their income, enjoy health and hospital care at no direct cost under the provincial health insurance plan. Physicians are now prohibited from demanding additional fees from their patients.

Quebec is currently the only province which integrates both health and social services at every level. It also offers universal access to insured services provided by the system. Eighty percent of total health expenditures in the Province of Quebec are publicly financed.

The health institutions in Quebec are operated and managed by local boards of directors, and members of the community play a key role on these boards.

Regional councils were a key element in the restructuring of health and social services that began in Quebec in 1972 with the passage of Bill 65. The regional councils, of which there are 11, develop regional objectives, measure need, establish priorities, are responsible for coordination of the sources of health and social services, and evaluate outcomes. To a variable but usually quite limited extent, councils approve capital and operating expenditures. Finally, they provide advice to the Minister as required.

The nature and role of councils (called the Conseil Régional de la Santé et des Services Sociaux Québec in French) is spelled out in the statute which created the regionalized network. The councils have 15 or more members representing post secondary educational institutions, voluntary agencies, municipalities, socioeconomic groups, the health and social service facilities (one from each of the four types), and professional providers of care. The executive director of the CRSSS is also a member. There are many mandatory committees and commissions (15 to 20) and other such bodies may be established. In the statute, great emphasis is placed on the need for objectives and plans.

Social Service Centers provide social services to institutionalized and noninstitutionalized persons and groups. A CLSC (local community health center), in theory, provides a broad range of primary health care and social services but often offers very few physician services. "Reception centers" include halfway houses, day care centers, rehabilitation centers, and long term care institutions. Of the hospitals, 32 have been designated by the ministry as sites for departments of community health (DCH), or, in French, département de santé communautaire (DSC). These departments do much of the public health planning for the region.

Figure 1.1

Regional Network of Health and Social Service Institutions in Quebec

Department of Health and Social Affairs
(Département de santé et des affaires sociales)

|

Regional Health and Social Services Council (RHSSC)
(Conseil régionaux de la santé et des services sociaux — CRSSS)

(There are eleven of these regional councils, each of which has responsibility for the following four major categories of institutions)

| Hospitals | Social Service Centres | Local Community Health Centers (Centres locaux des services communautaires -CLSC) | Reception Centers (Centres d'accueil) |

| Acute Care | Long Term Care | Special (e.g. psychiatric) |

All the councils make recommendations to the Ministry regarding new capital expenditures. In recent years the councils have been given the power to approve certain expenditures without provincial review and some councils have been given major control over regional expenditures or over selected special projects, for example, in 1982 the CRSSS for metropolitan Montreal was entrusted with the establishment of a coordinating center for emergency services. Operating budgets and staff complements of the regional councils in Quebec are many times larger than those of DHCs in Ontario. The councils play a major role in assigning functions to the various sources of care and in assuring coordination of these units. Only private practitioners are fully outside of their area of influence.

Quebec has over 900 health and social services institutions, divided into four categories: hospitals, social services centers, reception centers, and local community service centers. There are 230 short- and long term hospitals, with 28,000 acute beds and 15,000 long term beds. Of the province's physicians, half are specialists. There are 14 social services centers which provide mainly specialized social services for people in need of protection or placement (youth protection, young offenders, adoption, placement of young and elderly, and family mediation). Reception centers are divided into two categories. One is for the elderly, consisting of nursing homes and long term care (together a total of 40,000 beds). The other comprises 130 rehabilitation centers which provide institutional and ambulatory services to young offenders, alcoholics, drug abusers, physically and intellectually handicapped persons, and young mothers in need of support.

Finally, local community service centers provide ambulatory care to 15,000 people, and home services to 60,000. These institutions give basic health and social services, preventive as well as treatment services, with an emphasis on prevention and education in order to reduce health care costs. Included in these centers, or CLSCs, are psychological counselling, STD clinics, marriage counselling, soup kitchens, pre- and post-natal services, crisis intervention and day care. CLSCs are especially efficient in dealing with those with multiple problems. Most physicians at these centers work for a salary, although the salary may be supplemented by hospital and private clinic work. These are the centers (the CLSC) referred to in the September 1990 issue of *Consumer Reports*.

Quebec also has community health organizations, each serving a population of 100,000 to 500,000 people. These are similar to Public Health Units in English Canada and are responsible for conducting epidemiological studies, providing immunization, monitoring infectious diseases and epidemics, assessing occupational and environmental risks, and evaluating health program impact.

Quebec is divided into regions, each headed by a regional health and social services council, which, up to 1992, have maintained a consultative role to the ministry concerning service and resource needs of the region. At the provincial level, the Ministry of Health and Social Services is responsible for all services in the province.

The annual global budget in Quebec is currently 12 billion dollars, 30 percent of the total expenditures of the Quebec government. Expenses are typically growing faster than inflation, by 2.5 points over the consumer price index. Per capita expenditures are less than those of most other provinces and lower than in the United States. From 1985 to 1990 the rate of increase in overall public expenditures was 6.8 percent annually, compared with 10.9 percent in Ontario and 8.3 percent for all of Canada. Finally, the percentage of GDP allocated to public health expenditures has decreased in the past years, from 7.5 percent in 1983-84, to 6.9 percent in 1988-89.

In April, 1989, the Province of Quebec, under the auspices of the Ministry of Health, published a report entitled *Improving Health and Well-Being in Quebec*. It establishes a future direction for their health care system, and identifies some of the current reform issues in Quebec.

1. The system has been co-opted by producers of services.
2. The central planning body, the Department of Health and Social Services, has neglected to define clear policies and orientations, and rarely evaluates programs.
3. There has been a lack of cooperation between the various institutions withing the public sector, and between these same public institutions and the private sector, including community groups.

4. There are still deficiencies in terms of accessibility, quality, and adaptability of our services, especially with regards to the needs of elderly, of native communtities, of people living in remote areas, of the emerging and growing problems (like AIDS), of child and elderly abuse, and of homeless people.
5. Quebec faces some common problems: too much paperwork, deficiencies in human resources management, difficult working conditions for some categories of personnel, and lack of training and investment in human resource development.
6. The province also faces reduced transfer payments from the federal government, so the fiscal burden on the province increases.
7. The financing of services is in no way related to performance. Support continues for programs that may not have been evaluated.

Current Issues in the Organization of Health Care in Quebec. As a result of Bill 120, passed in August 1991, Quebec is enlarging the responsibilities of existing Regional Health and Social Services Councils, which will change from consultative bodies to associations responsible for the organization of health and social services within each region. Responsibilities will include budgets to all institutions and community organizations involved in the provision of health and social services, expenditure control, and evaluation.

Board composition will change at both local and regional levels, from members who are professionally involved in the health and social services sector to a majority of members from outside the sector.

Until 1992, resources were allocated to each institution by the ministry in the form of a global budget, based mainly on its past budgets. Now, under Bill 120, envelope funding will be given to the regional council, which will allocate resources to its respective institutions and community organizations, or to programs such as mental health.

A program would include all services and resources related either to a category of health problem or a specific population group. It would cover prevention, treatment, and rehabilitation services related to a specific health problem, an ambulatory service, or to institutional care.

The regional body will have the authority to reallocate resources within a program from treatment to preventive services, from institutional to ambulatory services, and from institutions to community organizations.

The program envelope would be determined based on the population to be served and the most efficient ways of providing services.

New Orientations All Across Canada

During the last five years, several Canadian provinces have appointed commissions to examine how health systems might be improved while costs were contained. All commissions recommended implementation of similar measures.

First, **health policy oriented to healthy outcomes** is an essential requirement in order to change the functioning of our systems from input-oriented strategies and dynamics to outcome-oriented ones.

Second, **citizens and providers should participate in the planning and management of the health system** at the same time as it is being decentralized and regionalized. Twenty years ago, centralization of decision-making at provincial levels was necessary in order to set up the health networks now in existence. At present, however, most commissions recommend that local communities become more involved in decisions and the setting of priorities in order to achieve the outcomes we desire.

A third principle, **accountability**, is also necessary, both for the prudent use of limited resources and with respect to outcomes. Commitment to both of the latter make possible, with some adjustment in our concepts of programs in the health sector, real accountability in all levels of decisions, from the legislature to the local manager and provider of services. Although aspects of accountability already exist in some of our systems, they have been primarily directed toward resources to the detriment of patient outcomes.

Fourthly, **provinces must match their resources to their health needs**. The recommended solution is to maintain the public financing approach as a strategy to control the increase of total costs and to maintain the partnership in financing of both federal and provincial governments. This needs to be done while controlling expenses and increasing efficiency through a new focus on results and outcomes, rather than just the allocation of resources.

Summary of Historical Trends and Organization

In the years prior to World War II, health care was a personal or a charitable function. Following World War II, Canadian governments quickly selected health care as an area for public policy and their interest has been sustained. In the 1950s and 1960s, the top priorities were the removal of financial barriers to health care and the expansion of human and institutional resources. By the end of the 1970s, cost containment was the top priority. The numbers of hospital beds and of newly licensed foreign medical graduates were sharply curtailed but the number of long term care facilities and domestic medical graduates proved hard to control. Regional planning was well established. The 1980s brought great interest in better costing, further constraints on the licensing of foreign medical graduates, timid reductions in medical school enrollments, and abolition of physician extra-billing. They also saw the introduction, in British Columbia, of controls on physician location, an expansion of collective bargaining by physicians, some cutbacks in the range of insured services, an expansion of noninstitutional services, especially in long term care, and, perhaps, the real beginnings of acceptance of the importance of new areas of prevention such as controlling smoking and other substance abuse.

Canada has opted for more public administration, more universality, less competition and a smaller private sector role than the United States, and a smaller government role in administration of the delivery of care than in Great Britain. Canada, like the United States, has a mixture of government, nonprofit agencies and institutions, and for-profit agencies involved in care delivery.

The source of the preoccupation of Canada's health services with physical health rather than mental health is difficult to pin down. Does our system shape public values and priorities or vice versa? Does society give its highest priorities to physical health care and the elimination of physical health hazards because that is the orientation of our technocratic professionals and bureaucrats? Do the health professionals and bureaucrats have their current preoccupations and skills because they reflect the society that produced them?

People in the United States, as well as other countries, have been looking to the Canadian health care system for a solution to their own system's problems. As shown here, however, Canada has its own problems and inequities to solve as it grows and matures. It is not a perfect system, simply a different system. Some elements of it work, and some don't. The challenge, now, is to study these elements and work out other systems to deliver health care in the most efficient and effective way possible.

References

Alberta, Premier's Commission on Future Health Care for Albertans (1990). *The Rainbow Report: Our Vision for Health, Volumes I, II and III.* Edmonton: Premier's Commission on Future Health for Albertans.

British Columbia, Royal Commission on Health Care (1991) *Closer to Home.* Victoria: Government of British Columbia, Queen's Printer.

Gosselin, R. (1984). Decentralization/regionalization in health care: The Quebec experience. *Health Care Management Review, 9* (1), 7-25.

Hurl, L.F. and Tucker, D.J. (1986). Limitations of an act of faith: An analysis of the Macdonald Commissions' stance on social services. *Canadian Public Policy, 12* (4), 606-621.

McCready, D.J. (1986). Privatized social service systems: Are there any justifications? *Canadian Public Policy, 12* (1), 253-257.

Saskatchewan, Commission on Directions in Health Care (1990). *Future directions for health care in Saskatchewan.* Regina: Government of Saskatchewan.

Taylor, M.G. (1986). The Canadian Health Care System 1974-1984, in *Medicare at Maturity*, R.G. Evans and G.L. Stoddart (eds.). The Banff Centre School of Management.

CHAPTER 2

Costs and Financing

Social Expenditures

Although health services are not the largest component of social spending in Canada, they will be a $70 billion industry for 27 million citizens in 1992. Health expenditures represent 33 percent of total provincial government budgets, and three-quarters of these expenditures are for institutional and physician services. In 1992, Ontario spent $17 billion on publicly financed health care for about eight million residents. These costs are not typical of other parts of the world. Canada is the most costly publicly funded system on earth. Table 2.1 shows the comparison in per capita spending.

When Canada introduced national universal health and hospital insurance, a variety of critics warned of runaway costs. Costs did, indeed, rise rapidly in the 1960s, but during the 1970s, Canadian health expenditures stayed close to 7 percent of Gross National Product (GNP) while the percent of GNP consumed by health services continued to climb in the United States. During the prolonged recession of the early 1980s, when GNP in Canada rose very slowly or not at all, hospital and physician costs continued to rise and, therefore, consumed a rapidly increasing percentage of the GNP. By 1983 health care costs in Canada had risen to a peak of 8.8 percent of GNP, and by 1992, 11 percent. It had become clear that the policies that kept costs at a constant percentage of GNP in the 1970s did not work in periods of economic stagnation. The growth of health services costs continues whether or not the GNP also grows. The financial demands of institutional and personal providers of care have, to date, been politically unmanageable.

Table 2.1

Per Capita Health Expenditures, Life Expectancy and Infant Mortality, 1987

Country	Per Capita	Life Expectancy	Infant Mortality Per 1,000 Live Births
United States	$2,051	75.0	10.1
Canada	$1,483	76.8	7.3
Sweden	$1,233	77.2	6.1
France	$1,105	77.1	7.8
Germany	$1,093	75.9	7.5
Netherlands	$1,041	77.1	6.8
Japan	$915	78.9	5.0
United Kingdom	$758	75.4	9.0

Source: 1987/88 O.E.C.D. and World Health Organization data.
Note: All in U.S. dollars.

Despite the increase in the percentage of GNP devoted to health care, the pressure for additional funds for health services continues to increase. The critics of universal programs no longer complain about the threat of uncontrollable costs. They speak, now, of underfunding. User fees are being vigorously proposed and hospital fund-raising campaigns have once again become common.

Table 2.2

Health Expenditures as Percentages of Gross National Product, Canada and the United States, 1960-92

Year	Canada	U.S.A.
1960	5.5	5.3
1965	6.0	5.9
1970	7.1	7.3
1975	7.3	8.3
1980	7.5	9.2
1985	8.7	10.5
1986	9.1	10.7
1987	9.0	10.9
1988	8.9	11.2
1989	9.0	11.6
1990	9.5	12.2

Source: National Health Expenditures in Canada 1960-92; Policy, Planning and Information Branch, Health and Welfare Canada, March 1992.

Per capita health expenditures in Canada grew from $357 in 1972 to $1,220 in 1982 — an increase of 240 percent. In constant 1970 dollars the growth was from $340 to $445, an increase of 31 percent. In the same period, total national health expenditures grew, in constant dollars, about 48 percent, and population grew about 14 percent. In actual dollars, national expenditures on health grew almost 300 percent. Although health costs continue to rise, the federal government has, through the *Established Programs Financing Act* (EPF) of 1977, stabilized the federal contribution to those costs. After introduction of EPF, federal transfer payments (the amounts of cash or "tax points" that the federal Department of Revenue agrees to return to those provinces whose people actually paid federal income tax) to the provinces fell from 4.7 percent of GNP in 1975 to 4.3 percent in 1980, with a rise to 4.4 percent in 1983. Since 1988, the transfer payments have been declining and are expected to be eliminated early in the next century.

Sources of Health Funding

Health care costs are met from five sources, with the importance of the five sources varying by province. The contributions, by source, are

- ☐ 27 percent to 36 percent from the federal government,
- ☐ 38 percent to 50 percent from the provinces,
- ☐ 0 to 5 percent from local government,
- ☐ 0.4 to 1.3 percent from Workers Compensation Boards, and
- ☐ 17 percent to 29 percent from private sources (Table 2.3).

Interprovincial variations are not predictable. Alberta, the bastion of individual responsibility, has the lowest contribution from private sources. Quebec and Alberta, at 49 percent and 50 percent respectively, have the highest provincial contributions. Figure 2.1 shows this breakdown for Ontario in 1991.

Figure 2.1

**Revenue Sources: Percent of Total
1987-88 to 1991-92**

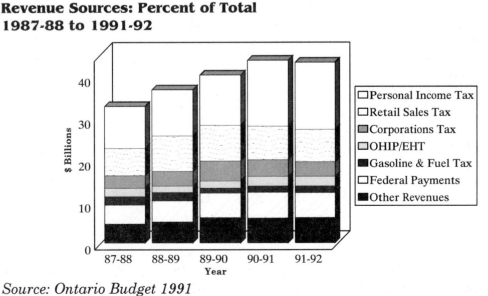

Source: Ontario Budget 1991
Note: Percentages estimated by author.

Table 2.3

National Health Expenditures by Source of Funds

	1975	1980	1985	1988*	1990*
Total Expenditures In Millions					
	12,267	22,704	40,408	52,003	61,753
Public Financing					
-Federal Direct	398	582	1,153	1,413	1,603
-Transfer to Province	3,391	6,869	11,199	13,597	14,870
Provincial	5,328	8,942	16,990	22,306	27,108
Local	132	363	451	602	751
Workers Compensation	121	211	389	405	442
Private Expense	2,897	5,737	10,226	13,681	16,980

* Provisional estimates.
Source: 1992 Policy, Planning and Information Branch, National Health and Welfare, Canada.

Notes: The breakdown of expenditures by source of funds provides a sectoral categorization of health care expenditures on the basis of where funding for health originates. **Federal direct** expenditures refer to outlays by the federal government in relation to health care services for special groups such as natives, armed forces personnel, and veterans, in addition to expenditures on research, health promotion, and protection services. Federal **transfers to provinces** include both cash and tax transfers for insured health services under Established Programs Financing, and the health portion of Canada Assistance Plan transfers. **Provincial** expenditures on health are reported net of federal transfers but include transfers to local governments. **Private expense** includes various uninsured and privately insured services provided by physicians, dentists, and other specialists, as well as non-funded institutional care costs and drugs and appliances.

Table 2.4

National Health Care Expenditures by Category

	1975	1980	1985	1987	1989*	1990*
Hospitals	5,443	9,294	16,228	18,809	21,770	23,592
Other institutions	1,194	2,638	4,259	4,946	5,984	6,616
Physicians' services	1,927	3,448	6,333	7,679	8,720	9,412
Other health professionals	731	1,578	2,745	3,255	3,917	4,332
Drugs	1,091	2,027	4,230	5,553	7,208	8,239
Capital	612	1,234	1,863	2,133	2,287	2,389
Other	1,269	2,485	4,751	5,562	6,555	7,172
Total	12,267	22,704	40,408	47,935	56,440	61,753
Hospitals	44.4%	40.9%	40.2%	39.2%	38.6%	38.2%
Other institutions	9.7%	11.6%	10.5%	10.3%	10.6%	10.7%
Physicians' services	15.7%	15.2%	15.7%	16.0%	15.5%	15.2%
Other health professionals	6.0%	7.0%	6.8%	6.8%	6.9%	7.0%
Drugs	8.9%	8.9%	10.5%	11.6%	12.8%	13.3%
Capital	5.0%	5.4%	4.6%	4.4%	4.1%	3.9%
Other	10.3%	10.9%	11.8%	11.6%	11.6%	11.6%

* Provisional estimates, in Canadian dollars.
Source: Policy, Planning and Information Branch, NHW, 1992.

Notes: Growth in private expenditures outpaced that of public expenditures by 3.3 percentage points, resulting in a slight increase in the private sector share of total expenditures from 26.9 percent in 1989 to 27.5 percent in 1990. Provincial/territorial expenditures on health care grew by 8.9 percent, including a 2.8 percent increase in federal transfers under Established Programs Financing (EPF) and cost-shared programs. Expenditures by municipal governments and workers compensation boards increased by 9.2 percent.

Expenditures on drugs exhibited the highest level of growth among categories of health care expenditures, increasing by 14.3 percent from 1989 to 1990. Expenditures on "other professionals" and "other institutions" increased slightly faster than total outlays, whereas hospital- and physician-related expenditures increased at a slightly slower rate. Capital expenditures increased by 4.8 percent.

Continued high growth in health care expenditures coupled with slow economic growth has resulted in a substantial increase in the share of national income devoted to health care. Estimates of health care expenditures show that they have increased from $56.4 billion, or 8.7 percent of GDP (a measure of the gross economy of the country, including foreign multinational), in 1989 to $61.8 billion or 9.2 percent of GDP in 1990. The year-over-year increase in health care expenditures was 9.4 percent for 1989-90, compared to 8.5 percent for both 1988-89 and 1987-88. Per capita health expenditures increased from $2,148 in 1989 to $2,318 in 1990, an increase of 7.9 percent.

Hospitals and other institutions account for about half of total health expenditures. Over the period from 1975 to 1987, a decline in the proportion of total spending by hospitals was partly offset by an increase in the spending by other institutions.

Part of the shift in relative costs between hospitals and other institutions was the result of reorganizations and reclassifications carried out by provincial governments.

The proportion of total health expenditures associated with physicians' and dentists' services and with drugs increased somewhat during the period, while the proportion associated with capital expenditures showed a moderate decline.

Costs of noninstitutional and institutional services can be expressed as costs per day, week or month of care, or as costs per unit of service. A home visit by a nurse, for example, costs $20-40; each client visit to a senior citizen or drop-in center costs $5-10; a day at a detoxification center costs $60-150; costs of an Ottawa psychogeriatric clinic are in the order of $150 per client month.

Institutions still consume the largest portion of new dollars available for health care. In the period from 1975-85, hospitals received 38.6 percent of the increase, while other institutions received 11.9 percent. Physicians accounted for 15.7 percent of the increase and drugs 10.7 percent. The growth from 1985 to 1989 is shown for Manitoba in Figure 2.2. In this figure all expenditure is labelled "100" for 1985.

Expenditures on physician services in the period 1970-82 gradually decreased as a percentage of total health expenditures (down to 14.9 percent) and then rose again to match 1975 levels (15.7 percent). In the period 1970-85, the proportion of the health dollar assigned to dental care increased until 1980 (at 5.7 percent), and has now fallen slightly. Drugs represent about 10 percent of total health service costs, and this 10 percent is quite evenly divided between prescription and nonprescription items.

Figure 2.2

Manitoba Health Expenditure Index for Major Programs, 1984-85 to 1988-89

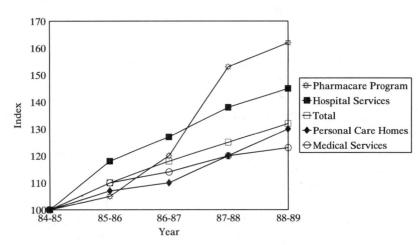

Source: Manitoba Health

It is useful to remember the relative sizes of different areas of expenditure when discussing cost control or resource reallocation. A 5 percent reduction in institutional expenditures could, for example, allow a 100 percent increase in public health expenditures, and a 10 percent reduction in expenditures on drugs would allow a doubling of our expenditures on research. Two forces may accelerate such reallocation, namely, the pressure of AIDS and the evidence produced by cost effectiveness studies.

The Health and Welfare Canada budget for 1987-88 was $29.21 billion, up 5 percent from the previous year. Old age pensions and family allowances accounted for $17.22 billion, up 6.6 percent from the previous year. Although there were budget increases for most areas of health expenditure, there were reductions in the budget of the Centre for Occupational Health and Safety (down 1 percent with staff down to 130 from 143) and in Medical Services Branch (budget down 4.1 percent and staff down from 3,040 to 2,710). Transfer payments for provincial and territorial insurance programs rose 3.1 percent to $6.84 billion.

The expenditure patterns in individual provinces often vary significantly from the national pattern. Some of the variations arise from provincial organizational and reporting differences. Comparisons are, therefore, hazardous. Reported home care expenditures varied from zero to 1.2 percent, but the inaccuracies become obvious when we note that Quebec and Alberta report no expenditure on home care when both offer this service extensively.

Provincial health insurance plans are major sources of income for most physicians. Physicians receive 93-94 percent of Ontario Health Insurance Plan (OHIP) payments to professionals (Table 2.6). Of these physician payments, 3 to 4 percent are for out-of-country services and for physicians on salary or capitation. Physicians also receive payments from WCB, private patients, and a variety of other third-party payers.

Health-related costs tend to rise faster than can be fully accounted for by inflation. For example, in 1986 the health care component of the Consumer Price Index (CPI) rose 5.6 percent, while the total CPI rose only 3.9 percent, and this was a year in which health cost increases were smaller than usual.

Table 2.5

Annual Percentage Rates of Increase in Health Expenditures Per Person For Various Categories of Care, Canada, 1960 To 1970 and 1970 To 1982*

Category	Per Capita 1960	Per Capita 1970	Per Capita 1982	Yearly Percent Increase 1960-70	Yearly Percent Increase 1970-82
	($)	($)	($)	(%)	(%)
Homes for Special Care	6.85	21.03	166.99	11.9	18.8
Dentists	6.12	12.43	68.24	7.3	15.3
General and Allied Special Hospitals	33.59	107.45	488.49	12.3	13.4
Capital	10.99	17.11	64.29	4.5	11.7
Physicians	19.82	48.81	179.02	9.4	11.4
Drugs and Appliances	17.33	36.55	132.83	8.1	11.4
Total**	199.30	293.37	1,220.18	9.4	12.6

* 1982 data are preliminary
** Total includes all categories

Source: National Health Expenditures in Canada 1970-82, Health and Welfare Canada, page 14.

Table 2.6

Payments by OHIP by Type of Service and by In and Out of Province 1984-1985

To Ontario Professionals		95.4%
Physicians*	90.2%	
Dental	0.4%	
Chiropractic	2.2%	
Optometric	1.7%	
Physiotherapy	0.7%	
Chiropody	0.2%	
Osteopathy (less than 0.1%)	—	
Out of Province Payments (including some payments to hospitals)		4.6%
	100%	

* Primarily fee-for-service (FFS) payments but includes capitation payments and payments from V.D. clinics and other minor sources of care.

Source: Practitioner Care Statistics, OHIP, 1984-85 (Pre-Audit), Ontario Ministry of Health.

As discussed, the federal government, through a number of mechanisms, provides provinces with funds equivalent to less than half of the costs of hospital and physician services. The provinces differ in how they finance their share of health care costs, but general revenue is the source of the majority of funds for most insured services in Alberta few provinces.

Alberta and British Columbia (and other provinces to a lesser extent) had always had, until the *Canada Health Act* and its associated penalties appeared, a number of hospital user fees. In British Columbia these fees represented 7.6 percent of daily hospital costs in 1955, but this figure had dropped to 2.6 percent of total costs in 1983. The 1984 fees included a charge of $4.00 for attendance at a hospital emergency department, $7.50 for an outpatient visit or day surgery, and a $7.50 daily fee while in hospital. These fees have been eliminated.

Alberta, British Columbia, Ontario, and the Yukon have had health insurance premiums; only the former two have retained them. Alberta premiums in 1990 are shown below. Those in B.C. are higher for the higher income families, with a $28,000 net income contributing $744.00 per year in premiums. There is more protection, however for lower income families whose rates are lower.

Table 2.7

Alberta Medicare Premiums, Couple with Two Children, 1989-1990

Taxable Income	Adjusted Taxable Balance	Annual Premiums
$16,000	$5,474	$ 0
18,000	7,400	153.00
20,000	9,327	306.00
22,000	11,253	463.50
24,000	13,179	463.50
26,000	15,105	463.50
28,000	17,042	463.50

Source: Health, Health Care and Medicare, a report by the National Council of Welfare, Autumn 1990. Document CAI HW60 90H23.

Note: Families with adjusted taxable balances of $6,000 or less paid no premiums at all. Families with balances above $6,000 but not more than $10,000 got partial subsidies. Those above $10,000 paid the full rate.

After the introduction of universal hospital insurance, municipalities felt they were permanently relieved of responsibility for hospital capital and operating costs. However, in response to pressure from hospitals, some municipalities are once again contributing to hospital costs. This trend is likely to continue, although it should not. The residential property tax is fully needed for other expenditures that are also important to health including recreation, urban planning, police and fire protection, sewage, water and garbage services, daycare and low income housing.

Tables 2.4 and 2.5 illustrate the cost of various types of health care. There is ongoing discussion of whether further expenditures on institutions and physicians is a reasonable way for society to spend its money, and the basic conclusion is that to improve or maintain the health status of the nation, money should be directed to activities and workers other than hospitals and doctors. Figure 2.3 shows the Manitoba response to growing expenditure on physician services and Figure 2.4 shows the percent growth in physician numbers in Manitoba.

If the costs of hospitals and physicians are controlled, there will be continuing complaints about longer hospital waiting lists and the absence of the latest technology. There is increasing evidence that Canada should accept these problems, however, because expenditures in other areas will produce greater improvements in the health status of Canadians, and will bring more social return per dollar spent than hospital or physician expenditures. It is reasonable to conclude that these two sources of traditional health care are already overfunded (in relative terms) rather than underfunded.

Insurance Programs for Hospital and Physician Services

Most Canadians take hospital and medical care insurance for granted. When any health service (or any other kind of service) is being insured, there are a number of quite different options available, and only a series of historical accidents coupled with a large measure of social concern led Canadians to have this kind of health insurance. A look at some of the options available to policy makers in 1946 (at the time of the introduction of Saskatchewan's hospital insurance) and in 1962 and 1968 (when medicare was born and expanded), will allow Canadians to consider whether there are other arrangements they would have liked better, or whether they should be thankful for choices made earlier.

Figure 2.3

Growth of Physicians in Winnipeg and the Rest of Manitoba (1980-1991)

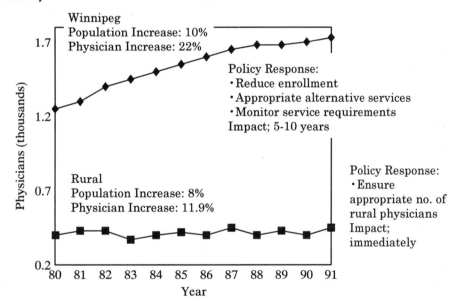

Source: Manitoba Health

Figure 2.4

Percent Increase in Manitoba Physicians Relative to Population

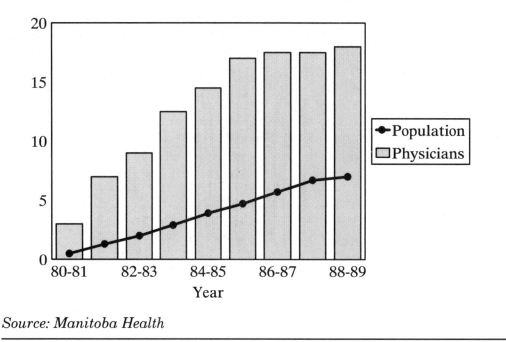

Source: Manitoba Health

The policy writers who create insurance programs have to decide who will be beneficiaries or be eligible to be beneficiaries. Health care insurance can be sold the same way fire insurance and dental insurance are sold today. Those persons who pay the premiums, or have the premiums paid on their behalf, are covered. The rest are not. Forty years ago this *laissez-faire* model applied throughout Canada. Premium costs might be paid by an employer as part of a collective bargaining agreement or by government on behalf of selected populations such as the elderly, the young or the poor, or by individuals alone or as part of a group. However, the picture began to change when Saskatchewan introduced universal hospital insurance in 1946.

In 1962-64, when the Hall Commission was preparing the report that introduced national medicare, many briefs from medical associations, insurance companies and others recommended that government should only pay the premiums of persons who could not afford to pay the premiums themselves. The Hall Commission chose to recommend the Saskatchewan pattern in which essentially the entire population was covered regardless of age, income or state of health. Under private insurance sold by for-profit insurance companies, it was routine for the company to refuse to renew health insurance contracts if the health of the beneficiary was deteriorating. Canadian arrangements assure that, regardless of whether a Canadian gets sicker, there is no danger that health insurance will be cancelled.

Besides deciding who is the beneficiary, policy makers must decide what kinds of services will be insured. Early private insurance sometimes listed all the things that were covered. If a particular problem or operation was not on the list, the patient had to pay his or her own bill. Sometimes there would be a cash payment to the patient when he or she had received a particular type of care. This was and is known as indemnity insurance. (If you had two or three insurance policies you could make money being sick, and having all your childrens' tonsils out was a financial godsend.) The better insurance plans, however, including most of the nonprofit plans in place before the universal plans arrived, covered most of the services that are covered now. Almost all admissions to hospital and almost all physicians' services were insured. The insurance did not then, and usually does not now, pay bills for which someone else was or is responsible. For example, it did not pay for injuries for which someone's car insurance would pay, or services covered by WCB. Other uninsured services theoretically include medicals to go to camp, or to renew a driver's licence. Such examinations, however, are often disguised by some kind of diagnosis and, thus, can be billed to the public insurance plan.

The issue of uninsured services is once again becoming important as provinces seek ways to control medicare costs and as a few physicians react to their loss of the right to extra bill. These physicians are beginning to charge for such services as writing referral letters, giving telephone advice, and ordering repeat prescriptions because these services are not considered to be within the list of insured services.

The definition of terms is important even terms which appear quite well understood may require clarification. **Hospital services** may mean only inpatient care, may mean inpatient and outpatient care, may exclude psychiatric care, or may be defined as "care which cannot be provided anywhere but in a hospital." They may or may not include care in the emergency room and the day surgery unit. Outpatient x-rays or laboratory work may or may not be covered. In the United States, where there are literally hundreds of different kinds of insurance policies, very complex computer programs are used to tell the hospital, the patient, and the provider of care which services are covered by a particular insurance policy.

By 1986, five of the Canadian provincially operated health insurance programs covered at least a portion of chiropractor, podiatry/chiropodist, and optometry costs. The services of osteopathic physicians were usually excluded. There was variable coverage of services provided by private physiotherapists and acupuncturists. Services provided by dentists tended to be covered if they were also commonly provided by physicians. Maxillofacial surgery is an example of such a service.

Coverage outside of one's province of residence is routine in Canada although Quebec, in 1982, reduced its coverage to emergencies only. Payment is usually made, as a maximum, at the rate that would have been paid if the services had been provided in one's home province. Special contracts or arrangements sometimes apply in communities such as Ottawa-Hull, where tertiary care for the residents in one province is routinely sought in another province, or in Lloydminster where a provincial border bisects the town.

There have always been provincial variations in the range of insured services, and the number of these has recently increased. In some provinces immunization in physicians' offices is not an insured service. Families are expected to receive these services from public health personnel or to pay for them privately. Cosmetic surgery may be fully or only partially covered.

Policy makers designing insurance programs must make choices regarding direct patient payment at the time of service. These direct payments are, at various times, called utilization fees, deterrent fees, co-insurance, user fees, deductibles, extra billing or balance billing. Objections to physician extra billing, as shown by the widespread support for the *Canada Health Act*, would suggest that Canadians are fundamentally opposed to these payments. These fees are still quite common, however, and include

- resident fees in long term care institutions,
- client payments towards drug costs in Saskatchewan,
- extra billing by chiropractors,
- extra billing when physicians provide services to patients from outside their province, and
- charges for ambulance services.

Arguments used to support the use of direct patient payments, (instead of first dollar coverage), include the following.

1. **These payments reduce premiums or taxes**. This argument is sound as long as the co-insurance fee is subtracted from the total payment or fee that would have been paid to the provider. For example, if the fee for an ordinary house call by a physician is $18, and the patient is expected to pay $5, then the insurance plan would pay the doctor $13. If the patient cannot pay or if competition makes it wise for the physician not to charge the $5, then the total cost of health care goes down. Either way, the funds required to operate the insurance program are reduced by $5 per visit.

2. **People will not appreciate the care they receive unless they pay something for it**. This is an entirely political/philosophical argument which the voters of Canada have largely rejected, but which is still supported by a minority of the population.

3. **Payments at the time of service will keep people from seeking unnecessary care**. This is an argument that is not defensible for most medical care. For people with a modest amount of disposable income the deterrent fee is of no consequence. For the working poor the fee becomes a barrier to care and, for those in selected groups such as the very poor and the elderly, the fee is of no consequence because it is routinely waived. When Saskatchewan had such fees in the 1960s and early 1970s, the use of services by low income residents decreased. In 1987, New Brunswick reported a 12 percent increase in outpatient and emergency room visits after the removal of a user fee. Experience in other countries indicates that demand for eye glasses and drugs is altered by a requirement for patient payment. Deterrent fees can be best defended for services shown to be likely to be seriously abused and in situations where the patient has control over choice.

4. In the special case of long term institutional care, **people should have to pay for their room and board wherever they live**, especially when they are receiving publicly financed pensions. Thus, a monthly payment is collected in long term care facilities in all provinces.

In Canada, because insurance is provided by a single payer, that payer would simply reduce the fee-for-service to doctors by $5.00. We have an excess supply of doctors, so any patient who could not, or would not, pay the user fee would just doctor-shop until he/she found a doctor who had too few patients to make a living and would work for less. Perhaps this process was developed first by Medicare in the U.S.

The form of co-insurance in which patients pay all or part of costs to some sort of maximum per year can be administratively cumbersome. A full refund may be paid to users when a prescribed ceiling per person or per household is reached. A continuous co-insurance fee of a fixed amount per prescription, or a fixed percentage of costs, is much simpler. Protection beyond an annual maximum is known as catastrophic coverage. It can apply to a broad range of services or to one service only.

Co-insurance fees sometimes have a more noticeable effect on utilization when they are first imposed or removed than they do later on. They appear to have no effect when the patients pay the fee but physicians make the decisions. British Columbia and Alberta had hospital fees for 20 to 30 years and their patterns of hospital use were no different from those of other provinces where there were no patient payments. Roemer's Law applies: "A built bed is a filled bed." Roemer is an economist well-known for cryptic remarks.

Participation in health insurance plans run by government can be voluntary or compulsory. When it is voluntary, some people will not join because they choose to pay their own medical bills. Some will not join because they cannot pay the premiums, and others will not join because they have no assets and assume they will get needed care anyway (which they will). The voluntary versus compulsory argument can be completely avoided by paying for health care out of taxes and offering the same set of health services to all residents.

Single Versus Multiple Carriers of Insurance

Competition is in the public interest if it reduces price without lowering quality, but when many companies compete in the health insurance market there are increases in price and, at best, no effect on quality. When physicians and hospitals set the rates and insurance companies compete for clients (and this is the case when a variety of for-profit companies are selling health insurance) the consumer is the loser. Several arguments favor having all health insurance (including WCB medical care functions) handled by a single public agency.

☐ The government is best able to represent the public (the consumer) in discussions with the providers of health care services on such questions as price, quality, and distribution.

☐ Administration in both the physician's office and in the central insurance program is simplified. Administration costs in the United States, with multiple carriers and contracts, are many times those of the Canadian system.

☐ There is better capacity in the insurance agency for evaluation and research.

☐ There is more uniform and more complete statistical documentation of patterns of service.

☐ The use of a single program covering all of the population eliminates all discussion about whether people should be rejected, or charged higher premiums, because they are likely to consume a great deal of care.

The choice of a single carrier usually settles the question of whether the insurance program should be run by government or a for-profit agency. Monopolies should, to the extent that they are the rational choice, be in public rather than private hands. Either way they invite inefficiency and insensitivity to users, but in public hands there is, at least, some degree of accountability. Deciding whether to operate the public plan from within a ministry or through a crown corporation (such as The Manitoba Health Services Commission) is less important, but the political accountability of a department is greater than that of a crown corporation. Many special purpose bodies which formerly administered health insurance programs, in Canada have now disappeared.

Many of the above comments apply only to an insurance arrangement that must adapt to the fee-for-service method of physician payment. When capitation is a real option, as it is with the health maintenance organizations in the United States, then multiple competing carriers can lower costs. In capitation, the providers (or an agency representing providers) agree to deliver a prescribed spectrum of care for a fixed amount per person per year and competing agencies can lower the price. When fee-for-service is the method of physician payment, the volume and value of services that will have to be paid for is unknown. The same principles apply to hospital insurance, where global budgeting is a better approach than per diem or fee-for-service payments.

Features that Canadians Wish to See in their Health Insurance Program

☐ No payment by the patient directly to the providers of service at the time of service.
☐ Coverage of a broad range of services provided by a variety of providers in a variety of locations.
☐ No loss of coverage when costs are high, and no cancellation of insurance when future costs are likely to be high.
☐ A program open to all persons.
☐ A reasonable quality of care with quality measured in terms of clinical adequacy, continuity of care, accessibility and acceptability.
☐ Freedom of choice of providers and receivers of care.
☐ Simple and inexpensive administration with a minimum of red tape. Consumers want a program designed to keep things simple for the patient and the doctor.
☐ Continuous coverage on moving from one province to another (portability).
☐ Good value for money spent.

Utilization

Age and sex are closely correlated with the use of health care services. Babies, the elderly, and females aged 15 to 45 are heavy users of health care. Before age 5, males use more health services than females. From 5 to 14 years and after age 45, males and females consume relatively equal amounts of care per capita whether measured in number of services or cost in dollars.

In most provinces, 80 to 85 percent of the population see a physician at least once a year. For optometrists and chiropractors the figures are 10 to 20 percent and 5 to 15 percent respectively.

Utilization of health services is usually expressed as numbers of contacts per person, per 1,000, or per 100,000 per year. The number of physician contacts per person per year in Canada has risen from less than 3, 30 years ago, to around 10 to 12 in recent years. The increase is continuing.

Charges to the System

Canada is presently in the midst of a recession, but physicians are billing more in provinces such as Alberta. The 1990-91 Alberta annual report shows that doctors services rose 8 percent ($60 million) to a record $836 million, while the population increased less than 2 percent. Twenty-six specialists billed over $800,000 each, while the average for specialists was $236,000. Dermatologists bill $389,000 on average. General practitioners billed on average $137,000. These billings are gross payments from which doctors pay office expenses and are not necessarily the total income. Uninsured services and Workers Compensation Board fees are also available.

Alberta has 560 patients per doctor, and data show that a 15 percent increase in utilization occurred in 1991. In May 1992, the government set the global budget for doctors at $867 million. (Alberta Health Annual Report, 1991).

The number of admissions to hospitals per 1,000 is falling steadily. The number of days of acute hospital care per 1,000 is also declining, but the amount of the decrease is not easily identified because of the mixing of acute and long term days of care since many hospitals provide both types. The number of hospital admissions per 1,000 involving surgical procedures and treatments is rising despite a reduction in the availability of surgical beds. Shortened lengths of stay for inpatient surgery have more than made up for the reduced bed supply. In addition to the increase in hospital surgery there has also been a steady increase in the number of surgical procedures performed as day surgery, outpatient surgery and office surgery.

Utilization of long term care institutions is increasing steadily per 1,000 total population, but there is not much recent change in utilization if expressed as use per 1,000 population over 65, and in some locales such as Ottawa-Carleton, there has been a decrease in the percentage of those over 65 who are in institutions.

Home support services have grown rapidly from their formal beginnings in the 1950s. Emergency visits and the use of ambulances continue to grow.

Even the rates of established individual procedures are rather unpredictable. In 1968, less than 5 percent of Canadian births were by caesarian section; this statistic rose to 12 percent in 1977 and now to 20 percent or more in many centers. There is now a national effort, led by the Society of Obstetricians and Gynecologists of Canada, to reverse the trend.

Physician approaches to common ailments also vary greatly and bring quite different levels of utilization and cost. Examples include hemorrhoids (where therapy options include high fiber diet, ligation, injection, topical medication, cryosurgery, and surgical removal) or mild to moderate seasonal allergies (where the choices are long term desensitization with injections or use of medication during the allergy season). Use of diagnostic procedures is also unpredictable. The volume of Pap smears varies with the source of advice followed and the habits of the practitioner, as does the use of ultrasound in pregnancy, the use of fetal monitoring during labor, the volume of mammographies, or the frequency of CAT scans for patients with headaches. In at least two of these cases — fetal monitoring and the use of ultrasound in pregnancy — the patterns of use are inconsistent with the recommendations of the Society of Obstetricians and Gynecologists of Canada. In cancer treatment there is immense disagreement regarding when to use radiation, radical surgery, chemotherapy, or conservative surgery for a plethora of types of cancer, and the costs and side effects vary greatly as therapy changes. Manitoba studies found regional hysterectomy rates varied by as much as 100 percent. In the management of hypertension, overtreatment is frequently reported.

Excluding obstetrical and newborn days of care, half of total hospital days in are consumed by females. Persons 65 years or over account for over one-fifth of hospital separations and over one half of all hospital days. Persons 75 years and over, who represent 4 percent of the population, account for 10 percent of separations and almost one-third of hospital days. The age group 45 to 64, which make up approximately 20 percent of the population, account for approximately 20 percent of separations and hospital days. The volume of use of hospitals by the elderly has increased primarily because this age group has become larger, but partly because they were using hospitals 38 percent more per 100,000 in 1982-83 than in 1961. Dr. Robert Evans, in 1988, reported a major concentration of care in the year before death, regardless of age.

Major provincial variations in average hospital length of stay are, to a significant extent, merely a reflection of the degree to which acute treatment hospitals in the various provinces operate long term care beds. Table 2.8 lists the hospital costs in the provinces. Table 2.9 demonstrates expenditures on public health and home care. Since 1986 home care has grown in response to shorter lengths of stay in hospitals as well as a consumer interest in early discharge.

The number of reported abortions in Canadian provinces per 100 live births varies from 5 percent to 26 percent, with British Columbia having the highest rate. In the last 10 years while the total number of abortions performed has slowly increased, the percentage performed in the first 13 weeks of pregnancy has decreased, and the percentage performed on persons less than 20 years of age has gone down by one-quarter.

The extent to which health services utilization is a product of mental or emotional problems is uncertain, but many primary care health workers have identified psychosocial problems as the cause of over half of their patient contacts. This pattern applies to all socioeconomic classes.

Table 2.8

Ratio of Hospital Expenditures Per Person, Per Patient-Day, and Per Separation, Provinces, Territories and Canada 1985-86

	Hospital Expenditures ($ Millions)	Hospital Expenditures Ratio			
		($) per Person	($) per Bed	($) per Patient-Day	($) per Separation
Canada	16,227.7	644.43	95,054	329	4,409
Newfoundland	346.7	607.33	97,883	357	3,819
Prince Edward Island	68.1	540.63	90,438	311	2,783
Nova Scotia	603.4	693.25	103,748	370	4,033
New Brunswick	450.0	633.56	87,294	276	3,698
Quebec	4,550.8	698.38	87,311	299	6,037
Ontario	5,612.3	622.32	111,703	373	4,279
Manitoba	685.7	644.93	105,525	385	4,060
Saskatchewan	545.0	540.24	74,180	275	2,643
Alberta	1,619.9	689.85	89,502	320	3,853
British Columbia	1,680.1	584.69	80,138	287	3,933
Territories	65.8	871.18	—	—	—

Source: Institute for Health Care Facilities of the Future, 1990: A-110.

Note: The figures are for 1985-86, except in the case of Hospital Expenditures $ Millions and $ per person which are for the year 1985. As a result of the source of the numerator, cost ratios may be higher than traditionally published ratios from Statistics Canada; however, the trends are the same.

Table 2.9

Public Health and Home Care Expenditures as a Percentage of Total Health Care Expenditures, Provinces, Territories and Canada 1975 and 1986

	Public Health		Home Care	
	1975	1986	1975	1986
Canada	4.2	4.4	0.3	0.7
Newfoundland	3.6	3.0	0.0	0.2
Prince Edward Island	5.2	4.9	---	0.9
Nova Scotia	4.0	2.4	0.2	0.1
New Brunswick	3.3	4.1	0.1	0.1
Quebec	5.3	5.2	0.4	0.0
Ontario	3.1	3.1	0.3	1.2
Manitoba	4.2	5.2	1.0	1.6
Saskatchewan	6.3	5.6	0.3	1.3
Alberta	5.6	7.1	0.2	0.0
British Columbia	4.0	4.7	0.0	1.4
Territories	13.9	16.1	---	0.0

Source: Health and Welfare Canada (1990), National Health Expenditures in Canada 1975-1987, unpublished data.

Summary

Health care in Canada is financed through a variety of taxation strategies including income tax, excise tax, sales tax, and lotteries. About 25 percent of health care costs are paid by private sources including direct payment by consumers and private insurance. Each province has the authority to implement revenue generating policies and to determine resource allocation.

Health care costs in Canada are now rising faster than resources can be generated. Because health policy is developed explicitly in Canada, the public debate over choices in health care has become a prominent part of the political and policy agenda.

CHAPTER 3

Social, Political, and Structural Factors in Canadian Health Services

Philosophy

he current philosophical underpinnings of Canada's health services are, to a large extent, a product of former decades. Canada has, in theory, opted for

☐ an egalitarian rather than elitist or market-based access to health care;

☐ the right of every individual to approve or reject recommended care, or to approve or reject a healthy or an unhealthy lifestyle, or to approve or reject almost any form of risk;

☐ greater societal response to physical ill-health or injury than to mental or psychosocial difficulty;

☐ protection of children against public or individual decisions which are not in their best interests; and

☐ collective priorities and practices determined increasingly through public policy rather than by providers.

Canadians are uncertain about the extent to which access to services should be linked to the potential benefit to the patient. To date, the decision has usually been to provide unlimited service if such is prescribed by a physician. Patients have the freedom to choose a physician and have access to any number of physicians. Physicians have the freedom to reject any patient except in selected situations. It is current practice to give much greater weight to the needs of people who are already receiving services than to those who are waiting in line. The rationing of health care is regularly mentioned, and usually condemned, although the practice is with us and always has been.

Social Factors

The overall goal of a civilized society should be the highest possible health status for present and future populations. This global goal does not imply that the highest quality or the maximum consumable amount of health care or health protection will be routinely available to everyone . . . or to anyone. It does not mean that the life of everyone will be the longest it could possibly be, or that every hazard will be eliminated.

This social goal, if it is accepted, implies that there will be a collective willingness to share risk and resources in such a way that the health patterns of the total population will be as good as they can be. As one part of the vast social and economic network of activities that affect health, health services should contribute to the attainment of that global social goal to the maximum extent possible with the resources that are available. Health services should also avoid seeking more resources when those resources will have a greater positive effect on health status if they are consumed elsewhere.

The goal of the publicly funded health services network is therefore to exert influence and provide services that are consistent with the priorities assigned by society, the total availability of resources and the citizens' wishes. The Canadian population has repeatedly reiterated, in elections and in opinion polls, its wish for equal and excellent access of all Canadians to those health services that are publicly funded. Services privately funded will, as with other services purchased in the marketplace, reflect the wishes and wealth of a buyer and the willingness of a seller subject to legal and regulatory constraints.

Global goals are easy to write because they rely on the rhetoric of motherhood and apple pie for impact. Unfortunately, what they mean and how they should be transformed into specific policies and actions with specific objectives and targets is not so clear. Several governments have recently attempted to respond to the current need for better defined national and provincial health objectives. Ontario has health goals and Alberta has a blueprint for change, for example.

Health objectives need to be translated into services which support health. These can include social services, recreation services, transportation, education, income assistance, vocational rehabilitation, and/or help with household chores or maintenance. It also is difficult to decide how to categorize care provided by oneself, by household members, or by friends.

The Major National Models

There are three basic national or provincial approaches to the organization of health services. These are the national health services model, the public insurance model, and the entrepreneurial/market model.

In a national health system (NHS) model, a government, usually through a ministry of health, organizes and delivers health services. Great Britain has chosen this model. An NHS tends to be centralized but it may sometimes be quite decentralized as in Sweden and Finland.

Canada has a few examples which illustrate the NHS model but they represent only a small part of the health services network. Examples include the major psychiatric facilities which in most provinces are still owned and operated by the province, public health services in some provinces, the provincial laboratory networks, provincial ambulance systems (financed, organized, planned, evaluated, and delivered by a government) and the childrens' dental services program in Saskatchewan, which operated from 1974 to 1987. At the federal level, the armed forces' medical services and the services to Indians and Inuit are also examples of the NHS model. Most Canadian health services, however, are not organized this way.

Most Canadian health services are publicly financed but are administered and delivered by someone other than government. Canada, in general, has chosen the public insurance model. The Canadian public insurance umbrella, through which services are paid for by a provincial government, universally covers physician and hospital services. Ambulances, dentistry, chiropractors, optometrists, podiatrists, long term care, drugs, private physiotherapy, and home care thus have differing degrees of coverage in different provinces. Governments usually finance, regulate, and sometimes plan health care services, but delivery is usually carried out by nongovernmental for-profit or not-for profit agencies. The agency and the workers who actually deliver the services are not a part of, or employed by, the Ministry of Health or any other ministry.

The third health service model is the entrepreneurial model in which the government does not play a role as a major provider or a funder of health services. The United States is probably closer to this model than to the public insurance model but in the United States, as in Canada, there are elements of each of the three basic models.

The Federal Government

The *British North America (BNA) Act* of 1867, and subsequent interpretations of it, gave the provinces jurisdiction over most health services. The federal government was given jurisdiction over health services only for those specific populations mentioned in the *BNA Act*. These include native peoples, the armed forces, the RCMP, immigrants or refugees at certain stages in the immigration process, those living in the Northwest Territories and the Yukon, and a few other small groups.

Several federal departments are involved in the planning and delivery of health care. The Department of National Health and Welfare (DNHW), also called Health and Welfare Canada (HWC), through its Medical Services Branch provides services to one-third of a million Inuit and status Indians. HWC has financed many special studies, including the Royal Commission, whose 1964 report helped establish national medicare. Through an Ottawa production center and warehouse, HWC offers emergency health supplies (including portable hospitals) and maintains regularly updated emergency equipment and supplies stored throughout Canada. HWC also provides

☐ specialized laboratory and epidemiological services through its Centre for Disease Control (CDC);

☐ drug and equipment testing through its Food and Drug Directorate and its Bureau on Medical Devices;

☐ occupational health services to a broad network of federal government employees;

☐ consulting services in many environmental, occupational, and health care fields;

☐ expanding programs in the field of health promotion; and

☐ research funding of over $240 million annually to the Medical Research Council (MRC).

Through its welfare side, HWC delivers old age pensions and other income maintenance programs that are frequently fundamental to independence and good health. In 1974, a health minister, the Honorable Marc Lalonde, published a book, *A New Perspective on the Health of Canadians*, which received worldwide recognition because of its call for a reorientation of health services towards health promotion.

The Department of National Defence (DND), through facilities on military bases or at the National Defence Medical Centre in Ottawa, provides services to the armed forces, the RCMP, veterans, members of parliament, senators, foreign students funded by Canada, visiting dignitaries and selected senior civil servants, and representatives of the crown. At one time, the Department of Veterans Affairs (DVA) had a network of veterans' hospitals, but these have now largely been converted to civilian hospitals. DVA is now more of a paymaster than a deliverer of service.

Atomic Energy of Canada (AEC) controls the use of all radioactive equipment and supplies. Correctional Service Canada (CSC) spends about $50 million a year providing health care for the inmates of federal custodial institutions. Partly for health inspection purposes, the Department of Manpower and Immigration maintains immigrant stations at major ports and airports as well as in selected locations outside Canada. Other federal ministries such as Labor and Environment have functions closely or directly related to health care delivery, and Statistics Canada is a major producer of and repository for a broad range of health and health services information. The Canadian International Development Agency (CIDA) and the International Development Research Centre (IDRC) provide a variety of health programs and services as part of their assistance to less developed countries.

The above list mentions most federal health service activity, but it does not begin to list all of the ways in which federal activities directly affect health, nor does it fully illustrate the difficulties inherent in determining federal versus provincial jurisdiction. For instance, the transportation of toxic materials can be interprovincial and, therefore, is controlled by the federal Ministry of Transport. To a constitutional expert, the activity is transportation but people and municipalities tend to think of it as a health and safety matter.

The health services over which the federal government has constitutional jurisdiction serve over half a million Canadians, and other services provided by HWC and Statistics Canada are also of national importance. The influence of the federal government has perhaps been most felt, however, when federal money has been used to affect policy in areas of provincial jurisdiction.

In 1867, when the provinces were given jurisdiction over education and social services, they were not very expensive. Costly functions such as defense and transportation were assigned to the federal government and, therefore, the most lucrative revenue-producing taxation methods were reserved for the federal government. As the cost of education, health, and other social services increased, they became increasingly unaffordable for the provinces and the federal government became able to influence provincial policies through offers of financial aid.

The withholding of financial aid was not the first choice of the federal government as a tool to influence national health. World War II had shown that an unacceptably high percentage of Canadian recruits were medically unfit for military service, and both the Beveridge Report in Britain and the Marsh Report in Canada that studied the levels of fitness and health, had recommended the establishment of national health systems. At the Conference on Reconstruction during World War II the federal government proposed a national approach to health services funding and planning, a proposal that required provincial support and an amendment to the constitution. The provinces, however, would not agree to give up their control over health services.

Constitutional amendments which allow the federal government to act in an area of provincial jurisdiction are not always rejected by the provinces. In 1940 and 1951, for example, the provinces consented respectively to federal implementation of national unemployment insurance and universal old age security.

Having lost its bid for a federally operated health insurance program, the federal government then sought other ways to contribute to and influence health services and their costs. The following three devices have been most commonly used.

First, federally financed and operated services which are useful to the provinces, laboratories, and health promotion were established. **Second, conditional grants**, which are available only if used for specified purposes and in specified ways, were created. There are two main types of conditional grants.

1. Funds available without provincial government expenditures (although various other conditions must be met). The Canada Assistance Plan (CAP) is one example. Through CAP, 50 percent federal funding is available for a broad range of rehabilitative, social support, and community based-programs as long as the other funding is provided by other than a federal source. Many programs which are funded through CAP have the second half of the necessary funds raised locally, with the provincial government contributing nothing. The vocational rehabilitation of disabled persons arrangements and the new 1987 drug abuse expenditures are also in this category.

2. Funds available only when there is an associated provincial government expenditure and when other conditions are met. Such arrangements are known as **cost sharing**. Hospital insurance and medicare were in this category from their inception to 1977. The *Hospital Insurance and Diagnostic Services Act* (HIDSA — Bill C-60) was passed in 1957 and came into force on July 1, 1958. It required

☐ that a minimum but broad range of hospital inpatient services be insured, with outpatient coverage being optional;
☐ that there be standardized national reporting;
☐ that services be available on equal terms and conditions; and
☐ that basic standards be met.

In return, provinces received a per capita payment for each insured person. The payment was a composite of 25 percent of national per capita costs plus 25 percent of provincial per capita costs. Through this formula, high cost provinces received less than 50 percent of their program costs. The opposite held true for low cost provinces.

The medicare legislation which came into force in 1968 required public administration, coverage of a comprehensive range of physician services, coverage of at least 95 percent of the population (later raised to 100 percent), portability between provinces, and reasonable compensation for physicians. These were all principles put forward in the 1964 Royal Commission report chaired by Justice Emmett Hall which set in motion Canada's medicare program. The financial formula was slightly different from that applied to hospital services and was once again designed to assure that poor provinces would be more generously assisted that the wealthier provinces. The provinces had all joined medicare by 1971.

The third device used by the federal government to help the provinces is the **unconditional grant**. These funds increase provincial revenue and have no strings attached.

The *Hospital Insurance and Diagnostic Services Act* of 1957 and the *Medical Care Act* of 1966 are still seen as the vehicles through which universal health insurance was brought to Canada. They are, perhaps, our most famous pieces of health legislation, but they are now largely historical documents. Federal-provincial fiscal arrangements in the two famous statutes were replaced in 1977 by the *Federal Provincial Fiscal Arrangements and Established Programs Financing Act*, (EPF), and by the *Canada Health Act* of 1984. These two acts spell out the terms and conditions prerequisite to receipt of federal financial assistance subsequent to 1977 and 1984 respectively.

The unconditional transfer of federal funds to the provinces is not new, but under EPF these unconditional transfers were sharply increased. Actually, it can quite properly be argued that transfer payments under EPF are not unconditional because of the conditions stipulated in the *Canada Health Act* in particular. Nevertheless, the degree of federal control certainly decreased significantly in 1977. EPF terminated federal responsibility for a fixed portion of provincial expenditures for selected health services, and for practical purposes eliminated federal control over provincial medicare and hospitals. It also reduced federal financial risk. As compensation, the provinces were given a per capita block grant, per capita payments tied to the gross national product, 14 additional points of personal income tax, one additional point of corporate income tax, and full flexibility to financially support various health services to whatever extent they wished.

From 1977 to 1984, predictable sums were transferred from the federal government to the provincial treasuries, with the provincial governments being, for practical purposes, able to spend these monies in any way they wished. The amounts transferred continued to rise, but not as rapidly as they would have risen if the 1977 cost-sharing arrangement was still in place.

Bill C-69, *The Federal Restraint Law*, was passed in 1991 and has created a rapid withdrawal of federal contributions. For example, federal transfer to Ontario for post-secondary education and health care has fallen from 52 percent of the cost in 1979-80 to 31 percent in 1991-92. In dollar terms, Ontario has lost an expected $12.3 billion in expected revenue.

Thirty-five years ago about two-thirds of personal income tax points (revenue) came to the federal government. As part of the process of helping provinces, the federal government had regularly increased the provincial share until 1991.

The *Canada Health Act* (1984) once again required certain performance from the provinces if all promised federal funds (under EPF) were to be received. Requirements included coverage of 100 percent of the population and direct charges for insured services only under a limited number of circumstances. User fees and physician extra billing became tied to provincial penalties. The province lost one dollar of EPF payment for every dollar of user fees or extra billing.

Federal legislation can also significantly affect delivery of health care without any change in federal/provincial fiscal relations. For example, the 1971 bill legalizing abortion had a direct effect on hospital functions, medical staff organization, hospital board decisions, health care costs and the emotional and physical health of many women.

Health Services to Native Peoples

There are various interpretations of the statutes and treaties which establish federal responsibility for health care to the Indians and Inuit, and there is disagreement about the range of responsibility and who is entitled to care. However, a relatively unchallenged relationship based on a combination of contract, precedent, legal decision, and acceptance of obligation, exists between the native peoples and the federal government. This relationship includes an obligation for health and other social services, although the federal government continues to regularly seek devices through which native peoples can, at least for the purposes of health care, be seen as provincial residents. Provinces have varied in their willingness to accept natives as regular beneficiaries under provincial medical and hospital insurance, but in most provinces this administrative absorption has occurred.

For the last 40 years health services to native peoples have been financed and delivered by the Medical Services Branch (MSB) of the Department of National Health and Welfare. This branch maintains nursing stations, health stations, health centers, clinics, and small hospitals. MSB also trains and employs indigenous health workers, and pays directly for care provided by health workers and institutions outside of the MSB network.

Services operated or funded by MSB include a wide range of preventive, diagnostic, treatment, and educational programs in the fields of dentistry, medical care, public health, and environmental health. Some programs such as the National Native Alcohol and Addictions Program (NNAAP) are operated by national and local native organizations, and there is currently a major push towards transfer of administrative responsibility for health services to bands or native councils. The transfer of function is being impeded by

- disagreement over the amount of money that will be available to the native authorities,
- uncertainty regarding the role of provincial governments,
- the lack of skills in some native communities, and
- the question of how much federal control will remain after transfer.

In several provinces, medical schools contract to supply services to northern communities. For example, since 1969 the University of Manitoba has been responsible for maintaining medical services in Churchill, Norway House, Hodgson, and a number of other smaller communities in northern Manitoba and in the Northwest Territories. The federal government, as a partner in national health care, influences the health of Canadians through the programs described above. These programs can be summarized as

1. health services within its jurisdiction,
2. healthy public policy in all areas of federal jurisdiction, and
3. pressure on the provinces to meet national standards.

Provincial Governments

Each province can, almost to the extent it wishes, be directly responsible for all priority setting, policy selection, planning, financing, regulating, administration, resource allocation, evaluation, standard-setting, and delivery of any type of health service. These services include physician services, dental services, ambulances, hospitals, and public health. Provincial jurisdiction is absolute, subject only to rights enshrined in the *Charter of Rights* and other components of the Canadian constitution, and to the exclusion of the limited areas of federal jurisdiction. Theoretically, each province could choose any of the macro-organizational models discussed earlier. To varying degrees, the various provinces have chosen, by act or omission, to delegate certain managerial and delivery functions to quasi-governmental, voluntary, professional, or commercial entities, but all provincial governments now have also chosen to be directly active in most major aspects of health care.

All provinces, through one or more departments and statutes, take a direct interest in the standards and costs of most health care, with hospitals, physicians' services, public health, home care, long term care institutions, and ambulances being most routinely under scrutiny and control. Drugs, dental services, and the supply of health manpower receive varying attention. Some activities such as chiropractics and optometry receive funding but are otherwise largely ignored. In the smaller provinces, most public health programs are administered by the provincial department of health or its equivalent. Psychiatric hospitals are primarily provincially owned and operated as well. Provincial governments tend to require standardized reporting with respect to selected aspects of institutional or other operations and care delivery.

Health Insurance Programs

All provinces operate health insurance programs either from within a ministry, which is the commonest approach, or through some separate agency very closely linked to the Ministry of Health. The public insurance agency always covers hospital services and physician services because public administration was a condition of federal financing, but it may also cover drugs, ambulance services, long term care, dental services, prosthetics, glasses, home care, optometry, and chiropractics.

Health care insurance operates within the same principles as any other insurance. It is a means whereby people replace unpredictable major expense with predictable regular expense. A beneficiary facing a risk makes regular payments to an insurer, who agrees to meet the unpredictable costs if they materialize. Public health insurance differs somewhat in that it is usually compulsory and the beneficiary usually makes all payments through the tax system. When health care costs are paid out of general revenue, the payments made by each person vary with their level of taxation rather than their level of risk.

Public insurance systems have major advantages for most taxpayers. Their administration costs are very low compared to those of private and competing insurance companies. Multiple carriers, on the other hand, are inefficient and bring no more benefits to users. Because Canadian health insurance programs have public service as their motive, the user need not worry about losing insurance coverage if costs are high. The insurance will not be cancelled. The likelihood of major expenses falling to the user, as was common with the exclusions, deductions and indemnity payments in profit-based plans, are much reduced. Because billing forms are standardized and computerized, physician payment is rapid as well as inexpensive. With the abolition of extra billing, the patient reimbursement mode of payment is now almost a thing of the past.

Provincial and federal governments affect health programs and institutions through many statutes and regulations other than those administered by the department of health. Laws and regulations governing such things as minimum wages, vacation pay, affirmative action, equal pay for work of equal value, the rights to and process of certification, collective bargaining and conflict resolution, payroll deductions, discrimination, collection of sales taxes, quality of construction, Workers Compensation Board (WCB) participation, and public safety apply throughout the health services network unless specifically exempted.

All provinces are more dominant in planning and financing health services (both capital and operational) than in administration or evaluation. Provinces usually standardize statistical, financial, and other reporting, and these provincial data are sometimes also nationally standardized, as with hospital data. Governments have excellent data which increases their ability to identify unreasonable billing patterns. Governments, as the only major paying agency, are in a better position to regulate payment amounts and patterns of practice by using negotiation as well as statutory powers. All provinces define, by statute, the status and the self-governing powers and responsibilities of the various professions. One such statute is the *Health Disciplines Act* in Ontario, soon to be replaced by broader umbrella legislation, the *Health Professions Regulation Act*.

Provincial governments all have one or more departments directly related to health care organization, financing and delivery. Some provinces, like Ontario and Saskatchewan, have only a ministry of health which deals with all health services and little else. Other provinces, such as Quebec and Manitoba, have combined health and social services in one ministry. Other provinces have more than one department dealing with health, with one or more of these departments usually also responsible for social services. Departmental titles and functions regularly change. Within a ministry, the deputy minister is the senior bureaucrat or manager of the department, while the minister is the elected official held accountable for the policy and operations of the department.

In almost all provinces, there are also a series of quasi-public bodies of varying importance. These bodies usually report to the minister or deputy minister and, occasionally, to the cabinet. They perform tasks which could be, and which in other provinces often are, carried out from within a department of government.

The Quebec Model

The organization of health and social services in Quebec is sufficiently different from the rest of the country to merit separate attention.

In the 1960s under Premier Lesage, the quiet revolution converted the Quebec education system from a primarily parochial system to a system similar to that in other provinces. In the 1970s this quiet revolution was applied to the health and social services systems, but the product was unlike the systems in other provinces.

In 1970, the second and enlarged version of the Castonguay-Nepveu Report on health reform was published, and before the year ended Castonguay was Minister of Health. In the same year, the Quebec Ministries of Health and of Welfare were combined to form the Ministry of Social Affairs (Ministère des Affaires Sociales, which was later renamed Ministère des Affaires Sociales et de la Santé). This 1970 amalgamation of ministries was the first step towards implementation of the Castonguay-Nepveu Report.

In 1972, Bill 65 reorganized and regionalized health and social services. It established a province-wide network of 12 regional councils, later to become 11, each with 21 members. Four of these members were to be elected by the mayors of the municipalities of the region, two would be named by the Ministry as representatives of regional socioeconomic groups, three representatives would come from universities and community colleges and three would be from each of the four categories of institutions within each regional system.

The four categories of health and social service organizations into which most existing and future institutions would fit were the local community service centers (Centre Local des Services Communautaires or CLSC), the social service centers, the hospital centers, and the reception centers (Centres d'Accueil) which included group homes and halfway houses.

Bill 65 described the composition of the boards of the four categories of institutions. In each case the boards included one or more representatives of neighboring institutions, the regional council, the professional staff, the other staff, and the public. The public representatives are elected at an annual meeting. The spirit of the Castonguay-Nepveu Report, which had recommended a high degree of local participation and of regional control, was not fully evident. Bill 65 opted for a minority role for unaffiliated local representatives on all boards and gave regional councils very little power. The government clearly believed, probably correctly, that a radical redistribution of function and the introduction of new structures would be more likely to succeed if there was a strong central hand at the helm.

Among the hospitals within each region there is one or more "designated" hospital centers which, through departments of community health (départements de santé communautaire or DSC), was given responsibility for epidemiological studies and planning. These functions in other provinces usually rest with the public health departments. There is no separate public health agency in the Quebec system, the functions having been merged with other functions and carried out primarily by the DSC in designated hospitals and by the CLSCs. Some functions, such as those of public health inspectors, were transferred completely out of the health agencies and into such departments as environment, agriculture, and fisheries and food, or to agencies dealing with such things as work safety.

The Quebec system is a network of population-based facilities and programs, each with a specific population for which they are responsible and to which they are at least somewhat accountable. Each institution and program has a responsibility to offer a specified range of services to its targeted population. The situation is analogous to a police force, an Ontario public health unit, or a school with a designated service area. It is quite different from the usual hospital or grocery store which provides services to those who come in, rather than having a mandate to serve a specified population. The boundaries do not restrict client access to other physicians and hospitals, but they do give the institutions an obligation to be available to the population in their area.

Quebec created a network of agencies responsible for

- social services;
- primary, secondary, and tertiary health care;
- home care;
- public health;
- emergency care;
- health planning;
- health promotion;
- long term care;
- episodic care;
- physical health; and
- emotional health.

In the Castonguay concept, the regional network measured local needs, set local priorities, and delivered a broad range of services to the extent possible given the resources available. Unfortunately, the private practitioners were sufficiently entrenched and powerful enough to resist merging. Therefore, the integrated network is incomplete. The merging of mental health with other services was not immediate, but has been accomplished.

Other provinces have implemented, in a less comprehensive way, similar integrated regional systems. Many parts of rural Manitoba are served by long term care facilities, public health services, home care services, and community hospitals all under one board. Alberta has a small number of rural communities, the town of High Level being one example, with a similar arrangement. Quebec, however, is unique in its province-wide plan and the breadth of the health and social services integration.

The current role of the federal and provincial governments has been determined by tradition (and provinces do not all have the same traditions), by law (in particular the *BNA Act* and its successors), by experience (for example, the failure of the private sector to deliver health care to the high-risk part of the population), by the imbalance between provincial responsibilities and financing capabilities, and by public demand. There is no typical provincial or municipal role. Role varies with political philosophy and with culture, with population characteristics, with economic capacity and other factors.

Municipal Governments

Municipalities are the creatures of provinces. Their roles in health care can therefore be defined and constrained by provincial decisions. Most provinces have not assigned major health care functions to municipalities, but municipalities have contributed to the Canadian pattern of publicly controlled, rather than privately controlled, health care. Many western municipalities had municipally-based doctor and hospital plans in the early part of the century, and many major urban municipalities in Canada have always directly administered public health services through a public health department. This organizational pattern may yet become more common. In Ontario, several large municipalities including Halton, Toronto, and Ottawa have, in the last decade, taken over public health functions that were formerly under the control of a separate public health board.

Up to 15 percent of total municipal expenditures in any single municipality are for health and social services, but was mostly for social services. The amounts and the emphasis on health and on social services vary greatly from one area to another.

Prior to universal hospital insurance, many municipalities regularly contributed to the operating and capital costs of hospitals. Contributions to operating costs largely ceased in 1958, but municipal contributions to capital costs continued in some provinces, and this practice is currently expanding. Toronto City Council, in 1987, voted $3 million a year for health services and earmarked all of it for hospital capital costs.

Quasi-Governmental Agencies (also sometimes called Crown Corporations)

Quasi-public agencies are created by governments of all levels to perform some specific regulatory, educational, policy-making, evaluative, or managerial function that government prefers not to do itself. The function is moved outside of the government bureaucracy, although usually not fully beyond government influence. Quasi-public agencies are usually created by statute, although some, such as the District Health Councils in Ontario, are created by an Order in Council.

Moving functions out of government is often said to be a good thing because it removes political influence, the implication being that political influence is a bad thing. Not only is political influence usually still at work, but there is also often a reduction of accountability to the public and an increased insensitivity to outside concerns. The proposition that separation from government will reduce bureaucratic characteristics is seldom borne out and coordination is apt to be more difficult.

There is, in organizational terms, only an invisible line between quasi-public agencies or special purpose bodies, and voluntary agencies. These two categories are best thought of as a spectrum rather than two distinct organizational forms. The spectrum covers the entire range and variety of ties to government, ability to generate revenue, degree of public accountability, degree of public visibility, spending ability, and dependence on government financing.

A number of quasi-governmental agencies that once had major operating responsibilities have been abandoned. Two examples are the Ontario Hospital Services Commission and the Saskatchewan Medical Care Insurance Commission. Others, including the Manitoba Health Services Commission and the Quebec Health Insurance Board (La Régie), still remain. Many governments and electorates see these special purpose bodies as an inappropriate transfer of public policy and administration functions to the control of non-elected persons.

Some agencies, such as The Addictions Research Foundation in Ontario, have only advisory or educational functions. Councils of this type have a history of self-immolation. They tend to eventually become sufficiently critical of government to be disbanded or lose funding. They function best, and survive longest, when their area of advice is clearly defined, their mandate is clearly stated, and their mandate is primarily education or research. Prior to appointment to the boards of these agencies, nominees should be clear about the agenda they are expected to deal with, the level of governmental contact available to them (the Minister, the Deputy Minister, other staff, the cabinet), the resources that will be available (for instance, can special studies be done), and the expected schedule of meetings and payment. Members can then know whether the agency is likely to exert the kind of influence that is consistent with their wishes.

Provincial Colleges of Physicians and Surgeons and equivalent other professional organizations are also quasi-governmental agencies. They are created by statute to perform functions which are delegated to them by the province including the licensing, regulation and discipline of their members. They are funded by fees paid by their members.

The Private Nonprofit Sector

Boards of the private non-profit agencies may be elected or appointed. They usually manage a corporate entity and are responsible for planning and/or operational decisions for a hospital or community health center. They are legally independent, although often considerably controlled by government regulation or financing arrangements, as well as being less formally constrained by precedent, public perception, and social values. These boards operate agencies that usually provide either health services or health and other social services. Examples include Alcoholics Anonymous, community health centers, group homes, long term care placement agencies, Childrens Aid societies, senior citizen centers, and halfway houses. A small number, such as Social Planning Councils, exist primarily or exclusively to plan. Hospital boards are similar to other independent boards in many ways, but operate under an unusually high degree of ministerial control.

Private nonprofit agencies or facilities can be quite parochial and, therefore, are less easily fitted into an overall regional or community plan. On the positive side, they may be able to mobilize local support in the form of volunteers and money. Efficiency is seldom measured. Quality is also seldom evaluated except in hospitals through the accreditation process.

Workers Compensation Boards (WCB) are health-related agencies that don't fit well into any of the listed categories. They have their own statute, but a minister is usually politically responsible for their activities. They exist to provide aid to workers suffering from work-related injuries or diseases. They were created in the early part of the twentieth century to protect employers from the hazard of being sued by workers who were injured on the job. They have a history of being technocratic, bureaucratic, and autocratic, although they have, over the years, become somewhat more worker-oriented. Workers have, until recently, been unable to sue for damages arising from negligence at the workplace, but they are eligible for long term care and income support even if the negligence is theirs. Recent senior court decisions giving workers or their families the right to sue employers may bring about major changes in the entire WCB operation.

A WCB is financed entirely by employers (and, therefore, to some degree by workers through deferred wages) who pay a percentage of payroll (up to 20 percent), depending on the accident experience of each category of employer. There may or may not be experience rating of individual employers. Rates may or may not be higher for employers with a bad safety record. One-quarter to one-third of WCB expenditures are for health care.

Voluntary agencies are non-profit and non-governmental. They range from quite organizationally complex (the Canadian Red Cross) to very simple (an unincorporated self-help group). They can be small and local (Meals on Wheels) or large and national (Canadian Cancer Society, Victorian Order of Nurses or VON). They may be largely publicly funded (Canadian Red Cross) or receive no public funding (Alcoholics Anonymous). Their function may be primarily or entirely education and research (Canadian Heart Foundation), service delivery (group home) or political action (anti- and pro-abortion groups or the Canadian Health Coalition). They are often concerned with a specific disease or condition such as cancer or heart disease. They may be clearly identified with health services, or may have health matters as only one part of a broader mandate (the Canadian Labor Congress and the National Anti-Poverty Association). This vast network of nonprofit agencies is important and powerful in the Canadian health services mosaic.

Charitable institutions were operating hospitals and institutions for the disabled and the dying hundreds of years ago, and their example is perpetuated in religious and voluntary institutions and programs. Before national compulsory hospital or medical care insurance was introduced, the hospital associations and the physician organizations were the largest carriers of hospital and medical care insurance respectively. They were, in a competitive market, quite easily able to offer more attractive insurance than the for-profit sector.

Non-governmental boards and agencies organized at the federal or provincial level are likely to have separately incorporated regional or local chapters. These local or regional chapters usually have some degree of management autonomy, but also have close structural ties with the central body (VON, Canadian Red Cross, Planned Parenthood).

Public policy has altered the nature and role of several national voluntary agencies. Publicly operated home care programs altered the role of the VON, of previously existing cancer treatment programs, and of the Arthritis Society, for example. Further conflicts and changes are likely to emerge. Changing disease patterns have produced changes in some diagnostically specific agencies; the Anti-Tuberculosis League, for instance, became the Canadian Lung Association. The emergence of the consumer age, with a reduction of acceptance of paternalistic programming, altered the power balance in organizations such as the Canadian National Institute for the Blind (CNIB).

The Private For-Profit Sector

In Canada, the private-for-profit sector has been much less dominant than in the United States. It has played a particularly small role in hospitals and health insurance. This restricted role is much more a product of experience and of culture than of political ideology. Even before the appearance of government sponsored universal insurance, most insured Canadians used a not-for-profit carrier.

The for-profit sector, however, remains active in the Canadian health services network. The extent to which its role should be expanded — that is, the extent to which health care should be privatized — is under active examination. For-profit involvement is usually in one or more of the following ways.

☐ An outsider who has a contract with a specific institution or program to provide a specified service
   1. **Advice**. This is the role played by most consultants.
   2. **Management**. A for-profit firm may be hired to manage a total institution or program, or any part of it. When management of a total institution is contracted out it may be combined with an infusion of private capital, as in Hawkesbury, Ontario, and Wetaskiwin, Alberta, although there may be no financing associated with the management contract.
   3. **Hotel services** such as housekeeping, laundry, dietary, and parking.
   4. **Administrative services** such as payroll management, occupational health, and fund raising.
   5. **Clinical (patient care) services**. A small number of community agencies buy nursing and other care from for-profit sources. In theory, a hospital or other health care agency could contract out its laboratory, pharmacy and radiology department, and probably others.

☐ Owners and operators of sources of health care such as nursing homes, ambulances, special hospitals, pharmacies, agencies providing services in the home, laboratories and the manufacturers and fitters of orthotic or prosthetic devices.

☐ A banker who provides the capital which is, as has been noted, sometimes tied to an ongoing management role. In other cases payback is based on a share of revenue rather than an interest rate. An example is the construction by Extendicare of long term care beds at the Queensway General Hospital in Toronto. When the private sector provides capital for hospital construction, there is weakening of one of the provincial government devices for control of institutional costs. The government is less able to control the timing of the construction.

☐ Partners with non-profit agencies in some other mutually advantageous arrangement such as the agreement between University Hospital, London, Ontario and Hospital Corporation of America (HCA). In this agreement the hospital gains access to the purchasing power of HCA, and HCA gains preferential access to the hospital for care for selected patients. Patient care costs in Canada are significantly lower than in the United States and HCA saves money by having some of its patients come to the London hospital for elective care. In 1986, the Toronto General Hospital entered into a similar, mutually advantageous arrangement when Travenol Canada financed a $750,000 intravenous drug administration center within the hospital in return for a fee-for-service contract to deliver the 300,000 intravenous drug doses. In 1985, this cost $4.5 million. This type of arrangement has also occurred in the supply of infant formula to hospitals.

There is, within the chronic care system, one recent transfer of function from the non-profit or governmental sector to the private sector which has gone relatively unnoticed, but which would have major impact if extended. Institutionalization was, until a few years ago, the standard solution when the level or complexity of care required by any individual exceeded what was available from household members or home care programs. This is still the practice for the disabled elderly, but younger, severely physically disabled persons, such as quadriplegics, now routinely live in their own residential units and receive 24-hour services from staff who are somewhere nearby. The health and social support services are publicly funded, but the disabled persons are tenants with leases who obtain their housing through the same arrangements as the rest of us. A few years ago, this housing would have been part of a long term care institution, but may now be provided by the private sector.

The extent to which health services should be provided by the for-profit sector is uncertain. Profit is most clearly a hazard when competition, useful to the consumer is absent, when quality is very difficult to measure, or when caseloads or service mix can be manipulated to avoid unattractive components, which must then be borne by non-profit providers. Profit is most defensible when competition exists that is useful to the consumer and when product specifications can be clearly written. Health services do, after all, buy large quantities of supplies and services from the private sector (food, equipment, linen) but this is not usually referred to as the privatization of health services.

Whether or not private practitioners (dentists, physicians, chiropractors) should be included in this listing of for-profit sources of health care is a matter of opinion, but in this chapter they are not included. Physicians and dentists may be sole proprietors but their income is generated from professional fees for services rather than resale of goods. Dentists can make a profit from the sale of dental hygiene services, charging customers more than the actual cost. The most distinguishing characteristic of the profit sector is the concept of return on investment. Fee-for-service practitioners are distinguished from other workers by their method of payment, but it is inappropriate and sometimes unnecessarily provocative to consider their offices to be equivalent to places of business.

Provider Organizations

Major health worker groups (nurses, physicians, physiotherapists, laboratory technicians), some facility types (hospitals), and most major service areas (mental health, public health) have national, provincial, and often regional or local organizations. The most important of these organizations are at the provincial level because health is a provincial matter. Provincial professional associations are of two types: those which perform licensing/ certification and regulatory duties as assigned by statute, and those which perform trade union functions. Not all professions are represented by both types of organizations. Provincial institutions and programs are in some provinces served by a single umbrella association, usually called a health association. In other provinces the various associations such as the hospital association and the public health association remain separate.

Provincial institutional associations can be active in many ways. The Ontario Hospital Association, for example, offers a provincial hospital computer service, and a hospital purchasing program. Regional organizations like the Hospital Council of Metropolitan Toronto (HCMT) operates, or has initiated, a consulting service, group purchasing, a drug information service, laundry service, an instructional media service, a nursing registry, a specialty food shop, a high technology maintenance program, and a research support service.

The Ontario College of Physicians and Surgeons has, for almost a decade, conducted a peer review program in which physicians are visited by a review team. This ambitious program has statutory backing so participation is not voluntary. Although provincial provider organizations have the broadest range of functions, there are a number of important national organizations. Almost all physicians, for example, buy their medical malpractice insurance through a physician-operated nonprofit insurance company, the Canadian Medical Protective Association (CMPA). The CMPA has always been dominant in Canada, but in 1986 enrollment increased to almost all practicing physicians because of a withdrawal of private insurance from this market. In recent years the CMPA has moved to variable fees. Prior to that all types of doctors paid the same fee.

Most professional and institutional organizations have a code of ethics or conduct. This code is voluntary in such organizations as hospital, or hospital administrator, associations and is mostly window dressing. The codes can, however, be of importance in those self-governing professions who have been assigned responsibility for public protection. The vigor with which professions enforce their ethical codes through member discipline varies from absent to moderate. Physician organizations now probably perform (after years of concentrating on advertising practices and whether members talked to chiropractors) with the degree of professional rigor seeming to be at least somewhat related to the degree of governmental and public scrutiny. Professions about which few questions are asked, such as chiropractors and optometrists, appear to be quite internally unregulated. Some physician organizations now have active and expensive programs to detect and respond to drug and alcohol abuse, public complaints, aberrant billing, unusual practice habits, and the quality of office records and equipment. Some professional organizations such as the Canadian College of Health Service Executives and the College of Family Physicians of Canada require evidence of involvement in continuing education if there is to be continued membership. The latter organization is also currently developing a software package for evaluation of a physician's practice, and this evaluation may become part of the recertification process.

Governments, at least in principle, seek professional regulatory arrangements that protect the public by enforcement of professional standards and by describing the scope of activities that are within the competence of different professionals. The regulatory arrangements often assign responsibilities to the professionals themselves. The public interest would seem to be best protected by professions that work cooperatively with other professions, and that encourage cost control as well as good patient care. Unfortunately, independent professions more frequently oppose cooperation and vigorously defend their turf, even when tasks would be better and/or more cheaply, performed by other workers.

Communities and Consumers

The consumer age has changed health services. Consumers increasingly believe the health services network exists to work for them, and the services have been obliged to be more responsive, less paternalistic, and more sensitive. Changes have occurred in patients' rights statements and legislation, in obtaining access to records, and in the composition and roles of boards of trustees. Through influence on public policy, consumers could, if they chose, limit resource availability and utilization, control professional supply and function, determine rates of pay, and directly influence a broad range of professional decisions.

Consumers have always been able to complain to caregivers, institutions, the police, the media or anyone else, but historically, they seldom complained and were seldom listened to if they did. Complaints now are not only more apt to receive attention, but they are being delivered in more ways. Patient satisfaction surveys and questionnaires are routine. Institutional ombudsmen are increasingly available to help identify patient problems or abuse and to implement acceptable response. Self-help or advocacy groups are now common. Insurance is usually obtained through a public agency, which may be more apt to investigate and react to a consumer complaint. Legislation and court decisions have spelled out the rights of patients to information and choice, and professional complaints committees and higher appeal mechanisms have public members. The existence of these devices encourages institutions and individual caregivers to be aware of the wishes, preferences, and values of patients. Boards, discipline committees, payment agencies, and courts now routinely decide whether professional or institutional service and conduct is adequate or merits discipline.

The rise in public participation and influence can be endorsed as a means of strengthening democracy through the production of a more informed and less cynical population, and because the process identifies indigenous leaders. It also can counterbalance the power of professionals and bureaucrats and more decisively insert the priorities of users and payers into the decisionmaking process. However, despite all of the above changes and optimistic verbiage, the professionals still often manage to ignore, intimidate, or co-opt the consumer process.

Throughout this chapter the focus has been on the history, politics, societal role, and organization of Canadian health services. One significant fact should be remembered. Health care is under provincial jurisdiction. This jurisdiction includes resource allocation, the management of health professions, and the ability to influence provider organizations.

Provincial governments are influenced in turn by their electorate, making health care in Canada a political act, rather than a rational act.

References

Brown, M.C. (1991). *Health Economics and Policy: Problems and Prescriptions.* Toronto: McLelland and Stewart Inc.

Evans, R.G. et al. (1989). Controlling health expenditures — The Canadian reality, *New England Journal of Medicine*, 320(9):574-576.

Green, D. (1986). *Challenge to the NHS: A Study of Competition in American Health Care and the Lessons for Britain*. Institute of Economic Affairs, London, p. 48-55.

Managing Health Care Resources: Meeting Ontario's Priorities, Supplementary Paper to the 1992 Ontario Budget. Queen's Printer, Ontario, p. 27.

CHAPTER 4

The Role of Physicians

Introduction

The last half-century has seen a large portion of health care become increasingly multidisciplinary and technological. The all-purpose physician working with an all-purpose nurse is no longer dominant. Most care is now delivered by a physician who works with a particular set of problems or patients, a nurse who works in only one clinical area, and a continually expanding cadre of other specialized health workers.

Some things, however, have not changed. Physicians still often work alone. Nurses still usually have little if any specialized training. The workers within the traditional medical team still have minimal contact with the caregivers who are outside the medical model. Much health care remains relatively uncomplicated. Health workers who, in previous decades, were exposed to tuberculosis and septicemia, and then to hepatitis, as a condition of work, must now in the same way, deal with exposure to AIDS.

The specialization of physicians has had many effects. Medical care insurance statistics suggest that one quarter to one half of all primary care is now provided by specialists, and this percentage is much higher in pediatrics and in obstetrics. The rate of participation of the family physician in obstetrics has been falling for decades. Major increases in liability insurance for physicians performing deliveries has recently accelerated the trend. Two thirds of routine obstetrical care is now provided by specialists. Major surgery in large urban centers is now done almost exclusively by specialists, and the trend is pronounced even in rural and small urban centers.

Most formal health care is delivered within the medical model, a model in which the physician is the monarch. Other professionals who routinely work within the medical model almost always do so with the understanding that the right to diagnose and to prescribe is legally a physician's prerogative. This situation shows little likelihood of changing, although the Royal College of General Practitioners in Britain recently proposed that nurses working in association with family physicians should have the authority to prescribe or alter the dosage of a very limited list of drugs and biologicals.

Many health workers are anxious to climb the ladder or, at least, to defend their rung. Physicians staunchly pretend chiropractors and optometrists do not exist, and equally vigorously continue to believe that nurses, physiotherapists, psychologists, and pharmacists are merely useful responders to the orders of doctors. Dentists continue to battle with denturists and dental therapists, and family physicians continue to struggle to preserve a meaningful — but perhaps shrinking — place in the health care team.

Physicians are much less dominant in health policy development and somewhat less dominant in patient care than they have been in the past, but their powers remain massive. They, and only they, can admit and discharge patients from hospital. They do almost all the prescribing and have almost total control over access to diagnostic and therapeutic tools, including most of the high technology tools. Patients perceive physicians as the primary holders of the key to life, despite the importance of other caregivers and the dominance of non-health factors and environments in the equation of health. Physicians have great financial ability to defend themselves. In 1984, a small minority of right-wing physicians in Ontario quickly and easily raised $250,000 to support a legal challenge to legislation opposing extra billing.

Private Practice

Most physicians in Canada are **private practitioners**, a term which is also applied to a number of other health care professionals including dentists, optometrists, chiropractors, denturists, herbalists, osteopaths, podiatrists, chiropodists, acupuncturists, clinical psychologists, and a variety of other independent health care providers and counsellors. The term "private practitioner" is not usually applied to those professionals who, by law, are limited to providing services only under the supervision of, or on referral from, others. This large group includes most nurses, physiotherapists, occupational therapists, speech pathologists and speech therapists, audiologists, laboratory technologists, radiology technicians, respiratory technicians, dieticians, nutritionists, health educators, health inspectors, midwives, nurse practitioners, clinical nurse specialists, and dental hygienists. Although "private practitioner" can apply to many independent professionals, it will, for the remainder of this chapter, refer only to physicians. In some provinces in Canada, supervised groups are achieving independent or private practice status through legislative change; for example, in 1991, physiotherapists in British Columbia had a limited range of private practice services introduced by government.

Two features most strongly epitomize private medical practitioners. The first of these is their control of executive functions such as choice of location, hours of operation, hiring of support staff, choice of office procedures, selection of clients, keeping of records, and distribution of revenue. Medical practitioners provide services to the population of their choice from the locations of their choice on the days and hours of their choice. They utilize facilities and auxiliary staff, somewhat, in the way they choose and limit services offered in whatever way they choose. In earlier times, they billed whom they chose on a fee-for-service basis in the amount that they chose. (Since the enactment of the *Canada Health Act* in 1984 extra-billing by physicians has been banned.)

The second major distinguishing feature is the use of fee-for-service as the dominant method of payment. A small number of private practitioners, such as those in Ontario who practice in a health service organization, receive income via capitation. Others receive major income through sessional payments (flat fee payment for half days or full days) or by salary (when hired by another doctor or by a health agency such as a health center, a hospital or a university), but fee-for-service dominates and is considered by some to be fundamental to the concept of private practice.

A third important feature of private practitioners (both those in health and elsewhere) is the probability that they evaluate themselves. Governments are increasingly expressing interest in the quality and cost of physicians' services, but most fee-for-service professionals with executive control either are not evaluated or are evaluated primarily by their peers.

One product of the executive independence and the piece-work method of payment is the lack of opportunity or mechanisms for coordination between private practitioners and the many other sources of service. This lack of continuation is found both regionally and in communities. Coordination can be seen by private practitioners as both an impediment to the entrepreneurial concept and an intrusion into areas of legitimate personal control. Certainly coordination is unlikely to occur unless incentives or disincentives promote it. Whatever else can be said about private practitioners, it is abundantly clear that regional planning and the rationalization of community health centers (where several types of providers, including physicians, work together on salary) cannot be fully successful as long as one major and dominant component rejects coordination with the rest of the network.

The entrepreneurial features of private medical practice increase the difficulty of finding solutions to a number of health delivery problems including

☐ poor geographic distribution of health professionals;
☐ inadequate availability of certain kinds of services (for example, counselling, house calls);
☐ inadequate availability of services at certain hours of the day, days of the week or seasons of the year;
☐ uncertainty with respect to quality of services rendered or the usefulness of the services rendered;
☐ incomplete regional planning and coordination;
☐ lack of consumer influence over the way in which an essential social service is organized and delivered; and
☐ the need for greater development of health care teams with greater use of other health professionals;

Physician spokesmen regularly contend that physicians are the group best qualified to design and evaluate health services networks. At the provincial and regional levels, this position is fairly universally rejected, although physicians remain influential. At the institutional level, however, and especially in acute treatment hospitals, most priority-setting decisions still tend to be made by the medical staff rather than by the board or the administration.

Physicians in
Policy Roles

There was a time when ministers of health were almost always physicians. Now it is unusual to have physicians in that role. Physicians do, however, continue to lead important commissions and boards of enquiry with a mandate to recommend changes in the health system. Recent examples include Dr. John Evans in Ontario in 1986, and Dr. Jean Rochon in Quebec in 1985-86. Physician associations also continue to make submissions on most health policy issues and physician representatives are usually given special status in terms of access to ministries and ministers of health. Physicians continue to fill most senior positions in provincial psychiatric services branches or divisions and frequently lead branches dealing with emergency services and public health.

Among decentralized nongovernmental sources of service, such as hospitals, public health units, regional planning bodies and long term care facilities, only the public health units continue to prefer chief executive officers who are physicians.

In larger hospitals, the senior management team routinely includes a physician and the heads of clinical departments have important administrative as well as clinical duties. In recent years, the heads of clinical departments have, in some hospitals, acquired new budgetary and resource allocation roles.

Training Physicians

Canadian medical schools are all schools of **allopathic medicine**. The teaching in allopathic schools is based on a theory in which, for all diseases or body disorders, there is assumed to be an external neutralizer. These schools accept that something can be done from the outside to counteract the undesirable internal events. This external therapy model would appear inevitably to lead to major reliance on drugs and surgery and to be quite physical health-oriented.

Osteopaths need a special comment because their status in Canada is so different from that of osteopaths practicing in the United States. In the United States, osteopathic schools of medicine are common and their graduates usually have the same opportunity for hospital privileges and entry to specialty training programs as do the graduates of schools of allopathic medicine. Canada, in contrast, has no osteopathic schools of medicine, despite the attractiveness of some of their basic concepts, and an American Doctor of Osteopathy (DO) coming to Canada cannot be licensed except as a drugless practitioner.

Medical students are taught primarily by specialists and then, as interns and residents, work almost exclusively with specialists. The role of family physicians in Canadian health care has been protected somewhat by a widely established and governmentally encouraged network of family practice training programs that are based largely in university affiliated primary care (non hospital) group practices.

The theory of osteopathic medicine (osteopathy), holds that within the body, if it is operating well, there is the capacity to respond to many diseases and threats of disease. Osteopathy emphasizes strengthening the ability of the body to overcome disease through nutrition, exercise, manipulation, and lifestyle, although drugs and surgery are also regularly used.

Homeopathy is treatment or protection by use of minute doses of whatever makes you sick. Homeopathy is not usually thought of as consistent with modern scientific theory.

The Professional Organizations of Physicians

Most practitioner groups have provincial and national organizations. National organizations such as the Canadian Medical Association tend to have little power because health is a provincial matter and provincial governments tend to talk to their provincial counterparts.

In all provinces, physicians have a College of Physicians and Surgeons and a Medical Association or equivalent. The colleges carry out licensing and disciplinary functions in accordance with appropriate provincial legislation, and, in each province, were created by provincial statute to protect the public. They investigate complaints, conduct peer evaluation programs, and identify and work with physicians addicted to drugs or alcohol.

The provincial medical associations, syndicates or societies are fee setting/ collective bargaining/political organizations. They are the labor unions or quasi-labor unions of the medical profession. They exist to serve and protect their members, not society. They negotiate fees, lobby for legislative changes and may represent their members when in dispute with the licensing/disciplining professional society. In a number of provinces there has been open conflict between the medical association and the college. Conflict usually centers around the vigor with which the college pursues its quality review functions.

In Quebec, the trade union functions are performed by two syndicates, one for family physicians and one for specialists. The Quebec Medical Association has tended to have questionable importance in the past but, in recent years, its membership has increased and its role may expand.

As physicians have increasingly come to think of their provincial associations as their collective bargaining instruments, they have begun to accept other labor union practices. In four provinces (Ontario, Manitoba, Quebec, and Nova Scotia) physicians now have a closed shop. All licensed physicians must belong to both the College (the licensing body) and the provincial medical association (the trade union). In provinces without a closed shop, a physician must pay an annual fee only to the College, and a significant minority of physicians — frequently one quarter or more — do not join the provincial medical association. The change to a closed shop (in Ontario this is called the Rand Formula) significantly increases the funds available to the medical union.

Physician Incomes

Physicians, as a group, have always had high incomes. For decades, their average incomes before taxes and after expenses have been the highest among the professional groups. Despite this fact, they usually consider themselves underpaid.

Frequent reference is made to the fact that physician incomes consumed a decreasing percentage of the total health dollar in the period 1973-82. The early 1970s, however, were peak years which were the culmination of 15 years of steady improvement in doctor incomes. This 1956-71 income trend was unlikely to continue; 1973-80 was, therefore, merely a period of adjustment. The relationship between physician incomes and other professional incomes was, by 1978-

80, approximately the same as in 1956. Since the early 1980s, the relative income of physicians has risen steadily to the point where, in some provinces, the peak relative position of the early 1970s has been matched or exceeded.

Most Canadian doctors are fee-for-service practitioners. Some academic and clinical teaching physicians are giving up their right to bill the province's health insurance plan and accepting a global budget or salary instead. This strategy allows specialists to devote more time to difficult procedures and research without a drop in income. (*Globe and Mail*, p. 1, June 9, 1992, Rod Mickleburgh).

The decade of the 90s is a time of increased attention to physician incomes. In April 1992, the British Columbia Minister of Finance stated in his budget address that

"over 20 percent of all health spending goes to physicians... a total of almost $1.4 billion during this coming year." He added, "We will be taking steps to eliminate the doctors' pension plan, cap the overall growth of physician billings, and reallocate these savings to other high-priority health-care areas." The Minister argued that "such action is essential if we are to maintain the viability of our health-care system."

Doctors in Quebec Under Bill 120

Bill 120 is the new health legislation in Quebec that restructures health and social service delivery into regions.

Regional boards are seen as the tool for solving medical staff shortages in rural and remote areas, along with community health centers and homes for the aged. These boards would be able to deny hospital privileges in urban areas to young specialists. This is an extension of the fee differential currently in use to encourage doctors to work in under-serviced areas. Bonuses under this scheme can be as large as 40 percent above the average specialist earnings in Montreal (*CMAJ* 1991; 145(8)). The boards will include physician members.

A controversial $5 user fee — "ticket orienteur" — will be in place for those consumers who inappropriately use an emergency room in a hospital. The fee is in effect in areas where primary care is available and a public education campaign has been launched.

The Decreasing Autonomy of Physicians

Autonomy is hardly ever absolute, but physicians, in the past, came close to it. There were few limits on which diagnostic or therapeutic approaches were to be used, on where or how to practice, on which or how many patients to see or not to see, or on whom to charge or how much to charge.

Today, Canadian physicians have less autonomy than they previously had and the decrease applies to both individual physicians and to physicians as a group. In a relative sense, they remain quite independent, but to many physicians, the reduction in autonomy that has occurred is immense, unjustified, unacceptable, intolerable, and abusive. These terms and the fervor with which they are used represent an overreaction which is intellectually inappropriate, because the loss of physician autonomy in Canada has followed a predictable, understandable and defensible pattern and will probably continue to do so. Factors at work include technological developments, philosophical and political evolution, professional example, the appearance of new data and the increasing use of rationing.

Physicians, unfortunately, tend to pretend that the philosophical/political changes have not occurred, and they tend to have a less-than-adequate understanding of other factors. Physician spokesmen receive standing ovations for their attacks on "pinkos" and "weak-kneed politicians," but the loss of professional autonomy is occurring in all Canadian provinces and all developed countries regardless of the stature or stripe of the politicians.

Political/philosophical evolution has seen the emergence of consumerism and the acceptance of the idea that all Canadians should have access to publicly funded health care. Both of these events have made consumers or their representatives part of, and sometimes the most powerful members of, the decision-making team.

Technological developments have created physicians who usually work in very narrow clinical areas. They no longer see a broad mix of patients and cannot be expected to retain a balanced view of the role or importance of their part of health care versus that of others. As physicians have become more and more diverse and dissimilar in their skills and interests, it has become more and more necessary that others be accepted as champions of the larger picture. This role has been acquired by planners, administrators, and other primarily nonmedical persons.

Professional examples — that is, examples set by physicians themselves, and the appearance of new data — are factors which have, in an unplanned way, contributed significantly to the alteration of the role and autonomy of physicians.

It is not precisely known when information began to affect professional decision making, but the Hippocratic Oath contains the words, "I will not cut persons laboring under the stone but will leave this to be done by men who are practitioners of this work." This edict, which prohibited surgery for the removal of kidney stones, was the first of many which impinged upon the freedom of individual physicians, and it was promulgated by the medical profession as a group.

By the middle and late 1800s — the age of Lister, Pasteur, Semmelweiss, Koch, and others — information had definitely begun to affect physician choices. Semmelweiss, for instance, established that very modest levels of cleanliness sharply reduced maternal mortality. Numbers proved his point and physicians were frowned upon by their colleagues if they went from the autopsy room to the delivery room without washing their hands. Information had confirmed the need for altered physician practices although it would be many years before malpractice suits and the need for access to hospital privileges would make such alterations mandatory.

Seventy years ago, the intrusion into professional autonomy began to develop teeth. The Flexner Report in the U.S. had found that most physicians were poorly trained and most medical care badly documented, and shortly after World War I the American College of Surgeons founded the Joint Commission on Hospital Accreditation. This Commission and other professional bodies began to work with hospitals, universities and governments to upgrade the care of individual patients. These changes were a response to new information.

The second world war accelerated the evolution of medical specialists and the formalization of the process of appointing physicians to the medical staffs of hospitals. Studies increasingly confirmed the relationship between proper training and process, on the one hand, and good patient outcomes on the other. Medical Audit Committees routinely used medical records to assess the appropriateness of medical care.

Tissue Committees began to look for evidence of unnecessary surgery in hospitals, and the vermiform appendix became the first target. In very short order, at least in teaching hospitals with Tissue Committees, fewer normal appendices were being removed. By the 1960s, the physician-operated medical insurance plans had begun to study physician billing habits, and, where these habits were found to be excessively deviant, payment was adjusted downwards. Policies created and applied by physician-controlled bureaucracies were placing limits on the opportunities, choices and income of individual physicians, and data were the origin of these limits.

Hospital medical staffs have, for decades, regularly rejected or recommended rejection of new medical staff applicants because there were said to be too few beds to go around; that is, the hospital already had enough doctors. Through this process, physicians denied other physicians the right to choose their places of practice and they denied patients the opportunity to be hospitalized by the physician of their choice. Physicians, sometimes for self-serving purposes, used bureaucratic methods to limit the freedom of location of other physicians long before the governments of British Columbia and Quebec even discussed restricting physician access to medical insurance if they settled in communities with an oversupply of physicians.

Hospitals, many years ago, in an attempt to deal fairly with both patients and physicians, began to categorize patients waiting to be admitted to hospital. The categories of emergency, urgent, and elective emerged with the involvement of leadership from the hospital medical staff. In the early years of implementation of this categorization, the process was primarily subjective and was much manipulated and abused. Soon formal criteria were written, review procedures and committees were created, and data were collected. Rational people, including physicians, agreed that, in complex systems, fairness is unlikely if based only on collegial or professional statements of principle. The additional requirements are data and specific policy. Physicians did not foresee that, when policy and data replace professional judgment, physicians might no longer be the ones best equipped for making decisions.

In the 1970s, Canadian governments began to seek ways to reduce the extent to which physician decisions threatened government spending limits, and in the United States exactly the same objective was sought by the large corporate employers. Evidence both in Canada and elsewhere suggested, and some would say confirmed, that spending more on health care was a poor way to elevate the health status of the population. Data showed, in fact, that spending money in a broad range of other social sectors would be more productive. Other information showed that the costs of caring for apparently similar patients varied a great deal from hospital to hospital, from doctor to doctor, and between capitation and fee-for-service payment systems. When more than one clinical approach is professionally acceptable, and when outcome measurements are not available to indicate whether one clinical approach is better than another, it is financially prudent to promote the cheapest approach to care. Better data, in association with the acceptance of publicly financed and universally accessible health care (or, in the United States, the financial concerns of large corporate employers) allowed non-physicians to know more about "the big picture" than did physicians.

Physicians also led the march toward use of data in the evaluation of clinical care. More and more regulations and protocols obliged physicians to investigate, treat or refer within prescribed patterns. New medical audit programs which used preset criteria to evaluate care of a large number of similar patients, began to appear. Analysis of health records assessed the extent to which the habits of a physician met prescribed standards.

Prescribed policies have replaced individual professional opinion. Information systems analyze billing patterns, prescription patterns, surgical patterns, referral patterns, manpower distribution, and physician incomes. Data are available too and quite logically are used by all interested parties. Physicians in groups have, for decades, reduced the autonomy of individual physicians. Now consumer representatives or corporate representatives have been able to become parts of the controlling mechanisms because physicians laid the groundwork. The clock cannot be turned back now.

At various points in history, physicians, as a group, developed medical care standards and made them mandatory. They controlled physician access to hospitals, used doctor profiles to alter physician habits and incomes, wrote policies governing the admission of patients to hospitals, described the training requirements for specialty status and, through their recommended fee schedules, estimated the relative value of various professional acts. In the evolution of policies in each of these areas, the decision making process moved from a reliance on opinion to a reliance on data. Physicians, individually and collectively, should not have been surprised when other interested parties also began to use these same data for the same or for other purposes. When medical judgment was central to decision making, the physicians cornered the market. Now, individuals with data analysis skills have become able to intelligently favor certain choices because data show that one option is better than the other options.

The question now is not whether physicians like the sequence of events, but how they will choose to react. What role will they play, or be allowed to play, in the continuing evolution of rationing, resource allocation, manpower production, manpower distribution, and the pricing of services? In the days before data were available, the system could not operate without professional opinion; now it can. Decisions will not be as good as they should be if physicians are not participants in the decision making, but the decisions will be made whether or not physicians participate.

Physicians should not feel they are without power. They have a great deal of it. They need not feel they will be ignored, but they should recognize that their advice will not be taken if it is inconsistent with the evidence, or is unacceptable to too many of the other major players. If they cry wolf, as is common, no one will listen because they are not truly in danger and are not likely to become so. Even if physicians live in the past, the system will continue to examine the future and respond to new data (without physician input). If, however, physicians develop a cadre of informed and respected leaders and staff, they will be able to significantly influence the rules and protocols that will continue to affect every physician.

On the surface, the choice looks easy. One option means decreasing influence over policy; the other means greater influence. Hence, many persons, both within and outside the profession, find it difficult to understand why medical leaders so often opt for uninformed bombast, the option which reduces their influence.

Technological evolution has made the potential cost of health care almost limitless. Political/philosophical evolution in Canada has made health care an area for public policy. Examples provided by physician organizations and leaders have demonstrated the desirability of many of the current public policies and programs which limit the options of individual physicians. It remains for physicians to decide whether they will be among the users of existing data and of the data of the future, and among the major participants in the writing of new policy.

External controls over physicians, in the areas of both individual caregiving and the profession, will increase in the future. Society and policy makers cannot avoid limiting physician choices when certain of these choices are seen as threats to public budgets and public priorities. Physicians should, for their own sakes and for the sake of the system, continue to fill a seat at the negotiation table, even though their power at that table is less than it formerly was.

Fee Setting

In terms of current factors influencing the profession, the Royal Commission report in B.C. (Province of British Columbia, 1991) fingers "machines and medication" as the events eroding the physician's domain and replacing specific functions. Various physician organizations have disputed the constitutional right and even the moral right of society to decide how much physicians must accept as payment in full for an insured service. However, for the foreseeable future, physicians will be paid either what the government decides or what is negotiated.

In most provinces there are at least three fee schedules in use,

☐ the fee schedule set by the physicians,
☐ the fee schedule set by the government (and used in its medical insurance program) and,
☐ the Workers Compensation Board (WCB) fee schedule (of lesser importance).

Some provinces may also have fee schedules established by cancer foundations or other paying agencies. With the abolition of extra billing, which occurred in the three years following passage of the *Canada Health Act*, the medical association fee schedule has become of much less importance. Prior to the abolition of extra billing, the difference between the government fee and the medical association fee usually determined the amount of extra billing for that particular service.

Financial bargaining between physicians and government affects fees in two quite different ways. One set of decisions determines the percentage fee increase or the extent to which total physician payments will increase. The second type of decision deals with the relative worth of various physician services, and increases or decreases some fees relative to others. Over the years, such adjustments have significantly decreased income disparities between specialties. The price of a surgical consultation, for example, is now approximately one-half that of a consultation by an internist whereas many years ago they were the same. This second type of decision is, to varying degrees, assigned to the professional societies. Governments tend to dominate with respect to percentage increase of fees and in capping total payments to physicians.

There is increasing attention by government to the total increase in payments to physicians. Most provinces now do more than establish a percentage increase in fees; they establish a formula within which the fee increase will not be given if utilization changes or billing changes increase governmental costs to a level considered to be unreasonable. This interest in total payments to physicians rather than in individual fees is the product of experience.

For example, *The Medical Post* (May 19, 1992, p. 4) reported that

> "The Nova Scotia government brought down a $4.8 billion budget that will hit hard and fast at health-care services — and physicians' fees."
>
> A global cap was placed on total payments for physicians' services for the next two years, and fees have been frozen at their present level.
>
> "The restrictions on physicians' fees was by far the most significant attempt made by Minister of Finance and Guysborough County physician Dr. Chuck MacNeil to contain spiralling health-care costs in the province. The two-year cap will be followed by a 3 percent fee or utilization increase — at most — for physicians in 1994-95."

The 1992 budget in Saskatchewan proposed a 5 percent drop in payment to its physicians. The spokesman for the Medical Association acknowledged that a lower amount had been expected (*Medical Post*, May 19, 1992, p.2).

Changes in Physician Billing Patterns

The fee-for-service method of payment allows practitioners to alter income by altering service volumes and/or billing patterns, as well as through alterations in the fees themselves. In the period 1980-81 to 1983-84, the average annual increase in Ontario Health Insurance Plan payments to practitioners was 17.6 percent. The number of claims rose 5.7 percent per year. The average number of claims per resident rose 4.7 percent per year and the average cost per claim rose 11.2 percent.

The 1983 Report of the Federal-Provincial Advisory Committee on Health Manpower reported the same phenomenon.

> "On reviewing statistics on medical utilization in Canada (as measured by services provided by physicians under provincial medical care insurance plans) there were increases of per capita utilization of 3.3 percent per year from 1974/75 to 1982/83. Only about 0.5 percent could be explained by demographic changes. "

Explanations given for the 85 percent of the increase that was not due to demographic changes were

1. changing consumer expectations or demand;
2. changing practitioner practice and billing patterns, at least partly due to increasing numbers and availability of physicians;
3. changing medical technology, which also will be altering practice patterns; and
4. availability of a wider range of diagnostic and therapeutic modalities, which may be part of (3).

The report describes interprovincial per capita utilization differences which do not appear to have led to differences in health status. Physician over-supply and the fee-for-service method of payment each present a major challenge to those trying to rationalize the system and control costs.

Malpractice Insurance

The Canadian Medical Protective Association (CMPA) is the insurance plan that covers medical malpractice in Canada. All physicians are members of this self-insurance organization. Its differential fee system is underlaid by the two principles that state that fee by type of work should be commensurate with risk and that there should be stability in fees or fee change from year to year as much as possible. Establishing the fee structure involves both risk rating and fee setting. Up until 1992, the latter was directly linked to the former mechanism. As a result, fees were shown by risk group rather than by type of work within the risk group. However, this undermined stability in fees or fee change because of changes in risk rating of certain types of work.

In 1992, altered risk group typing was established based on purposes of actuarial and statistical credibility. In order to stabilize fee change from year to year, fees were set, not by risk group, but by type of work. This change in approach should enhance the ability to be responsive to variances in risk of types of work while allowing much greater stability in year-to-year fee change.

In comparison to rates in the U.S., CMPAs are lower. However, it must be remembered, that the average income for physicians in the U.S. is at least double that of Canadian physicians and that fiscal advantages in the U.S. are by far superior to those in Canada.

Table 4.1

C.M.P.A. Membership Fees by Specialty 1983-1986

	1983	1984	% (Change)	1985	% (Change)	1986	% (Change)
Category 1	$250	$200	(-20)	$200	(0)	$200	(0)
Category 2	400	300	(-25)	300	(0)	300	(0)
Category 3	400	500	(-25)	500	(0)	600	(20)
Category 4	400	600	(50)	600	(0)	800	(33.3)
Category 5	400	1,100	(175)	1,100	(0)	1,100	(0)
Category 6	400	1,200	(200)	1,200	(0)	1,400	(16.6)
Category 7	400	1,800	(350)	1,800	(0)	3,340	(889)
Category 8	400	2,800	(600)	2,800	(0)	4,800	(714)

Key:

Category 1:	Residents
Category 2:	Administrative, Laboratory, Public Health
Category 3:	General Practice without Obstetrics
Category 4:	Pediatrics, Neurology, Nephrology, Geriatrics
Category 5:	Family Medicine with Obstetrics, Anesthesiology, Emergency Surgery
Category 6:	Ear Nose and Throat Surgery, Emergentology, Cardiology, Diagnostic Radiology
Category 7:	Gynecology, General Surgery, Pediatric Surgery, Urology, Plastic Surgery
Category 8:	Anesthesia, Obstetrics, Orthopedics, Cardiovascular Surgery, Neurosurgery

Table 4.2

C.M.P.A. Total Litigation Costs* 1980-1986

Year	Amount	% Change
1980	$ 3,762,794.00	—
1981	5,376,840.00	42.9
1982	6,567,615.00	22.1
1983	7,631,739.00	16.2
1984	10,807,162.00	41.6
1985	13,121,167.00	21.4
1986	16,236,359.00	23.7

Increase over period: + 331.5 percent
Average annual change: 28.0 percent
* Defined as the sum of legal, administrative costs and fees paid to experts

Table 4.3

Litigation Costs as Percent of Payments to Plaintiffs*
C.M.P.A. 1980-1986

1980 - 107.7%		1984 - 66.7%	
1981 - 101.9%		1985 - 92.1%	
1982 - 110.2%		1986 - 90.4%	
1983 - 69.6%			

Average: 91.2%
* Calculated as follows:
sum legal, administrative, expert x 100
compensation paid

Table 4.4

Fee Schedule for 1992

Code	Type of Work	Annual Fee $	Code	Type of Work	Annual Fee $
20	Administrative Medicine	948	49	Geriatric Medicine	2,208
40	Allergy	2,208	84	Gynecologic Surgery (without obstetrics)	8,340
90	Anesthesia	7,116			
38	Anesthetic Practice without General/Spinal/Epidural Anesthesia	2,208	23	Hematological Pathology	948
			50	Hematology	2,208
			52	Infectious Diseases	2,208
21	Anatomical Pathology	948	53	Intensive Care — Full Time	2,208
33	Assistance at Surgery — no other professional work	1,284	54	Internal Medicine and its subspecialties not elsewhere noted	2,208
41	Cardiology	2,208			
75	Cardiology with Arteriography/Cardiac Catheterization	2,592	10	Interns and Residents, Clinical Fellows for the 24 months immediately following postgraduate training	600
91	Cardiovascular Surgery	13,668			
42	Clinical Immunology		24	Medical Biochemistry	948
28	Community Medicine (Public Health)		25	Medical Microbiology	948
			59	Medical Oncology	2,208
44	Dermatology		55	Nephrology	2,208
45	Diagnostic Imaging		56	Neurology	2,448
82	Emergency Medicine/Emergentology		26	Neuropathology	948
46	Endocrinology		92	Neurosurgery	14,796
35	Family Medicine or General Practice Including:	1,284	58	Nuclear Medicine	2,208
			39	Obstetrical Practice without Labor and Delivery	2,208
	- digital block and local infiltration anaesthesia only		93	Obstetrics	14,796
	- antepartum and postpartum care only		51	Occupational Medicine	2,208
	- minor office surgery only		60	Ophthalmology	2,976
	- assistance at surgery		94	Orthopaedic Surgery	14,796
	- emergency department: a physician with in-hospital care privileges may fulfill an emergency department commitment consistent with that Family Medicine or General Practice appointment		77	Otolaryngology	6,192
			85	Pediatric Surgery	7,116
			61	Pediatrics	2,208
			27	Physical Medicine and Rehabilitation	1,284
			86	Plastic Surgery	11,004
			36	Psychiatry	1,284
			62	Respiratory Medicine	2,208
80	Family Medicine or General Practice including Obstetrics/Anesthesia/ Surgery/Emergency Department Work not covered in Type of Work 35	2,796	63	Rheumatology	2,208
			64	Sports Medicine	2,208
			37	Surgical Practice without Operative Treatment	2,208
			65	Therapeutic Radiology/ Radiation Oncology	2,208
47	Gastroenterology	2,448	87	Thoracic Surgery	8,340
22	General Pathology	948	88	Urology	8,340
83	General Surgery	8,340	89	Vascular Surgery	8,340
48	Genetics	2,208			

The Effects of How a Physician Is Paid

The charge that physicians are unethical if they work for anyone but themselves or another doctor is not heard much now, although it was a common bit of rhetoric, especially in the United States, for three decades (1940-70). It emerged briefly in Saskatchewan in 1962 when doctors on the staff of community clinics were denied hospital privileges because they were employed by community boards and, therefore, were considered to be unethical.

The proposition that fee-for-service is central to a good patient-doctor relationship and to a high quality of care is quite unfair to the large number of practicing physicians who work on salary in community health centers, with a university, or elsewhere. Most workers, including most health workers, are not paid by fee-for-service, but there is no evidence that the way they are paid has reduced the quality of their services or the relationships they have with a variety of clients.

If method of payment can affect quality and the patient-doctor relationship, that fee-for-service is probably damaging to both. The physician gets paid the same amount whether a service is provided quickly or slowly, well or poorly. If one wishes a high income, one must perform many activities. A quickly done, and perhaps less well-done, examination is worth the same as one done more thoroughly. Keeping good records and writing good referral letters are not income-producing, so there could be a tendency to omit them or do them poorly.

All methods of payment have advantages and disadvantages. When considering income and how to provide it, it may be desirable to note that income is not the same as worth, and that both the amount and method of payment are set primarily by tradition and by market forces — not by any predictable or fair evaluation or any rational process. Preferred method of payment tends to be related much more to tradition and to net income than to altruistic principles.

One of the unfortunate products of fee-for-service in Canada is that, in most cases, it definitely does not reward excellent physicians as well as it rewards some mediocre or poor ones. It definitely does increase the number of patients seen per hour and it increases hospital use and surgical volumes.

Physician Power Over Other Professions

In Canada, professionals operating within the medical model, a group which includes nurses, physiotherapists, speech therapists, radiology technicians, and laboratory technologists, have few things they can legally do except when under the supervision of a physician. There is ongoing negotiation between nurses and physicians as to what procedures and duties can be appropriately and legally performed by nurses, but the power remains with the physicians. It is they who are, in law, allowed to "practice medicine." Of the professionals within the medical model, the physicians are legally entitled to diagnose and prescribe. Others carry out duties approved by physicians or make decisions delegated to them by physicians. This is legally the case, despite the fact that other health professionals have clearly described areas of expertise that are quite distinct from the expertise of physicians. Physiotherapists, nurses, speech pathologists, and others routinely diagnose and develop treatment plans, but almost all, in law, must act under the direction of a physician.

Some health professionals operate outside of the medical model. These include chiropractors, optometrists and osteopaths. These practitioners have usually, at some time, been in dispute with physicians, and sometimes the dispute continues. These health workers each have their own legislation and each can diagnose and treat within a prescribed spectrum. Physicians have no power over these professionals and play no direct role in determining what they can do.

Control Over Information

This is another area of interaction between government and physicians. In Quebec, information belongs to the patient, who is entitled to read anything written down by the physician or other health worker. In most provinces, however, information is still perceived to be institutionally or professionally owned and patients have no guarantee of access.

Programs Which Influence Location of Practice

Independent (private) practitioners can still open an office wherever they wish (including in their homes in most municipalities) but governments are using an expanding array of incentives and disincentives to influence physicians and dentists in their selection of locations for their practices. These programs have the intent of increasing availability of practitioners in selected rural areas and/or of decreasing availability in selected urban areas.

Programs to improve the rural supply of physicians have been used by most provinces and have been directed towards both medical students and physicians licensed to practice. Incentives directed towards graduates have tended to be more successful than those directed towards students. Half or more of the students buy their way out of their contracts after they graduate and few go on to provide long-term service to rural areas. An Ontario program directed towards licensed physicians has led to 400 to 500 physician placements and 7,090 dentist placements since 1979. Of the physicians, about one fifth have been specialists. The incentive payment takes the form of a tax free grant over a four-year period to a maximum (in 1985) of $10,000 per year. Quebec has considered requiring agreement to provide a minimum of one to two years of rural service as a condition for acceptance into a Quebec medical school.

Factors contributing to a disinclination for rural settlement include nonmonetary factors such as personal attachment to urban life, the lack of availability of medical colleagues, and the lack of availability of educational opportunities for children. Financial incentives must offset these nonmonetary disincentives. Quebec is experimenting with a twinning of rural and urban hospitals as a technique to reduce the isolation of rural practice.

Disincentives to locating in overserviced areas are usually monetary and range from reduced payments to exclusion from medicare. In Quebec, physicians who settle in underserved areas are paid up to 120 percent of the regular fees. Settlement in overserviced areas is discouraged by payment at a rate as low as 70 percent of the regular fees for the first three years of practice. Preliminary assessment suggests that this plan has had little effect on physician location patterns although it may have saved the province a bit of money.

Refusal by the public insurance system to assign a billing number to physicians who settle where the supply is considered to be adequate is a more aggressive approach to the use of monetary disincentives. Without a billing number, no payments will be made directly to the physician by the insurance plan and no reimbursement will be made to patients receiving care. Quebec considered this control of billing numbers several years ago but did not introduce the required legislation. British Columbia introduced the plan, but it was struck down by the courts.

Only tradition can explain why it is acceptable for government to decide how many teachers or police officers should serve a particular community at public expense, but offensive when government applies the same principle to physicians.

Efforts to date to influence location have been limited to correction of rural/urban imbalances. Inappropriate intraurban distribution, especially the aggregation of specialists in medical towers either downtown or adjacent to teaching hospitals, has not been given attention. The recent rapid growth in doctor supply and the associated competition for patients have led to a significant number of family physicians opening clinics in suburban areas. However, dispersion of specialists, including those such as pediatricians and obstetricians who are practicing primary medicine, is still often narrower than is reasonable.

The Professional Functions

The most formal point of contact of physicians and governments is through those acts that govern the profession. These acts describe the functions that are delegated to the profession as well as its responsibilities and powers.

The question of who licenses physicians is not as important as is usually thought. State licensing boards have, for decades, licensed physicians in the United States whereas, in Canada, physicians often believe self-licensing is a prerequisite to professional survival. In Canada, each province has delegated the licensing responsibility to a professionally controlled College.

For example, self-regulation is now seen to be a costly business in Newfoundland and is almost certain to become more so in future.

At the 1992 annual meeting of the Newfoundland Medical Association, when the registrar for the Newfoundland Medical Board was asked to estimate how much licensing fees in the province could cost in future, Dr. Young speculated fees could rise to $650 or go as high as $1,000 in the next few years.

Doctors in the province were hit with a licensing fee increase of almost 50 percent last year ($200) which raised the fee to $450. This is not out-of-line with the costs of other provinces.

Besides licensing, provincial laws make the profession responsible for the protection of the public against professional misconduct. This duty obligates the

Colleges to evaluate physicians; a task done with varying vigor but done much better now than a decade ago.

In 1992, the Canadian Medical Association adopted a new policy on the requirements for licensure for both practicing physicians and those in training. This policy is an effort to protect currently practicing but non-certified physicians from changes in the medical examination procedures of the Medical Council of Canada. By 1994, certification will be a prerequisite for licensure in most Canadian jurisdictions for most new Canadian graduates. Certification by either the College of Family Physicians of Canada or the Royal College of Physicians and Surgeons of Canada will be accepted.

Despite what may come into effect in other jurisdictions, the Newfoundland Medical Board will continue to recognize the old Licentiate of the Medical Council of Canada (LMCC) and successful completion of a rotating internship when deciding whether to grant a licence to practice.

Physicians are united in their objection to the direct intrusion of outside agencies, including government, into the way a physician deals with an individual patient. They have, historically, also been equally adamant about how physicians are evaluated. In both of these functional areas, physicians are usually aware of the extent to which their professional lives are becoming or have become bureaucratized by hospital limits on privileges, rules regarding referral, rules regarding billing, and regulations pertaining to the care of specific types of patients. The wish of physicians and other professionals to have a major influence over how they carry out their work is legitimate and usually respected, but physicians, in particular, tend to damage their credibility by being insensitive to the legitimate wishes of others who also wish to be involved. Questions of relative cost-effectiveness and of equity make external evaluation inescapable, and the availability of better data makes external evaluation possible.

For years, users have complained that the various professional committees set up to respond to public complaints and to evaluate professional conduct have not reasonably defended the public. In response to these concerns, most provinces now appoint non-physician members to those quasijudicial bodies that examine the conduct of physicians and investigate complaints from users.

The Bureaucratization of Medicine

Professionalism is, by definition, a decentralized and individualized concept with emphasis on personal responsibility and control. The term can also be used with reference to a self-governing profession in which there can be significant regulation and control of members by the profession itself. Having a professionally controlled bureaucracy which sets fees, controls professional training, determines specialty qualifications and designation, defines acceptable personal and professional conduct, sets penalties for misconduct, and applies these penalties as it sees fit is, therefore, consistent with the concept of professionalism. In a pure sense, a professional reports either to no one or to his or her peers, and a self-governing profession reports to no one.

A bureaucracy is, by definition, centralized, systematized, regulated and supervised. Individuals within a hierarchical authority structure write rules and collect data to be certain the rules are obeyed. Individual decision-making takes place only within the constraints laid down by the system.

The fact that there is a professionally controlled bureaucracy affecting physicians is illustrated by such things as the existence of the medical association fee schedules, the peer review program operated by the Ontario College of Physicians and Surgeons, medical staff support for regulations governing mandatory referrals or protocols, professional discipline committees, and procedures governing designation as a specialist. The presence of bureaucratization arising from external sources is illustrated by such things as

☐ the fee schedules of third party paying agencies (whether negotiated or arbitrarily applied),

☐ the banning of extra-billing,

☐ the mandatory reporting of certain diseases or events such as that required in suspected child abuse or in cases where pilots or automobile operators are thought to be unfit to drive,

☐ the application of income ceilings,

☐ the control by hospital boards of appointments to the medical staff,

☐ the mandatory provision of specified information to public insurance agencies, and

☐ the production and use by government insurance bodies of doctor billing profiles.

The increase in external bureaucratic influence and control is usually associated with an increase in the use of objective data. This use brings with it a rigidity which can be seen as, and (at times) will be, a threat to the clinical decision-making freedom of a physician. There will be continuing tension associated with the need, on the one hand, to prevent physician decision-making that is either clinically incorrect, culturally unacceptable, or not cost-effective, and the need, on the other hand, to leave physicians with a reasonable degree of flexibility as they deal with the individual variations in patient need and response.

The next few decades will see increasing intervention by governments, boards, committees, administrators and courts into the professional lives of practitioners of many types. Keeping three thoughts in mind may allow health administrators to make these interventions more rationally and fairly.

1. Physicians are simply one group of workers. Whether one agrees with their positions or not, they should be dealt with in basically the same way as one deals with other classes of workers.

2. Physicians are powerful. When an administrator goes to war with them too aggressively, the administrator is likely to be the one that loses, especially in a hospital. If the administrator and the medical staff are permanently at odds, it is unlikely that the hospital board will keep the administrator and go out looking for another medical staff. Physicians are not famous for seeing the big picture, but their ability to close ranks when the herd is threatened should not be underestimated.

3. Policy creators and administrators should be frequently reminded of the fact that care providers constantly, and on short notice, make difficult decisions. Administrative decisions may also be difficult and may often be much more important to the community than the decisions of caregivers, but the decisions which physicians and other health professionals must make are highly personal. They are often made in an emotional atmo-

sphere, often trivial to the point of annoyance, sometimes of great importance to somebody, and often emotionally draining. Policies should not be designed with only physicians in mind; rather, effects on communities must come first. In both policy selection and implementation, however, administrators should be sensitive to the occupational pressures regularly faced by a number of health workers, including physicians.

Future Directions in Physician Resource Planning

"Barer-Stoddart Report Toward Integrated Medical Resource Policies for Canada"

The Barer-Stoddart Report, Toward Integrated Medical Resource Policies For Canada, was prepared for the Federal/Provincial/Territorial Conference of Deputy Ministers of Health (June, 1991).

The project's three main objectives were

1. to bring as much as possible together on matters of relevance to physician resource policy in Canada;
2. to develop principles and a framework to guide future policy development; and
3. to make policy recommendations consistent with the principles and framework.

Report Themes

Of the eleven themes prevalent in the report, four are of primary importance. The first states that there is no agreed-upon policy objective, at present, for management of the Canadian physician resource sector. This objective according to the report, should be to meet those health needs of the population that can be most efficiently met by individuals with training as MDs.

The second theme is that we cannot define an "optimal" number of physicians by technical means. Ultimately, this judgement is a social rather than a technical one, and unwillingness to accept this fact unnecessarily delayed policy development while improvements in data collection or planning methodologies were awaited.

The third theme involves the tension that has arisen, since the inception of publicly funded health care, between the personal interests of physicians and the universal goals and objectives of the public enterprise in which they now work. This tension has gradually induced in physicians a greater appreciation for the collective public goals, but it has been a slow process. The report suggests that more attention should be paid to incentives and structures that increase the responsiveness of physicians and organizations to the collective goals and needs of the public enterprise, while minimizing coercion and regulation.

The fourth theme is that a national strategy encompassing specific policies to which all provinces and territories must commit is not feasible. Nationally coordinated provincial/territorial policies built upon a commonly understood policy objective and framework, on the other hand, may well be feasible. This approach must accommodate the reality that stakeholders will not agree on all issues, and that the nature of problems in this sector will vary considerably by region. There is, however, an important consensus among stakeholders that falling back on the status quo as a policy is not acceptable for most problem areas. Many of those interviewed during this project felt that "the time is right" for reforms to address physician resource management in Canada.

Several problem areas were identified.

☐ There are increases in physician supply in excess of population growth without any compelling justification.

☐ Numbers and mix of residency training positions and of specialists are disproportionate with population need.

☐ Academic medical centers have a poorly defined role and unstable funding of their activities.

☐ A significant geographic variation in physician supply is evidenced, which affects timely and/or convenient access to necessary services.

☐ A non-trivial amount of medical services utilization is being found to be ineffective, inappropriate, or inefficiently provided.

☐ There is a lack of uniform national standards of clinical competence for licensure.

☐ Inadequate attention to the self-regulation of practice to overlapping "scopes of capability" has been found, as well as the need for continuing competence review.

☐ There is significant dissatisfaction with processes for negotiating remuneration forms and levels.

☐ Conflict exists between fee-for-service payment and clinical, educational and public policy objectives.

☐ Deficiencies in both the amount and quality of basic clinical and management information, as well as incomplete use of information which does exist have been found.

Conclusion

Canadian physicians have a long tradition of dominance in the provision of health care services. The twenty-first century will see continued turf warfare, but more doctors on salary and probably more acceptance of practice standards designed to support the delivery of cost-effective care.

References

Barer, M.L. & Stoddart, G.L. (1991). *Toward Integrated Medical Resource Policies for Canada*. Report prepared for the Federal/Provincial/Territorial Conference of Deputy Ministers of Health. University of British Columbia.

Colligan, R.D. & Berglund, E. (1985). Changing roles of physicians, nurses and administrators. *Medical Group Management*, 32(2), 38-42.

Coburn, D. (1988). Canadian medicine: Dominance or proletarianization. *Milbank Quarterly*, 66, Supplement 2, 92-116.

Fulton, M.J. (1988) *The Regulation of Emerging Health Care Occupations*, Ottawa: Canadian Hospital Association.

Gamble, S.W. (1980). Changing roles in the '90s: Will R.N.s manage M.D.s? *Hospitals*, 63(22), 42-44.

Haddad, A.M. (1991). A source of support. *Health Progress*, 72(1), 60-63.

Hafferty, F.W. (1988). Theories at the crossroads: A discussion of evolving views on medicine as a profession. *Milbank Quarterly*, 66, Supplement 2, 202-225.

Haug, M. (1988). A re-examination of the hypothesis of physician deprofessionalization. *Milbank Quarterly*, 66, Supplement 2, 48-56.

Hollander, M. & Campbell, A. (1990). Conceptual models of the professions and their implications for the professionalization of health administration. *Healthcare Management Forum*, Winter, 21-27.

Institute for Health Care Facilities of the Future (1987). *A View of the Horizon*, Montreal.

Kenkel, P.J. (1989). Physician's changing roles. *Modern Healthcare*, 19(45), 48.

Light, D., & Levine, S. (1988). The changing character of the medical profession: A theoretical overview. *The Milbank Quarterly*, 66, Supplement 2, 10-32.

Magnee, D. (1991). So where do we go from here? *Physiotherapy Canada*, 43(3), 10-16.

Mechanic, D. (1991). Changing our health care system. *Medical Care Review*, 48(3), 247-260.

Miller, M.M. & Heine, C. (1988). The complex role of the head nurse. *Nursing Management*, 19(6), 58-64.

Nova Scotia Department of Health (1990). *Health Strategies for the Nineties: Managing Better Health*, Government of Nova Scotia.

York, Jeffrey (1987) *The High Price of Health: A Patient's Guide to Medical Politics*, Lorimer.

CHAPTER 5

Short Term Acute
Treatment Hospitals

What Is a
Hospital?

I n addition to being a source of essential health care a hospital is also a legal entity, an employer, an educator, a laboratory for research, a neighbor, a competitor, and a safety net for communities.

Hospitals as Determinants of Health Status of a Community

There is general agreement that the health status of a population is based on many factors. The four main determinants of individual and collective health are often given as

- environment,
- lifestyle,
- health services, and
- human biology.

The World Health Organization has recently added public policy as a fifth major determinant. **Environment** includes the physical, emotional, social, political, economic, occupational, and cultural environments. **Lifestyle** includes individual characteristics or habits over which the individual is considered to have some degree of control such as alcohol use, expectations, exercise patterns, response to stress and diet. **Health services** include all those preventive, diagnostic, therapeutic and rehabilitative services delivered through health facilities and programs. **Biological factors** include those human frailties and strengths, primarily genetic, which determine our susceptibility to and response to illness and injury.

Of these determinants, the genetic factors are currently beyond both individual and collective control, except in circumstances where prenatal screening is available. Some physical environmental factors are also unalterable. However, many of the environmental factors, most or all of the lifestyle factors, and all of the health services features are under human control.

Hospitals are a major subheading under one of the three areas over which we exercise control (Figure 5.1). Despite their psychological and financial importance, it is obvious that hospitals cannot affect health status more than is compatible with being just one part of health services. They also are only one part of the total network of factors or determinants that affects our health.

In an age in which hospitals, their fund raising, their technical miracles, and their requests for more money are in the media almost daily, it is difficult to keep hospitals roles in perspective. Community health agencies and other services, also very important to health (for example, social service agencies and employment programs), constantly struggle to be noticed in the face of the profile and clout of hospitals. Hospitals have most of the glamour, the greatest aggregation of clinical and administrative expertise, the longest history of public fundings, and they have the loyalty of communities.

Figure 5.1

The Determinants of Health Status

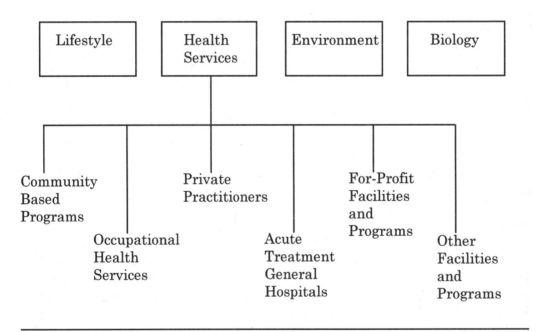

Hospitals are now of greater interest to provincial treasury boards, who must find money, than to health planners, who wish to improve community health status. There is preliminary evidence that if the supply of hospitals or physicians is expanded beyond a modest or even the current figure, there will be no further noticeable effect on the health status of the community or the nation. The only effect would be the change in availability of hospital-based services which would be of consequence to specific individuals.

Hospitals Classified by Ownership

In Canada, hospitals can be owned and operated by community boards, churches, municipalities, provincial governments, the federal government, and private-for-profit corporations.

Community Ownership

Most acute care hospitals in Canada are privately owned corporations, registered as charities under *The Income Tax Act*. They are often owned by communities but may also be owned by doctors or other special interest groups. Some of these hospitals have elected boards, while some have appointed members. Health Science Centres in universities and teaching hospitals may have academic members or government appointees on their boards.

Religious Hospitals

These hospitals may be individually incorporated or part of a multi-institutional corporation which may operate hospitals and other types of institutions.

Twenty to thirty years ago, organization charts of religious hospitals were very simple. A Sister Superior or equivalent in other religious denominations (who would now be called an Executive Director or President) would have executive authority, but would report to a higher level of religious authority.

In the last 25 years many religious hospitals, especially Roman Catholic hospitals, have been transferred completely to community boards and therefore are no longer classed as religious institutions. Those that continue to exist as religious institutions are often owned by the church and governed by a board whose members are selected largely or completely by the religious group. Prior to the appearance of an independent board with executive authority, it was common to have an advisory board working with the chief executive officer.

Municipal Hospitals

Municipal hospitals — for example, the Hamilton Civic Hospitals, the Civic and Riverside Hospitals in Ottawa and the Union Hospitals in the prairie provinces — are owned, but not operated, by one or more municipalities. Municipal operation of hospitals would be quite possible and reasonable (municipalities do operate long-term care institutions), but is uncommon. The boards of these hospitals tend to be appointed by the municipalities but have full executive authority. They do not report to the municipalities in any meaningful way. Since the introduction of universal hospital insurance, municipalities have usually accepted no responsibility for hospital deficits, except when required to do so by the province. This has, at times, been the case in Alberta.

Some of the municipal hospital boards have been replaced by boards who are also responsible for a mix of public health, hospital, long term care (LTC), and some other functions on an occasional basis.

Provincial Hospitals

Most provincial hospitals are psychiatric institutions that are part of the physical inventory of the Department of Public Works (or equivalent) and are administered by the psychiatric services branch of the Ministry of Health. All staff are provincial civil servants.

A few of these provincially owned psychiatric hospitals are administered by community boards (as in Alberta). In New Brunswick some of the acute treatment hospitals are owned by the province, but operated by community boards.

Canada does not have public hospitals, as America does. The state owns only a few institutions.

Federal Hospitals

The federal government operates military hospitals (Department of National Defense), hospitals for the native populations (Medical Services Branch, Health and Welfare Canada), veterans' hospitals (although these are almost fully integrated with provincial services), and small specialty institutions including quarantine stations.

Proprietary (for-profit) Hospitals

Most provinces have a *Private Hospitals Act* or equivalent. These Acts regulate institutions which are not governed by the *Public Hospitals Act*. These institutions tend to be fairly small and they provide specialized mental health or addiction-related services. They usually provide insured care to provincially insured persons but payment is on a fee-for-service or per diem basis rather than through a global budget.

Summary

There are significant variations in ownership and corporate structure of nonprofit hospitals, but these differences have little impact on services. In every case, the hospital serves basically the same functions, it has the same relationship to the Minister of Health, the same reliance on public funds, and it may or may not fit into a regional system. The options at the top of the hospital organization chart have been described because these affect the opportunities available to a citizen or a community for influence over an important community institution.

Relationships Between Hospitals and Ministries of Health

Ministries of Health or the Minister of Health (or equivalent) have, through their provincial hospital statutes, almost absolute legal power over hospitals. In dealing with ministries, hospitals must rely on tradition, public image, persuasion, and an awareness of the perceived importance of the services they provide in order to get what they want. The hospitals definitely have the edge in tactical terms, but in those instances in which hospitals do not have public support or do not have a reasonable rationale for their demands, the Ministry can flex its legal and financial muscle.

The Legal Relationships

Hospital-related statutes usually give the Minister final authority over

- whether a hospital exists (a list of approved hospitals is usually part of some Act),
- the range of services it provides,
- the wording of hospital bylaws,
- physical size and changes in size,
- capital and operating expenditures,
- the keeping and reporting of information,
- admission practices,
- volume of and price of preferred accommodation,
- medical staff appointment and appeal procedures,
- patient consent procedures,
- quality review processes, and
- whatever other things the Minister chooses.

In recent years, ministers have expanded the *Public Hospitals Act* to include procedures by which the power and function of hospital boards of trustees can be formally transferred to a Ministry appointee when the Minister and/or cabinet considers this transfer appropriate. This unusual degree of intrusion by the Ministry into trustee functioning, has, to date, occurred in response to inadequate financial control, inadequate quality control, a combination of administrative and financial problems or inappropriate interest group control such as an anti-abortion stand. This intrusion usually occurs as a series of steps with each additional step being more restrictive.

In Ontario, the confrontation between the Ministry and hospitals, and the subsequent amendments to the *Public Hospitals Act*, followed directly from a decision by a substantial number of large hospitals to refuse to operate within the funds allocated by the Ministry. These hospitals set budgets that anticipated large deficits, some in the range of $15 to $20 million. The hospitals, in essence, dared the Ministry not to provide the money. It was a situation in which the government either had to let the hospitals write the provincial budget or act quickly and firmly. It chose to act. The hospitals then decided they would rather operate in a fashion acceptable to the Ministry than be operated by someone named by the Ministry. Hospitals have more or less accepted the fact that they, as well as schools and other kinds of public institutions, must operate within an assigned amount of public money. Ontario, for example, made proposals for a new *Public Hospitals Act* in May 1992 with such mandatory features as cost-effective care, utilization management, community input, and a social contract. The social contract is a document that sets out the services a hospital will provide, the community served, and the financial obligation of the government to support those services.

Financial Relationships

Financial control of hospitals by the Ministry is less complete than legal control, but is equally effective. For most public hospitals, 85 percent to 95 percent of operating funds come from their provincial ministries or from Ministry-financed hospital insurance commissions. Hospitals receive additional operating income from preferred accommodation and from revenue producing activities such as TV rentals and parking. Income is also generated from third-party payers such as Workers Compensation Boards and from investments, donations, direct-pay patients and payment for out-of-province patients. Revenue from these last two sources can be substantial in hospitals on an interprovincial or international border or with a multiprovince function. Through the budget allocation process the Ministry can support or discourage the establishment or expansion of patient care or educational programs. The Ministry can also determine the involvement of the hospital in regional or joint ventures.

The Business Oriented New Development (BOND) program in Ontario also merits comment. This program, introduced in response to the idea that hospitals should be more businesslike, invites hospitals to raise money through business ventures. Money raised is kept by the hospital. As part of the program, Ontario hospitals were allowed to keep all income from preferred accommodation (rather than only a portion of it as was previously the case) and to set their own rates for this accommodation. Rates for private and semiprivate rooms immediately rose by 30-100 percent producing a major financial windfall.

A recent fleeting aberration in the hospital financing scene is a practice whereby hospitals sell assets to private corporations and then lease them back. The hospitals get immediate capital above the amount which is reserved to pay all lease-back charges and the private investor gains tax write-off benefits. The net result is an increased cost of hospitals to taxpayers.

Other Areas of Ministry Impact on Hospitals

Ministries also affect hospitals by making available, or failing to make available, other health services such as long term care beds and home care programs, and by making or allowing changes in health manpower. Decisions of the Ministry regarding the presence and power of regional planning bodies affects hospitals because these regional bodies may interfere with or support direct hospital/Ministry discussions over planning options. In some provinces, collective bargaining with hospital-based unions is a Ministry function.

Hospital Organization

Figure 5.2 illustrates one possible organizational skeleton of a teaching or non-teaching hospital. The organization chart would, in the corporate model, show a president and a number of vice-presidents. The more common organizational chart has the positions of executive director and a number of assistant executive directors. In the corporate model the president is a member of the board of trustees. The two models have no other significant differences.

Note that the medical staff has two quite distinct organizations with different functions and status. The chief of staff and the **Medical Advisory**

Committee (MAC) are an integral part of the hospital organization, whereas the organized medical staff with its president and other executives is very much a free-standing organization.

Figure 5.2

The Organization of a Typical Acute Treatment Hospital

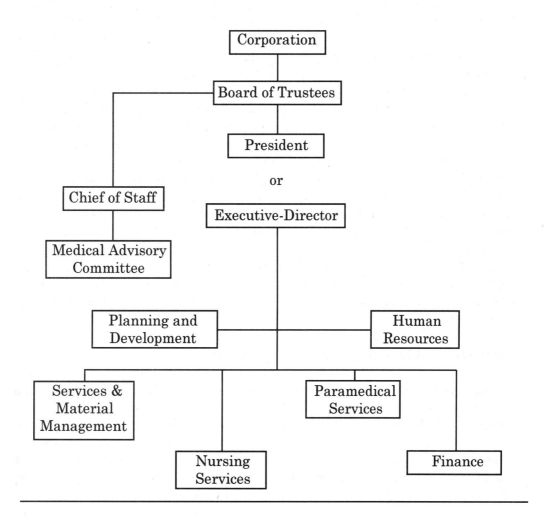

The MAC is currently, in Ontario and in some other provinces, given major statutory responsibilities. It must, in many situations, provide advice to the board. The board is, in turn, obligated to consult this advice. The present *Ontario Public Hospitals Act* states: "The Committee shall advise and collaborate with the administration in all decisions affecting patient care including the allocation of space, the allocation of beds by department and the development of facilities," and the Committee shall "approve plans and priorities for the use of funds in all departments and divisions." MAC members in Ontario teaching hospitals are appointed by the board; in other hospitals, the MAC is elected. The MAC is composed of all chiefs of clinical departments and major sub-departments or divisions, which in a large teaching hospital results in a membership of 30 to 60 physicians. The MAC may also have nonvoting members from the administration, the board, the nursing department and occasionally from other departments. By law, in Ontario, the chief of staff is the chairman of the MAC. The chief of staff is usually appointed by the board, and therefore is, in theory, its agent rather than being primarily a representative of the medical staff. MAC advice and decisions are received by the board via the presence of MAC minutes as part of the agenda of board meetings.

The medical staff, acting through its elected executive, may be active in institutional politics and in producing institutional policies, or it can have primarily social/professional functions. Whereas the MAC represents the medical staff elite (the department heads plus chief of staff), the elected medical staff executive directly represents the entire active medical staff.

The medical staff consists of all physicians and dentists who have been approved by the board. The medical staff usually consists of active staff, (physicians and dentists whose primary affiliation is with this hospital), consulting and courtesy staff (physicians and dentists who usually have a closer affiliation with another hospital), and special categories of staff.

It must be emphasized that individual hospital organization charts may vary quite markedly from the brief description and the single diagram given. There are frequently, for example, multiple separate service units under one board of trustees and possibly one executive director. There can also be two or more separate corporations with very close operational ties. The Ontario cancer clinics, for example, are operated by a provincial board but day to day delivery of services is functionally integrated into that of the hospital to which the clinic is attached.

Physicians in Management

The role of physicians in hospital management is unusual and, as such, has been the subject of study and comment by administrative theorists. Physician decisions are usually the primary determinants of resource consumption by patients, but they are outside of the administrative line of command. This situation frequently leads to conflict regarding costs, use of staff, and allocation of resources. One of the devices commonly used to help resolve this type of conflict is the Joint Conference Committee (JCC). The JCC is composed of equal numbers of representatives from the administrative staff and the medical staff, and reports to both the board and to the medical staff. Its agenda consists of all issues of interest to both administration and the medical staff, and some authors believe it is essential to reasonably harmonious relations between the two camps.

The JCC may be more necessary in nonteaching hospitals, where there is not a cadre of joint university/hospital appointees. These people, by virtue of their fixed incomes and their administrative, teaching, *and* clinical functions, can act as major points of contact between clinicians and the administrative staff. The JCC may also be more essential when there is a large nonteaching medical staff with a great deal of power, and considerable competition for available beds. These factors make it more likely that there will be major disagreement both within the medical staff and between it and the administration and/or board. The JCC is not in common use, however, and other devices for conflict resolution appear to be preferred.

For several years, there has been accelerating discussion of how, to what extent, and with what payment should medical staff be involved in administrative decisions. In some budgetary experiments, clinical chiefs have been given a significant degree of actual control over the manner in which their departmental budgets are spent. In this model a number of cost centers have mini-global budgets. The institution, through an institution-wide priority setting exercise, determines the size of the departmental allocation, but priority-setting within the department is determined, within institutional guidelines and controls, by the department.

The concept is, of course, not new. Departments such as dietary and admitting, which are under the direction of department heads employed by the hospital, have always operated within an assigned budget. The new wrinkle is to give budgetary control to a clinician, who is primarily a caregiver. Both the old and new approach share one overwhelming problem. In the absence of an understanding of the cost-effectiveness of various activities, the choices between different expenditure patterns must continue to be intuitive.

Hospital Foundations

Many hospitals have recently created charitable foundations as legally separate but organizationally affiliated fundraising arms. Funds raised by the foundations are not hospital funds until transferred from the foundation. This arrangement gives the hospital greater flexibility in the ways it can use the collected funds and greater assurance that these donated funds will not be seen as part of the basic operating or capital budget of the hospital.

There are two levels of regulation of charities in Canada. The federal *Charities Act* primarily allows organizations to become registered with Revenue Canada (the department of the federal government that collects tax) so as to be able to issue tax receipts for donations. There are some 65,000 registered charities in Canada and nearly 30,000 of these are in Ontario. The provincial charities and trust legislation in Ontario is administered by the Public Trustee under the *Charities Accounting Act*. A foundation is a special classification of charity because it only dispenses money rather than actually providing or performing a charitable service or act. Foundations may be classified as private (eg, a family foundation) or public (eg, in a community). Technically, there are some tax differences between them but they operate in very similar ways. A charity is not required to be incorporated, but many are. This includes most hospitals. Incorporation provides protection for Directors against liability in case of an action or omission by the organization or one of its employees.

Under the federal and provincial legislation governing charities, some basic rules apply. These rules stipulate that

- □ political activity and direct contributions to a candidate or party are prohibited,
- □ organizational activity focused on changing government policy must be limited,
- □ benefits of the charity must be available to more than just a small number of persons,
- □ the income recieved by a charity is tax free, and
- □ receipts may be issued for donation of money or property.

Charities are exempt from some prohibitions against conducting a business for profit if the business activity is performed by volunteers, and some limitations exist on the kinds of fundraising that can be undertaken.

Charities, including foundations, are obliged to issue financial statements for public information in addition to a private one for Revenue Canada. Failure to disclose this information leads to deregistration. An organization cannot issue receipts for charitable donation and, obviously, the number of donations falls dramatically. For example, the Red Cross was recently deregistered for failure to comply to the rules of Revenue Canada.

The *Charitable Gifts Act* prohibits the holding of land by a charity if the land is not used for a charitable purpose. Ontario has the most comprehensive and constraining provincial legislation in Canada for enforcing such rules. An Ontario charity is also prohibited from operating a business, with the exception of a business directly related to a charity such as a for-profit cafeteria in a hospital. The other exemption, as mentioned above, would be a volunteer running a business for a charity, such as selling greeting cards. These exemptions are found in the *Income Tax Act*. Such restrictions apply because government believes that it is unfair for a tax-exempt enterprise to compete with those who must pay tax.

In Ontario, the Ministry of Health has traditionally required the approval of the Public Trustee in the construction of new buildings or the use of land owned by a hospital. A recent ruling by the Ontario Supreme Court (June 13, 1989) has altered this procedure. It was the opinion of the judge that the *Public Hospitals Act* was intended to "provide an exclusive statuatory scheme for the supervision and regulation of public hospitals." (Ontario Hospital Association report no. 782, vol. 29, no. 11, p.11)

The decision in this case takes Ontario public hospitals out of the jurisdiction of their incorporating legislation or under the *Public Hospitals Act*. However, if the hospital receives a bequest for a specific purpose, the funds must be used only for the designated purpose, and these funds then fall under the regulatory control of the *Charities Accounting Act*.

Under the regulations of the federal *Charities Act*, a hospital foundation may raise money in order to perform charitable acts. A charitable act is one designed to relieve pain and suffering. Philanthropy is defined as an activity to change the cause or circumstance that leads to pain and suffering. Clearly, hospital services can be seen as charitable acts and the transfer of funds from a foundation to a hospital is a ligitimate transaction.

In 1978-79, when the provincial government of Ontario began to impose fiscal constraints on hospitals, many created foundations to move assets away from possible interference by the government. Income from these assets would go to the activities of the hospital. One Ontario hospital foundation included other uses for the income in its registration in order to prevent government from getting access to the funds. This foundation offers scholarships to local students who want to enter a health care occupation.

Recently, the Auditor General of Ontario charged hospitals with hiding money in their foundations, but no follow-up has occurred on these charges. The development of hospital foundations may be seen not as a tax exercise, but a budget protection exercise by hospitals.

Because foundations are supervised by the Public Trustee, and not by the Minister of Health, they are relatively independent of the constraints of direct reporting placed on hospitals who attempt to raise money to augment either their capital or operating budgets.

The July, 1990, report of Fundraising Programs in Ontario Hospitals points out a number of interesting relationships between hospitals and foundations. This report shows that some hospitals and foundations are closely knit. Of the 196 hospitals reporting on their fundraising activities, 110 reported on their foundations. There was a 10 percent growth in fundraising within the foundation structure. Of those reporting, 95 percent said their foundations were active or being reactivated, 88 percent said that the boards overlapped between the hospital and the foundation. Full-time staff exist in more and more foundations. Some hospitals share staff with foundations. This sharing of staff is one way that allows hospitals to help their foundations.

Hospital Reporting

For the last 10 to 15 years there has been a steady reduction in the acute treatment hospital bed supply per 1000 population. This trend has occurred at quite different times and rates in different provinces, but has occurred everywhere. In 1982, British Columbia closed nearly 10 percent of acute treatment beds and reduced provincial hospital expenditures by $60 million. The 1984 The Newfoundland Royal Commission on hospitals and nursing home costs recommended closure of at least 300 acute treatment beds from 5.0 (urban) and 5.5 (northern) per 1000 population to 3.5 (urban) and 4.0 (northern). In 1986 Alberta announced an objective of 4.0 beds per 1000 instead of the existing 5.2. In 1992, many provinces, including New Brunswick, reduced the numbers of hospital beds as part of the development of regional structures.

Hospital reporting and definitions are standardized across Canada. **"General" beds** are those designated medical, surgical, obstetrical (maternity), intensive or coronary care, pediatric, gynecological, ear-nose-throat (ENT or otorhinolaryngological), or eye (ophthalmological). **"Special" beds** (or hospitals) are those designated as psychiatric, chronic, extended care, auxiliary, mental retardation, rehabilitation, convalescent, contagious, isolation, orthopedic, and arthritic. There is considerable overlap between some general and special care categories — orthopedic and surgical, for instance. This ambiguity weakens the accuracy of the terms and the associated data. Bed totals do not include bassinets and incubators.

While there has been growth of chronic beds in general hospitals, there has been an even larger increase in the supply of chronic (long term) beds in long term care institutions. In keeping with this trend, the government of Ontario, in 1987, approved over 4,400 new institutional beds; of these, 1,375 (31 percent) were acute care beds and 3,081 (69 percent) were for chronic care. Approval of so many long term care institutional beds in preference to optional forms of housing for the chronically disabled is unfortunate at a point in time when the feasibility of the residential options has been proven and users often express a preference for noninstitutional living.

Besides hospitals and long term care facilities, institutional, and residentional resources also include detoxification centers, infirmaries in universities and correctional institutions, and a large number of group homes, halfway houses, and free-standing abortion clinics which are common and accepted in Quebec but struggling for existence elsewhere. Ontario has recently funded a 12-bed hospice in Toronto for AIDS patients. Emergency equipment includes vehicles, airplanes, boats, communication systems, and standby emergency supplies. Later chapters will look more closely at specific kinds of institutional resources.

Although there are many examples of the increasing sophistication of health care technology (lithotripters, MRI) there are also many examples of investigations being simplified by other technology. Small office-based laboratory tools are rapidly becoming cheap and reliable. More and more ciochemical, bacteriological, and hematology tests can be done immediately. A return office visit may be avoided. In the United States, 30 percent of lab work is now done in the doctor's office. Insurance agencies should be developing policies which will invite use of this new office-based technology without misuse. Reliable equipment for self-diagnosis is also rapidly appearing on the market. Although some of this equipment is of questionable quality at this time, the technology is rapidly improving. The ethics and medical implications of self-administered tests for a broad range of diseases including AIDS, gonorrhoea, hepatitis, and gout are under discussion. There is medical objection to these tests, even though there have been few problems with the availability of self-administered pregnancy tests, blood pressure examinations and urine tests for sugar.

Computers have also contributed to this change in health care and its delivery. They have brought better office procedures, easier and more accurate billing, faster handling of laboratory specimens and reporting of the results, on-line data bases that may make libraries redundant, and analysis of patterns of illness. The beginning of the biggest and most challenging clinical development — computer assisted diagnosis and treatment — has arrived. Computer-based simulations have, for some time, been a major part of medical teaching, but future diagnosis and prescribing will almost surely become partly a computer function. The computer will process data and evaluate alternative diagnoses and therapies with a skill equal to or greater than that of most health workers in many complex circumstances. The machine age is here, and many health workers, especially physicians, will have their work altered by it.

Organs for transplant are a new category of physical resources. The supply, whether of kidneys, hearts, or anything else that cannot regenerate, is routinely less than the demand. In 1992 due to improved control of motor vehicle accidents, the supply of organs for transplant was smaller even than in previous years, despite efforts to alter retrieval patterns. There are active campaigns to increase access to organs, including the Canadian Medical Association drive to encourage physicians to promote organ donation. Scholars are studying the "organ marketplace" and are evaluating various imaginative techniques to increase supply or optimally allocate what is available. In Belgium, as of 1987, organs could be taken for transplant without the consent of the patient or the family. Very sophisticated international organ matching services, such as the Multiple Organ Retrieval and Exchange Program (MORE) in Ontario, or the national Organ Waiting List (OWL) based in Winnipeg, have increased the likelihood that organs that are available will be used. There is, however, still greater need for public awareness and greater cooperation from physicians and hospitals. Kidney donations rose 300 percent in Ontario from 1976 to 1984, but patients who would be more economically and better served by a transplant continue to be on dialysis.

Hospital Bylaws

As already described, the hospital's charter sets forth general institutional goals and characteristics. As a source of operational guidelines the charter is not very helpful. The hospital, therefore, needs a more detailed set of rules describing such things as

☐ the responsibilities and functions of the board and of senior staff,
☐ the composition of board committees and the schedule of board meetings,
☐ financial control procedures such as the use of closed tenders,
☐ conflict of interest guidelines,
☐ appointments to and review of medical staff membership,
☐ duties and constraints associated with medical staff membership,
☐ the major organizational divisions of the hospital and the medical staff,
☐ the major health care services of the hospital,
☐ the process of patient admission, and
☐ other similar matters.

This detailed set of rules is known as **hospital bylaws**. Hospital bylaws tend to be divided into two major parts, one part deals with medical staff and the other part deals with all other matters.

Bylaws are in force when they have been ratified by a meeting of the corporation and approved by the Minister. The required content of many parts of the bylaws is often specifically spelled out in governing legislation such as a *Public Hospitals Act*. Provincial hospital associations, sometimes in collaboration with the medical association, produce model bylaws meant to assist hospitals as they create or revise bylaws for review by the Minister.

Medical Staff Bylaws

These bylaws describe the medical staff structure, including

☐ titles of medical staff leaders,
☐ how these leaders are chosen,
☐ the standing committees that will exist,
☐ the role of the MAC or other components of medical staff organization in various decisions,
☐ the process of review of applications from physicians and dentists for the right to have privileges in the hospital,
☐ the categories of medical staff and their rights and responsibilities,
☐ procedures for appeal if an applicant is not happy with decisions affecting his or her opportunity to practice within the hospital, and
☐ educational and research responsibilities and vehicles.

Central to many medical staff bylaws is the general principle that a public institution is expected to operate with rules that are clearly stated and are fair and non-discriminatory.

The functions of the medical staff fall almost entirely upon the active staff. In major urban centers it is now uncommon for a physician to have an active staff appointment in more than one hospital. Active staff members have voting rights, will be expected to participate in committee work, and are usually required to attend the regularly held educational sessions of the appropriate clinical group.

Medical Staff Committees

There is, once again, considerable variation among hospitals but common titles include

- ☐ the Admission and Discharge Committee,
- ☐ the Utilization Committee,
- ☐ the Credentials Committee,
- ☐ the Infection Control Committee,
- ☐ the Quality Assurance Committee,
- ☐ the Medical (Health) Records and/or Audit Committee,
- ☐ the Central Committee for the Assessment of Medical Acts (Quebec),
- ☐ the Tissue Committee,
- ☐ the Pharmacy and Therapeutics Committee,
- ☐ the Research Committee,
- ☐ the Therapeutic Abortion Committee,
- ☐ the Medical Education Committee,
- ☐ the Emergency Committee, and
- ☐ the Admissions and Length of Stay Committee (Quebec).

Not all of these committees will exist in any one hospital because the functions of some of them overlap, as is the case with the Quality Assurance Committee and the Infection Control Committee. The members of all medical staff committees tend to be named by the MAC.

The Process of Granting Medical Staff Privileges

Applications for medical staff membership or renewal are submitted to the hospital board. The application is referred to the MAC for assessment and the MAC makes a recommendation to the board. The recommendation is usually accepted, but the final decision and the legal responsibility for that decision rests with the board. Physicians who do not agree with the decision of the board may initiate an appeal process, which may end in review by a quasi-judicial body such as a provincial Hospital Appeals Board or a provincial court. It will be essential, in future, for appointments to be consistent with strategic planning and selected hospital programs.

Professional Staff Organization in Quebec Hospitals

The medical, dental and other professionals in Quebec hospitals are members of the Council of Physicians and Dentists (The Clinical Staff Advisory Committee). This Committee is quite analogous to the MAC but has a broader membership and shows some functional variations.

House Staff

The term **"house staff"** refers to all medical interns and residents and does not include other professional trainees or medical students in the hospital. Dental trainees might be a rare exception. These interns and residents are employees of the hospital and are not part of the medical staff. The term **"intern"** is usually reserved for persons in their first year of training following graduation with an M.D.

Residents are enrolled in specialty training programs, including family practice residencies. Residents may be licensed to practice outside, as well as inside, the hospital. They tend to be paid $25,000 to $40,000 per year and often work very long hours, a fact due more to historical precedent than to necessity. House staff are found only in hospitals which have been approved by the Royal College of Physicians and Surgeons or the College of Family Physicians of Canada as locations for training.

House staff members examine patients on arrival, write their medical histories, and, to the extent that their rank and experience allow, write patient care orders. They also assist during surgery, perform or order many diagnostic and therapeutic procedures, see the patients as often as necessary during their hospital stays, perform obstetrical deliveries, and accompany physicians on their rounds.

House staff members have recently achieved a more reasonable work week. This is similar to what happened to nurses, who 15 to 20 years ago went through an educational change in which student nurses ceased to be seen as sources of cheap labor. In the process, nurses became students, and therefore lost their access to free room and board and began to pay tuition. They also graduated with too little clinical experience to be able to work alone in many situations. Interns and residents are both employees and trainees.

The interest in having house staff is, at times, considerably greater than the interest in seeing them become practicing competitors. At various points in history, the failure rate among those taking exams for admission to specialty fields suffering from oversupply has been unreasonably high. Specialty exams can be taken after five years of approved training with the exception of family physicians who take them after three years.

Teaching Hospital/University Relationships

These relationships are made complex by legal, educational, quality of care and financial factors. They are, as a result, clearly set out in formal agreements.

Agreement is, in Canada, made more simple by the fact that most of the income of both institutions comes from government. Hospitals still, however, may wish to limit the extent to which their global budget supports costs which they think universities ought to pick up. There is a need to understand the extent to which each party will finance lockers, parking, uniforms, liability insurance and supervision for educational programs.

Territorial disputes can also arise over appointments to the medical staff and the selection of clinical heads of departments. Mutually acceptable candidates are sought although the universities hold the strongest veto. In a teaching hospital, it is essential that senior medical staff also hold a university appointment.

In the relationship between teaching hospitals and universities, the universities have become increasingly dominant through their control over department head appointments and their influence over development and staffing of residency programs. Clinical department heads in teaching hospitals usually have a university appointment as a geographic full time (GFT) professor and, therefore, university acceptance is a prerequisite to the hospital appointment.

Multi-Institutional Arrangements

The history of hospitals is filled with examples of multi-institutional arrangements. These include most psychiatric hospitals, some religious hospitals, Grenfell Mission hospitals in Newfoundland and veterans' hospitals (now mostly transferred to other management). These multi-institutional arrangements were a natural product of the nature and responsibilities of the owners. Since the 1950s, individual community (voluntary) hospitals have entered into collective solutions, either voluntarily or under direction from government, as a means of controlling costs and of improving the quality and/or the availability, of services. In essence, these arrangements always implement some form of centralization.

There are three common and successful multi-institutional models which do not seriously threaten the autonomy of the participating hospitals.

Model #1

Figure 5.3

One Master Provider and Satellite Users

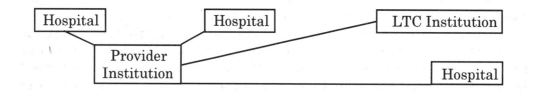

In this model, one provider institution supplies a service to satellite user institutions. The provider hospital (or other institution, program, or association) was chosen as the site of a central laundry, a computer center, a 24-hour pharmacy service, an in-service education program, a specialized maintenance staff, or a specialized laboratory service. The choice was made by virtue of the hospital's excess capacity, specialized skills, central location, or political or tactical skills.

The centrally produced service may be purchased on a flat fee or fee-for-service basis, or may be financed entirely within the global budget of the parent institution.

Model #2

A separate service center may be created (Figure 5.4). The center serves all member institutions but is not part of any of them. Examples include a data processing center, a food commissariat, and a separate regional laundry. All the users are equal in the sense that none of them perceives another institution to be in a position of excessive control or advantage.

When the new corporation or partnership is controlled by participating users, it is often referred to as a **joint venture**. The executive board may include community representatives and it may not include a representative of every user, but participation by all users is a popular model.

Provincial laboratories, or the federal virus laboratory, represent a variation in which the services of the laboratory are used by all who need them but none of the users have direct management influence over the service.

Figure 5.4

Shared Services Via a New Corporate Entity

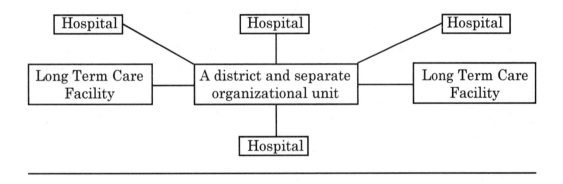

Model #3

In this model, which illustrates a cooperative and image- preserving style, parts of a major function are assigned to more than one institution.

This selective distribution model is ideal when a number of institutions each wish to retain a piece of the action and the service involved can be provided from several different sites, such as with surgical or pathology services. Dispersion of one part of the total range of services to each institution can preserve a role for everyone, while still concentrating a particular kind of equipment and expertise in one place. Figure 13.5 illustrates this approach to laboratory services.

Each hospital becomes a center of excellence, and each hospital must rely on all other hospitals. Operating agreements are needed to assure satisfactory service, rapid transfer of specimens and results when needed, and a method for resolving disputes.

The three models of multi-institutional services that have been described do not significantly reduce the autonomy of a hospital. Other models are more intrusive.

The most integrated model would be a regional hospital board as proposed in New Brunswick in 1992, and as exists in Great Britain.

Figure 5.5

Cooperative Dispersion

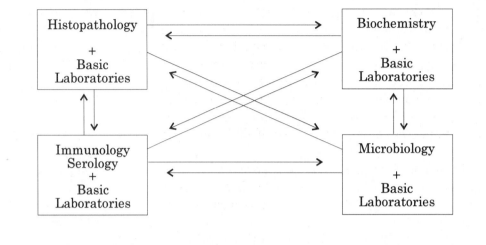

In British Columbia and Alberta, a number of hospital boards have been eliminated as a direct result of Ministry pressure and decisions, and most hospitals built recently in these provinces have been placed under an existing hospital board. This centralization process is usually politically unattractive, but appears to be proceeding without major confrontation.

Mergers

Mergers are sometimes seen as a cost-reduction tool, but there is no evidence they save money. They may serve another major objective; to make it easier to create a balanced and appropriately distributed network of regional resources operating in a coordinated and cooperative manner. The key to creating this network is a regional plan in which all major sources of health services, or, ideally, health and social services, are assigned an appropriate function and made to perform it. Having fewer hospital boards may not move Canadians closer to a regional system nor may this be necessary to achieve a regional system, but one argument presses the possibility that hospitals, in total, have less influence when each does not have its own organizational identity. The argument goes on to suggest that multihospital boards might move Canadians toward a balanced system.

Arguments that favor each hospital having its own board suggest that there would be an increased number of community leaders who would participate, and there would very likely be more charitable donations when institutions are clearly identified with their communities. The ideal situation would seem to be one in which community hospitals could continue to be specifically related to their communities, while at the same time hospital influence could be reduced to the point that ambulatory care, mental health services, long term care, health promotion, environmental hazards, and occupational health could receive attention consistent with their importance. Proposals in Ontario for a new *Public Hospitals Act* have recommended a community advisory board for each hospital, whil several hospitals share a regional governing board.

Multi-Institutional Management

Specific mention of a few Canadian examples of multi-institutional management may illustrate some of the models presented.

Three Vancouver hospitals — the Shaughnessy, the Grace and the Children's — merged, with each hospital keeping its own board and its own identity, but with each operating under an umbrella agreement, a master board, and a single senior executive body. The "super-board" is responsible for a fairly broad range of administrative and planning functions. There is only one staff, one set of collective bargaining agreements, and one set of personnel policies. Various major service functions such as radiology are concentrated in one place. The overall board acts as the policy and administrative controlling agency in all those areas where major conflict might occur or where the mass of all three hospitals is needed for reasonable efficiency and high quality of care.

This merger was expected by the government to save money, and it may have done so, though no overall assessment has been made. In the radiology department, however, costs went up. A larger unit attracted specialists who were closer to the state-of-the-art technology and more anxious to have it. The perception of adequate quality changed with the change from three 300-bed hospitals to a 700-800 bed complex.

In Kingston, a Joint Liaison Committee made up of representatives of Queen's University and four hospitals legally oversees the operation of the four hospitals. None can expand programs, alter functions, or build additions without the agreement of the group. Each institution continues to exist, but obviously not with the degree of independence it once had. This structure arose because in the early 1970s, when money started to become scarce, the Ontario government told a number of communities that, as soon as the community institutions got together and agreed on what actions were most collectively important to their community, the government would consider whether or not to fund them. The community institutions were obliged to agree upon local priorities and to cooperatively allocate many functions, including pediatrics, obstetrics, types of surgery and emergency services. Queen's University is also exploring the impact of salaries for university-based physicians, this perhaps to be implemented as early as 1993.

The Vancouver and Kingston examples demonstrate that some of the advantages of multi-institutional boards can be achieved while at least partly preserving the images of the individual institutions.

Mergers are less common in the east, but have occurred in both smaller communities such as Smith Falls, and in larger urban areas such as Toronto where the Toronto General and Toronto Western hospitals were merged.

Hospital Statistics and Reporting

Number of Beds per 1000 Population

The number of hospital beds is one of two major determinants of health services costs; the other is physician supply. Bed supply appears to be always slightly less than demand. Canadian centers have, or have had, a bed supply as high as 7-8 per 1000 and there were still calls for more. Ontario is now aiming for 3.5 beds per 1000 in urban centers and 4-4.5 in rural areas. Quebec has similar objectives. A number of other provinces are still apparently committed to a more generous formula, but the general trend during the last 10-15 years has been towards fewer beds per 1000 population.

Health planning has often been dominated by questions concerning hospital bed supply. Unfortunately, there is no body of evidence that clearly describes the relationship between bed supply and community health. Figure 5.6 describes two relationships, either of which may exist.

Figure 5.6

The Relationship Between Bed Supply and Community Health Status

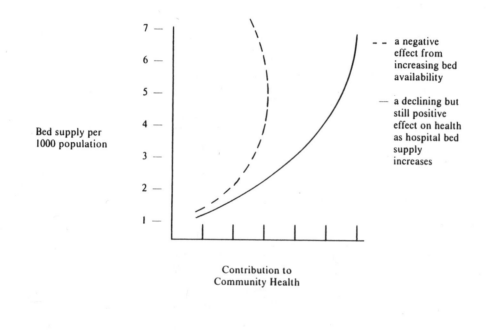

Figure 5.6 suggests that the first 2-3 hospital beds per 1000 population make a significant contribution to community health. The two curves vary in that one of them indicates that a bed supply in excess of 5 beds per 1000 has a negative effect on community health. This proposition can be defended on the basis of the undesirable trade-offs that would have been made to finance the extra beds.

Number of Separations or Admissions per 1000 (per year)

This figure has fallen steadily as the number of acute treatment beds has declined, and as more of the former short-stay patients are treated as outpatients or day surgical patients. Day surgery patients may or may not be counted as admissions, depending mostly on which is most financially advantageous to the hospital or what rules have been laid down by the Ministry. Normal newborns are usually not counted as admissions but the mother is counted, just as bassinets in the newborn nursery are not counted as beds while beds on the maternity unit are counted.

Average Length of Stay (ALS)

In calculating average length of stay, the day of admission is not counted and the day of discharge is counted. The ALS in teaching hospitals is usually about 10 days, with community hospitals ALS usually being about 8 days. ALS is now declining as more centers become integrated with home nursing services and early discharge programs.

Number of bed days per 1000 (total population per year)

This figure is obviously the product of average length of stay and the number of admissions per 1000. Provincial figures were, at one time, in the range of 1500-2000 but now they are more apt to be in the range of 800-1200 bed days per 1000 total population per year. Hospitals are measured in peer groups to evaluate the bed days per 1000 population. Funding is tied to performance being close to the mean.

Percentage Occupancy

Average daily census compared to a bed total gives an average occupancy. When working with this figure it is useful to know whether the bed total represents rated beds or beds set up. Occupancy rates in Canada tend to be well above 85 percent.

Annual Hospital Reporting

With the introduction of universal hospital insurance in 1958 under Bill 360, the *Hospital Insurance and Diagnostic Services Act (HIDSA)*, it became necessary for the federal government to know exact hospital expenditures. Consequently, two national hospital reporting forms, Hospital Statistics 1 and 2 (HS1 and HS2) evolved. Although the *HIDSA* requirements no longer apply, these two forms continue to be used.

HS1 contains descriptive data including type of institution, nature of services provided, patients by classification, volume of diagnostic and hotel services, and paid hours of work and staff costs by activity center. HS2 reports audited financial data including expenditures by activity center, income by source and amount, assets and liabilities, and other information required to indicate the financial stability of the institution.

Provincial psychiatric hospitals do not complete HS1's or HS2's.

Issues and Questions That Face the Hospital Industry

In a general sense this list starts with issues related to overall institutional goals and missions, and then moves to more limited issues such as those related to organization, money, and quality.

Responsibilities of Hospitals to Regional Planning or Service Bodies

Do hospital trustees and administrators, with their special skills and large budgets, have a responsibility to strengthen the total health care network? For example, should hospitals offer tangible and expert support to regional planning agencies, assist smaller agencies which lack educational or administrative expertise, and cooperatively accept decisions made at the regional or provincial level?

There is sometimes a tendency for hospitals, perhaps most marked in tertiary care hospitals, to wish to solve every community health-related problem that appears. When a problem is identified, the hospital may say "How can I (the hospital) respond?" instead of, "Who in the community is best suited to respond?" If the hospital takes the second approach then it may, by virtue of its highly developed capabilities and its capacity to find developmental funds, be the institution best suited to provide initiative and start up assistance for programs or functions that will become the responsibility of someone else. This second approach is more likely to lead to a balanced health services network with a full range of well-developed sectors.

When the parochial approach is avoided, it becomes more likely that the larger institutions will be aware of how difficult it sometimes is for smaller institutions to offer reasonable continuing education opportunities or fringe benefit packages to their staff. They also become aware of how difficult it is to create and maintain information systems, quality review mechanisms, or a variety of special services. The larger hospital could, without absorbing or threatening the smaller institution, sponsor a variety of multi-institutional cooperative efforts in which the smaller institutions may be the only major beneficiaries.

If the hospital accepts a responsibility for the strength and adequacy of regional agencies, then the hospital will not use end-runs to the Ministry when arguments are lost at the local level, and it will not actively seek to develop programs or levels of function that have been denied at the regional level.

Selection of Hospital Function

Should hospitals concentrate on and limit themselves to performing excellently in those functional areas which cannot be served by others, like major emergencies, major surgery, and all investigation and therapy requiring 24-hour supportive care? The alternative is to consider such things as home care, health promotion, long term care, and satellite ambulatory care units as fields which are appropriate for hospital attention or which are, perhaps, even seen as most desirably delivered under the direction of hospitals.

Traditional inpatient services are an important and high volume part of the health services network. They require highly specialized clinical personnel and equipment as well as sophisticated management. They operate in an environment dominated by high technology, high cost, high stress, and rapid patient turnover. Personalization and client involvement must often be compromised in the interest of efficiency and high technical quality.

Delivering and administering high quality institutional priority setting and patient care is demanding, socially important, and quite different from performing the same tasks in community-based programs. These differences make it undesirable for hospitals to become the managers of community-based services. This limitation is both in the interest of optimal hospital performance and in that of community or long term care programs that should not be required to accept the in-hospital environment and practices. It is preferable that the different parts of the health services network, like ambulatory care, hospitals, long term care, and health promotion, should each develop under their own set of specially trained and oriented workers and advocates. Coordination of the different sources of health related activities and services is the function of some regional umbrella organization that will not allow any particular service or need to be unreasonably dominant or unreasonably neglected.

Evaluation of Hospitals

Evaluation of hospitals and their activities is currently performed by the Canadian Council on Health Facilities Accreditation (CCHFA), provincial governments, professional and academic bodies, auditors, researchers, hospital associations, the Professional Activities Study (PAS) and Hospital Medical Records Institute (HMRI), legal tribunals, and users.

The evaluative role of each of these will be discussed in order.

1. The CCHFA accreditation surveys emphasize inputs (facilities, staff and their qualifications), process as documented in minutes of meetings and on patient charts, and departmental (intermediate) outputs such as completed charts and autopsy rates. They have emphasized, and still overemphasize, the environment in which care is delivered, but they are now exploring the use of outcome measures.

   In recent years CCHFA clinical review procedures have been markedly improved by the introduction of the prospective medical audit. This mandatory audit applies pre-established criteria and standards to all cases of a particular type, which is a much more objective and inclusive approach than that followed by the former retrospective medical audit. In this former audit, a group of peers individually and subjectively reviewed randomly selected patient files. Nursing audits are also routinely expected.

2. Provincial ministries of health or some delegated quasi-public body closely monitor approved budgets and monthly expenditure patterns. Through either regular monitoring or response to complaints, a variety of federal, provincial and municipal agencies or departments evaluate fire safety, the handling of noxious wastes, food handling procedures and personnel, exposure to radiation, and the process of awarding hospital privileges to medical staff.

3. The Royal College of Physicians and Surgeons and specialist organizations such as the Canadian Association of Pathologists regularly evaluate hospitals to determine whether or not medical internship or residency programs can be based there. Other professional associations, such as the Canadian Physiotherapy Association, evaluate the relevant departments of hospitals to determine whether internships should be approved in their field.

4. Auditors evaluate the acceptability of financial management and accounting practices, assure accuracy in reports and may comment on whether resources were used for purposes consistent with the mandate of the institution. Auditors usually report to the hospital board.

5. Researchers may evaluate individual institutions or the hospital industry. They analyze or report utilization patterns, production costs, service volumes, disease costs, and clinical outcomes. Either directly or indirectly, research findings may report the quality of the performance of institutions.

6. Evaluation of hospitals is not a primary hospital association function but these associations regularly collect information which allows institutional comparisons to be made. Examples of these data include the incidence of accidents, the presence of deficits, or the fundraising by foundations.

7. Almost all Canadian hospitals send an abstract of every discharge to either PAS, based in Ann Arbor, Michigan, or HMRI, based in Toronto. These programs report the aggregated discharge data to each hospital in ways which allow comparisons with similar institutions or with established norms.

8. Coroners' inquests and malpractice suits often include an evaluation of hospital care, and other judicial activities can also alter hospital procedures.

9. Patient satisfaction surveys are routine in many hospitals. Although patients are usually unable to evaluate the quality of the technical care received, they do provide valid evaluations of those aspects of hospital operations that are understandable or which pertain to values, courtesy, and caring.

Assessment of Hospital Evaluation Processes Currently in Use and Their Ability To Function With Future Issues

Evaluation requires an appreciation of objectives. The objectives of a hospital should include all of the following.

1. To perform those services that will, in combination with other health and health related services in the community, and keeping in mind the role assigned to the hospital, best preserve or elevate the health status of the community. The hospital will set priorities that optimally reflect community needs or wants and the hospital's role in meeting those needs or wants.

2. To provide patient care at the highest quality compatible with the resources available and the concept of best use of resources. The quality of one type of care should be reduced when the savings will serve the community better by being spent elsewhere.

3. To distribute available resources within the general principle that some degree of avoidable risk will have to be accepted by most, if not all, patients. The degree of risk that will be tolerable will vary with the consequences inherent in the relevant hazard and the volume of resources needed to reduce the risk.

4. To cooperate with and provide intellectual and tangible support to the regional and/or provincial planning and evaluation process, and to operate in accordance with regional/provincial decisions reached regarding function and expenditures.

5. To use resources efficiently.

6. To operate in ways that reflect the culture, values and priorities of the community, and to respect the individual values and culture of each user.

7. To contribute to research and education to whatever extent is compatible with the nature of the institution.

8. To be a good employer.

9. To be a good corporate citizen, including being a good neighbor.

10. To obey the law.

If these objectives are accepted, then evaluation of any hospital will need to report the extent to which each objective is being met. In examining the extent to which each objective is being met, it must be understood that various objectives may or will at times be in conflict. It must also be accepted that there may be major differences between wants (as expressed by clients) and needs (as expressed by professionals), and that deciding which to respond to may be difficult.

A matching of the current hospital evaluation activities and the list of objectives shows that the hospital accreditation process looks

☐ at patient care quality without giving much attention to the concept that quality should at times be consciously compromised in the interest of best use of resources,
☐ at the question of patient risk without providing many, if any, formal guidelines which describe an acceptable level of avoidable risk,
☐ at the extent of hospital sensitivity to patient values and priorities, and
☐ at selected other elements of hospital performance.

The activities of other sources of evaluation tend to relate to only one objective, and this seldom in a comprehensive way, although our rapidly improving production data does give us a preliminary feeling for efficiency.

It is clear that we do not know much about the extent to which hospitals are meeting most of the objectives listed. We do not usually know whether they have an internal priority-setting process or, if they have one, how well it is working.

No one regularly evaluates the extent to which a hospital supports or cooperates with regional agencies. Neither do we know which hospitals have effectively coordinated their activities with other institutional and community-based services — such as nursing homes or public health agencies — that are regularly used by the clients of hospitals. Indicators, standards, and a quality review process are equally lacking elsewhere.

There is need for refinement and expansion of what may be called the "social responsibility index." The terminology involved is not new (cost-effectiveness, outcome measures, community health status, quality of life, tradeoffs, being responsive to consumers, conflicting objectives) but movement towards a comprehensive, coordinated approach first appeared in the 1992 *Report of the Steering Committee*, Public Hospitals Act Review. The Committee has termed this a "social contract."

Can Improved Hospital Efficiency Solve our Financial Problems?

The answer is no. Canadian hospitals are already quite efficient. Much is written about how money can be saved (essentially, how available money can be better spent) through such activities as group purchasing, preventive maintenance and increased production. Some people would put lower labor costs, primarily obtained through contracting out to avoid unionization, in this list of efficiency measures. Many would not. Eventually, one must accept that, regardless of how efficient the system becomes, it will still face a public and a professional demand that cannot be fully met with the dollars allocated.

When it is fully recognized that efficiency improvements will not allow demand to be met, the system will then turn its efforts towards determining which service cutbacks will be least threatening to the health status of the community. Other alternative approaches to cutting back are available, but not as desirable. These include

- cutting services in ways that protect administration/medical staff relations or medical staff incomes more than community health,
- cutting back in ways that will make the most headlines so that government embarrassment or public pressure on government may lead to extra funding, or
- cutting back services to those populations with the least ability to fight back.

Physician Involvement in Decision-Making

There are frequently requests for greater involvement of the medical staff in hospital decision making and suggestions that there is greater need for physicians to recognize cost factors in their practice habits. These requests may not be realistic but they are regularly discussed. Some reasons why those requests are not being met follow.

- Physicians are not taught about budgets, costing or priority setting.

- Physicians, when delivering care, should have first loyalty to their patient, not to the institution; they are patient advocates.

☐ Physicians whose incomes are derived through fee-for-service only get paid when they are delivering care. They become charitable institutions when they sit on committees, evaluate each others' work, develop clinical protocols, prepare for accreditation, and carry out other similar activities. Teaching hospitals have a pool of salaried university-based physicians who can increase their involvement in management without loss of income, but most hospitals are not teaching hospitals.

☐ Fee-for-service physicians may see the whole process of institutional rationalization as a threat to their incomes as well as their autonomy.

Rationing

Hospital administrators and trustees are already occasionally blamed for delays in admission of urgent (not emergency) patients including, for example, those with cancer. This is not a fair criticism. The order in which patients are admitted has, until now, been almost entirely the product of physician-created priorities. If a patient waits, it is because other physicians have won the power struggles in the MAC. The number of urgent cases, especially those with proven cancer or a high degree of risk, is limited, and earlier admission of these patients would not seriously disturb the admission patterns of other patients. When physicians complain about their patients having to wait, it is fair to remind them that physicians, through their medical staff decisions, caused the delay.

The Use of and Cost of Preferred Accommodation

Preferred accommodation was described earlier as one source of income for hospitals. The current practices are, at times, coercive. One can, in some hospitals, be admitted earlier or more reliably on a particular day if one has insurance which covers preferred accommodation or will pay for a more expensive room. Charges for private and semi-private rooms are a form of extra billing which in Ontario has became an undesirable tool for hidden expansion of hospital income.

The Distribution of Beds Between Surgery, Medicine, Rehabilitation, Psychiatry, etc.

There has been a very rapid growth in the volume of surgical procedures. This growth is the product of the performance of surgery previously performed on inpatients in offices and day surgery units, and a shortened length of stay for patients who have their surgery performed in hospital. These improved bed utilization practices have, in practical terms, been the approximate equivalent of a doubling of surgical bed availability (with the effects upon different surgical specialties being quite different).

The Incentive to Promote Out-of-Province Income and Patients

When provinces allow hospitals to keep income from out-of-province patients, the hospitals are in an undesirable conflict of interest situation. This income should be considered when setting and revising global budgets.

The Granting or Continuance of Hospital Privileges

The Medical Advisory Committee, through the Credentials Committee, provides recommendations to the board regarding new additions to the medical staff. When the MAC feels that the hospital has enough psychiatrists, orthopedic surgeons, etc., it sends negative recommendations.

Boards and medical staffs do, usually, successfully refuse privileges on no grounds other than their wish for no more doctors of a particular type. The 1992 *Public Hospitals Act Review* in Ontario has reinforced the hospitals' ability to manage its physician resources based on a strategic plan.

As doctor supply increases and bed supply does not, there will be greater competition for beds. At some point in time, the community and/or its agents will demand evaluation on the basis of previously established criteria, which are fairly applied to all applicants. This practice will increase the likelihood that qualified physicians whose clinical field requires hospital access will not be excluded from hospital use by colleagues defending their established positions or favoring their friends.

A Reduction in the Number of 24 Hour Emergency Departments

The community hospitals in large urban centers are resisting closure of their emergency departments at night, even though this closure is desirable. Good evidence supports any decision to operate only one major 24-hour emergency service for each 500,000 people or more. Such a center can offer immediate availability of high-quality life support teams of all kinds, and can also handle the semi- or non-emergency walk-in patients during the night shift.

Objections come primarily from physicians who derive a significant part of their practice from the major emergencies which will seldom come to their hospital when the emergency service is downgraded. Institutional pride may also be a source of objections.

Changes in Birthing

Midwives in Ontario now have legal status as caregivers during pregnancy and childbirth. Other provinces are expected to follow. For those who prefer it, midwifery can combine the full safety of hospital back-up services with a personalized, family-based and less technical experience. Users and their supporters should not allow hospitals or physicians to inappropriately make it seem that the only choices are either home births or case room stirrups. There is a practical and attainable middle ground now available in cities such as Ottawa.

Summary

Hospitals have been described as the cathedrals of modern society; they are institutions of awesome power in that they are seen to be a source of medical rescue and the route to eternal replacement and renewal. To be unable to enter one when the need for one is perceived to be present (by doctor, family or patient) sometimes carries the anxiety-producing capability of excommunication in the Middle Ages. On the other hand, hospitals are also described as technocratic monsters, money-consuming preservers of the medical model, and the place where one leaves one's individuality at the door and becomes a test tube with a number on it. Hospitals provide important services, but there are many other kinds of equally health-preserving services.

References

Foreman, S.E. (1991). The power of health care value-adding partnerships: meeting competition through cooperation. *Hospitals and Health Services Administration*: 36(2) pp.175-190.

Evans, R.G. and Stoddart, G.L. (1988). *Medicare at Maturity, Achievements, Lessons and Challenges*. Calgary, Alberta: University of Calgary Press.

Porter, R.M.P. (1991). The Health Care System in Canada and its Funding: No Easy Solutions. Ottawa: Standing Committee on Health and Welfare, Seniors and the Status of Women, House of Commons.

CHAPTER 6

Community Health Services

Introduction

C anada's provinces are now allocating resources and supporting initiatives for health services that are provided in settings outside of a hospital or other institutional setting. This chapter describes these services as they exist in community health centers, care in the home, and public health services. Community mental health services are described in the chapter on mental health.

Community health services (CHS) are delivered from the broadest possible mix of nonhospital locations including

- [ ] homes,
- [ ] offices,
- [ ] clinics,
- [ ] the street,
- [ ] shopping centers,
- [ ] schools,
- [ ] work places,
- [ ] jails, and
- [ ] recreation sites.

CHS programs and workers deliver primary, secondary and tertiary care, and prevention. They deal with personal and collective problems. They respond to every type of medical problem, most types of social problems, and use most types of technology. Many programs in community health include an emphasis on health promotion and illness prevention.

CHSs are much more difficult to circumscribe than hospital services. Hospitals have a significant degree of control over the types of things they do. CHSs do almost anything. Hospitals are much more structured and are much more likely to admit and to discharge. In CHSs the users drop in, and out, at will.

Community health services merge imperceptibly with a number of other social networks, namely housing, employment, protective services, education, financial support, consumer protection, urban planning, recreation, transportation, and services for the learning disabled. All of these are, at various times, crucial to persons in need. Health workers and programs must regularly consider these primarily nonhealth services if multiproblem individuals and families are to be reasonably supported and aided. These other networks operate alongside community health services and should not be forgotten.

Although institutional services can be seen as different from community services, it is important to remember that the services provided in hospital outpatient clinics, as well as many services provided in the emergency department and "in day" programs, are very similar to those provided from various noninstitutional sources of care. In most communities only 5 to 10 percent of ambulatory care is provided by hospitals. The distinction being made in the various chapters is entirely for convenience, not because the different sources of care serve distinct clients or deal with completely different types of problems.

Community Health Centers (CHCs)

Community health center describes ambulatory care outlets which have a number of common features and which are quite different from traditional solo or group medical practice. They are reasonably recent developments that go back about 30 years in Canada and 50 years in the United States, although earlier precursors can be identified.

Community health centers are

☐ multidisciplinary and multifunctional,
☐ do not rely on fee-for-service payments as their primary source of income,
☐ are community-oriented,
☐ offer a broad range of services, and
☐ are known by many names.

Each of these features will be looked at in some detail. Despite their slow growth in Canada, CHCs continue to be seen as a desirable concept by a significant group of individuals and governments.

Methods of Financing

Fee-for-service billing is not the primary source of revenue although it tends to be used for certain clientele. Most CHC income is received in the form of either capitation payments or a global budget. The global budget is the most common in Canada.

The absence of fee-for-service as a major method of producing income is seen by many as the most fundamental CHC feature. The use of both capitation and global budgets is compatible with the development of multidisciplinary teams. CHCs have an integrated, holistic, and continuous (rather than episodic) approach to care and with an emphasis on health promotion. Capitation payments are made to the organization, not to individual providers of care. Physicians may be on salary or they may have a contract in which their income varies with the financial viability of the organization or with other factors.

The Multidisciplinary Team

Under fee-for-service, the physician is the only major income producer since work done by others will usually not be paid for by the provincial insurance plan. CHCs, however, are able to distribute work to the most appropriate worker because their income does not come predominantly from fees. Even in small CHCs, the team is likely to consist of social workers, nurse practitioners, public health nurses and/or registered nurses as well as physicians. In larger CHCs, the team can include dentists, optometrists, physiotherapists, community developers, mental health therapists and counsellors, health record analysts, dieticians, occupational therapists, pharmacists, psychologists, podiatrists or chiropodists, health educators, and chiropractors. The range of physician specialists will also expand as the CHC enlarges. Different CHC models emphasize or exclude certain types of workers.

The integrated multidisciplinary approach allows all health care workers

☐ to utilize their special skills,
☐ to share in the planning and delivery of care, and
☐ to share a common patient record.

Patients can receive services from a variety of workers without changing location or being uncertain about their central place of care.

A reasonably comprehensive team cannot be developed until the CHC has a population base of at least 10-15,000 people, and 20-30,000 is a more commonly quoted range. A population of 20-30,000 people is an optimum size because, once a reasonably complete range of services is available, further enlargement may increase patient travel and decrease the personalization of care without increasing the advantages of economies of scale.

Multidisciplinary care is not easy to deliver. Nonhierarchical teamwork is not part of the education of most professionals in Canada, especially physicians, and role models are scarce. Even the centralized multidisciplinary health record is not easy to introduce. The challenge is to encourage professionals such as psychologists, dentists, and social workers, each with their own terminologies and forms, to both share a record and understand one another. This is a particularly difficult challenge if the semantic and technical communication problems are worsened by interprofessional rivalry or negative perceptions.

One Stop Shopping

Fragmented and dispersed ambulatory care and other social services are inconvenient and inappropriate for the multiproblem person or family. The CHC attempts to reduce client difficulties by putting the required health and social service professionals in one place and having one integrated record. In this respect, the CHC is like a hospital.

Community/User Control

There is no universal management arrangement but CHC boards usually represent communities or consumers rather than providers. Boards differ in

☐ the way they are chosen,
☐ the extent to which they are accountable, and
☐ how they operate.

There is currently less legislation surrounding community boards than hospital boards.

The terms "membership" and "roster" are sometimes used. **Members** tend to be those persons who wish to have a say in the management of the CHC, at least to the extent of voting at an annual meeting. They may or may not be users of the CHC. **Roster** is a financial term applying to Ontario Health Service Organizations (HSOs). The roster consists of those persons who have indicated that they consider the CHC to be their primary source of care. Monthly capitation payments are made to the HSO for all rostered patients who, in that month, did not obtain from an outside source a service which could have been provided by the HSO.

The Planning of Ambulatory Care Networks

It is, as was stated earlier, difficult to create coordinated and regional networks when the regional agency is unable to significantly control private practitioner planning or operations. CHCs are nonprofit and their trustees might be expected to have an interest in area-wide and integrated programs. CHCs tend to deal directly with a government ministry with respect to such things as budgets, new services, productivity and reporting systems and, therefore, should have no difficulty cooperating with a ministry or regional agency on planning matters. CHCs are attractive to planners because they introduce an alternative to fee-for-service medicine. When one is seeking an efficient and responsive system and the one in use is uncertain on both counts, one ought to test alternative models. The CHC is such an alternative.

The Holistic Approach to Care

Many CHCs put great emphasis on holistic, continuous, and preventive medicine (including health promotion) rather than on the curative and episodic approach to care. To consider CHCs to be the only place where one can receive holistic care, or the only place one can find health workers interested in it, however, is unfair to those fee-for-service physicians who work very hard at seeing the patient as a complete person in an interactive environment. These physicians routinely practice preventive medicine and consciously contribute to health promoting lifestyles. Generally, physicians under all methods of payment can favor holistic and preventive care but the environment in CHCs is much more conducive to these emphases than is an environment dependent on fees as the major source of income.

A few other less uniformly present characteristics have, on occasion, been made part of the description of CHCs. Ontario CHC guidelines, for example, ask that CHCs direct their services toward underserved or disadvantaged populations. This is an undesirable limitation because, although CHCs are especially well suited to meeting the needs of groups such as the adult mentally retarded or alcoholics, they are also fully appropriate for the entire population.

Cost, Quality and Benefit

There is no universal agreement as to the relative cost, quality, and benefits of CHCs. After 30 years of valid and standardized data showing lower hospital use, lower surgical volumes, lower drug use, and lower per capita costs, the organized medical community still rejects the proposition that the fee-for-service model is more expensive.

If one examines client satisfaction, the CHC and the private fee-for-service practitioner may look much the same. If one uses the traditional productivity measure of cost per visit the fee-for-service unit may look best. This traditional measure, however, ignores the availability of extra services in CHCs and the lower volume of visits per person per year. Comprehensive cost studies have not yet been conducted. If the total financial picture including direct and indirect costs and savings were considered, documentation would include not only office costs and the costs of referrals, but also the extent to which CHCs and fee-for-service practices affect utilization of a broad range of community services. These services would include Children's Aid Societies, social service departments, emergency rooms, and mental health services.

Advantages of CHCs

For the consumer, a CHC provides one-stop shopping without fear of special charges. CHCs never indulged in extra-billing. Community and consumer control increases the likelihood of accountability to those who use the CHC. The average physician consultation is longer, meaning that there is more discussion and more patient involvement.

To the government, as the single funding agency, CHCs bring financial predictability. There are fewer units to deal with, more opportunities for regional planning and no incentive for overutilization.

For the doctors on the CHC staff, there are the pleasures of holidays with pay, regular working hours, sick leave, opportunities for continuing education without loss of income, and few administrative responsibilities. To other health professionals, CHCs offer the chance to make decisions and perform services beyond the range of opportunities available in fee-for-service settings. To the advantage of all concerned there appears to be, in the long term, more desirable patterns of health service consumption.

Disadvantages of CHCs

To a physician culturally accustomed to provider control over executive decisions, the big disadvantage is loss of that control. A board makes the management decisions and the chief executive officer reports to that board. There are two ways this loss of executive control can be perceived.

☐ Loss of administrative control over such things as hours of work.
☐ Loss of control over the personal practice of medicine. Concern with respect to this second factor was fundamental to the 1962 doctor strike in Saskatchewan. Doctors thought there was to be bureaucratic interference with their professional decisions.

Doctors object to nondoctors making decisions about how medicine will be practiced by physicians. Unfortunately, they do not always see how the concept of leaving a physician with considerable flexibility and discretion at the level of prescribing care for a specific patient differs from the concept of assuring political, board, or executive influence over the method and amount of care that is provided by groups of caregivers to classes of patients. When care is being delivered to one patient at a point in time, physicians still have a high degree of professional freedom. Overall patterns of resource allocation belong in the public rather than the professional domain. Some physicians quite honestly confuse these two concepts and, therefore, administrators and policy makers must spend whatever time is necessary to separate the two. CHC or hospital boards and the makers of public policy can, and should, decide what activities to finance. Physicians should be, within the limitations imposed by many factors including policy, relatively free to treat patients in ways acceptable to the profession, to themselves, and to their patients. This desirable degree of freedom is the same in a CHC as in a fee-for-service office.

Besides physician loss of executive control, the CHC also asks for team-work. Such cooperation may reduce physician control over how care is provided because there can be considerable negotiation in nonhierarchical teams. The potential for intrateam conflict can be seen as a disadvantage.

For the user, CHCs can be seen to carry the possibility of intentional underservicing. The provider no longer benefits when additional services are rendered and may gain if fewer services are rendered. There is no evidence that this practice is occurring in Canada but the potential is there, especially when payment is by capitation.

For governments, CHCs introduce the problem of evaluation. How does the bureaucracy decide the CHC is efficient and productive? Because a new method of delivery of care has been introduced with a new set of objectives and devices, new approaches to evaluation are needed. Unfortunately, there is a tendency to evaluate this new delivery model much more rigorously than the established fee-for-service model.

The increased delivery of health care by allied health professionals can also be seen by government as a disadvantage. Doctors in fee-for-service practice have considerable ability to control their incomes. Allied health professionals in CHCs may fully or partially provide services that would have been provided by the fee-for-service physicians if the CHC was not there. In this situation, the costs of the allied health professionals are add-on costs because the fee-for-service physician will find some other way to generate the expected income. Government may not wish to transfer physician functions to allied health professionals in CHCs or elsewhere unless it can control fee-for-service payments.

CHCs in Canada

Non fee-for-service ambulatory care alternatives have grown slowly except in Quebec. Even in Quebec, where there has been a rapid growth of CLSCs, over 90 percent of physicians are still on fee-for-service. Politicians have either been opposed to the new options, been favorably disposed to them but unprepared to aggressively promote them, or been seriously committed to the capitation or global budget options but unable to significantly reduce the number of physicians on fee-for-service. The private/public alliances that led to the rapid growth of health maintenance organizations in the United States are not present in Canada, and there does not appear to be much likelihood that CHCs will grow quickly here.

CHC Examples

For a small country, Canada has produced an impressive variety of community health center names and organizational arrangements. British Columbia has Health and Human Resource Centers. Saskatchewan has Community Clinics. Ontario has three similar models, Community Health Centers (CHC) and Health Service Organizations (HSO) and Comprehensive Health Organizations (CHO). Most HSOs have two features which are unique in Canada; they are most often controlled by physicians rather than consumers and they are funded through capitation. In Quebec, the CHC is called a **Centre Locale des Services de Santé (CLSS)** or Local Community Health Centre. These organizations offer some common characteristics.

- ☐ They are a single point of access for patients.
- ☐ They offer a coordinated, team approach to care.
- ☐ Their emphasis is on health promotion and disease prevention.
- ☐ They have an ambulatory care orientation and off non-traditional health services.
- ☐ They promote efforts toward effective use of limited resources.

The CLSC in Quebec is the only Canadian model that operates within a provincially planned regional network and under a comprehensive provincial statute that determines services, board membership, and relationships with other regional services. It is also the only CHC model that performs most of the functions performed in other provinces by public health units, and it is more closely related to a specific geographic area than most other examples.

A **Community Health Organization (CHO)** approaches care with a view to coordinate and manage a broad range of traditional health and social services. Payment by the funding organization is by capitation. The basic principles that form the foundation of CHOs and their American precursors — Health Maintenance Organizations (HMOs) — are care based on accepted standards and disincentives for over-utilization.

Health Service Organizations currently operating in Ontario focus on continuity of care, coordination of services, health maintenance, self-care, and home care. A multidisciplinary or team approach is common. HSOs are funded through capitation with incentives aimed to reduce hospital use. Patients are not prevented from receiving services outside of the HSO and if it is a specialist referral, the HSO is not penalized either. There are three types of HSO operating in Ontario:

1. the provider model (physicians in group practise, 63 centers);
2. the community board model (a non-profit corporation or hospital with an elected board, 5 centers); and
3. the family practice unit in a health science center (5 centers).

Many community health centers have been resounding successes. In the Sault Ste. Marie Group Health Centre, 45 to 50 doctors and many other health professionals provide a broad range of general and special services to 46,000 people — about half of the local population. One thousand of the members in this center are from Sault Ste. Marie, Michigan, just across the border. The Saskatoon Community Clinic is close to the size of the one in Sault Ste. Marie. Both operate a satellite unit as well as the original clinic and Sault Ste. Marie has a Women's Health Centre. Several Quebec CLSSs have received national attention, as has the Lac du Bonnet Centre in Manitoba and the James Bay Clinic in Victoria, B.C.

Perhaps the most puzzling aspect of CHCs is their failure to become more common. The answer lies in the lack of government support, the organized antagonism of the medical profession, the strong ties that tend to exist between the average Canadian and his or her physician(s), and the willingness of fee-for-service physicians to adapt when CHCs become a threat. When CLSSs, for example, offered easier access to evening and weekend care, the private practising physicians in Quebec responded with polyclinics offering more services over longer hours.

United States

Some mention of CHCs in the United States is desirable because of terminological confusion and because of the regularity with which reference is made to American experiences.

☐ **Health Maintenance Organizations (HMO).** This rapidly growing model includes many famous early names that proved the worth of the CHC concept such as the Kaiser networks, the Puget Sound Cooperative and the Health Insurance Plan of Greater New York (HIP). HMOs are all capitation based. They are owned and operated by a broad range of profit and nonprofit groups including labor unions, community groups, religious orders, universities, hospitals, physicians, and insurance companies. A number of HMOs have enrollments of half a million people or more and HMOs provide care to close to 10 percent of Americans. More than one quarter of all American physicians now have some relationship with an HMO.

☐ **Neighborhood Health Centers.** These centers were a product of the race riots of the 1960s and are less emphasized now. Their establishment was an attempt to reduce the social alienation of an underserved, ignored, and predominantly black population.

☐ **Social and Health Maintenance Organizations.** These organizations are an HMO variation in which the service spectrum is expanded to include social services.

☐ **Group Practices.** This term has a meaning in the United States that is quite different from its meaning in Canada. In Canada, it means merely a group of physicians (or other professionals) who cooperate or merge for mutual benefit. In the United States, it means prepaid, consumer-sponsored, non-fee-for-service, ambulatory care outlets and hospitals. The Kaiser-Permanente organizations were group practices before they became HMOs.

Care in
the Home

Health and Welfare Canada in its 1990 Home Care Report, states that all Canadian provinces and territories have home care programs. We have come from a time when care at home was normal, through a period of emphasis on care in institutions. We are now in an era of humanization and cost control in which care at home is again of increasing interest.

Care at home lost favor because the best care came to mean care in hospital. This trend toward institutional care was augmented when health insurance in Canada tended to cover the costs of institutional care or treatment in a doctor's office but not the costs of care at home. At the same time, changes in the nature of and dispersion of the family unit made home care more difficult. Care at home is now regaining favor, first, because it is becoming increasingly recognized that care at home is best for some patients. Second, institutional costs have risen sharply and care at home is seen as a way to economize. Third, services delivered to the home are becoming publicly financed, and, fourth, the concepts of patient control and protection of quality of life are most easily incorporated into care at home.

The Sources of Care in the Home

☐ **Public health programs**. Public health nurses were early sources of care at home, and their visits remain important. These visits now, however, make up only part of a broad range of services which are sometimes delivered through a "home care program."

☐ **Mental health programs** such as that in greater Vancouver.

☐ **Voluntary agencies** such as the Victorian Order of Nurses (VON), The Arthritis Society, the Canadian Red Cross Society and visiting homemakers associations.

☐ **Home care programs**. The organized home care program was created 40 years ago in the United States specifically to assist in the discharge of medically indigent patients who were tying up hospital beds. The basic function of these programs was to coordinate services from a number of community sources and provide care themselves only when it was not available from some other source. The model was obsolete in Canada before it was fully developed. Canadian home care programs quickly became major providers of care. Many provinces have made public health agencies responsible for home care. Manitoba has a provincial home care program which delivers home care to most of the province.

☐ **Community Health Centers**. Quebec, in the 1970s, largely eliminated the delivery of home care through separate home care organizations. Providing care in the home became part of the CLSC functions. Lately, however, home care is once again a separate program in some Quebec communities.

Some types of services provided at home or in support of care at home are

☐ **household maintenance services** including shopping, cleaning, laundry, meal preparation, meal delivery, snow shoveling, and furnace maintenance;

☐ **personal hygiene and care services** including assistance with bathing, grooming, dressing, walking, eating, oral medications, maintenance of dentures and glasses, and care of feet and nails;

☐ **health maintenance services** including diet care, physiotherapy, occupational therapy, podiatry, health teaching, and speech therapy;

☐ **health treatment services** including dressing wounds, drug care, catheterization, and irrigation;

☐ **individual and family social services** including the provision of information, counselling and referral, and financial, employment, and volunteer opportunity services;

☐ **community liaison services** including educational services, library services, visiting services, telephone assurance and telecheck services, child care, programs in seniors centers, and recreational activities;

☐ **facility care liaison services** including adult day care, day hospital care, and short term relief; and

☐ **support services** including diagnostic services, transportation services, home equipment services, home improvement services, wheelchair and prosthetic appliance services, health education and health promotion services, and nutritional counselling.

Factors Limiting Care in the Home

Certain patients require services which cannot adequately be delivered in the home. These include major surgery, complex intensive care, recovery room services, and the degree of supervision demanded by very aggressive behavior or severe dementia. The list of situations in which care at home cannot be adequate is not nearly as long as most people think. The suitability of home care may also be limited by several other factors. The patient may be unwilling to accept care at home. There may not be any responsible household members prepared to participate in the patient's care. Intelligence levels among patients and families vary, as well as the nature of the living accommodations. There may also be a limited range and volume of services offered by the home care program. While these factors are important to keep in mind, they do tend to be used too often as a basis for excluding consideration of home care.

Home care may or may not be less expensive than institutional care. It may be a substitute for care in other locations or it may be an add-on cost. The degree to which home care is being utilized can be undesirably reduced by administrative inadequacies such as taking several days to admit a patient to the program. A common criticism of the Canadian system is the lack of coordination in the continuum of care. The relationship between institutional services and home care is often a case in point.

Possible Determinants of Delivery of Publicly Financed Home Care

Client or agent willingness to receive care at home. If clients are to make informed choices among different types and volumes of support, they must understand the risks and benefits associated with the options. Canadian research has shown that health care providers were often hard to convince that an elderly person could be safely maintained in the community. Physicians were more likely to opt for institutionalization to reduce risk and uncertainty and to avoid perceived liability. (Shapiro, 1988)

Relative cost. Publicly financed programs might be expected to refuse to deliver care to the home, or to limit the amount and types of care, when it is feasible for that care to be obtained elsewhere at lower cost. In a large scale study of home care services, savings were not found to be common across programs. (Weissart, 1988)

Relative need. When demand exceeds the volume of home care services that can be delivered, some patients will be offered less than optimal amounts of care and some will be offered none at all. The interpretation of need will vary with the values of society and of the technocrats.

It is sometimes said that community care is always preferable to institutional care. This is not true. Care at home at public expense ought to be seen as undesirable when a mentally competent client prefers institutional care and public costs for institutional care are not significantly greater than for care at home. For institutionalization to occur, the needs of the individual also ought to be greater than the needs of other persons on the institutional waiting list or already within the institution. Institutional care is, therefore, appropriate if it is consistent with client wish, taxpayer costs, and resource allocation on the basis of need (a question of equity). Public safety is another factor which can make institutional care the preferred alternative. Care at home is less appropriate, although not ruled out, when the dependent person is not welcome at home. The preferences of professional caregivers should not dominate when deciding whether or not to provide care at home.

Whether a dependent person should remain in the community rather than be admitted to an institution is determined primarily by nonclinical factors. The nature of the dependency, especially among mentally competent persons, is not as important as the wishes of the client and other members of the household, the relative public cost, the willingness of other members of the household to provide care, and whether there are any other household members. A study in Manitoba 10 years ago showed that, out of 1,000 persons over age 65 and living alone, 166 were admitted to home care over a one year period. Only 66 out of 1,000 persons living with a spouse were admitted. Whether there was standardization by age is unknown.

Assistance to Caregivers in the Home

As already stated, the presence, competence, and willingness of household caregivers is usually more important in determining the viability of care at home than is the degree of dependency of the client. When planning to help these caregivers, one should consider

- [ ] financial assistance,
- [ ] respite care,
- [ ] personal and professional services delivered to the home,
- [ ] help with domestic chores,
- [ ] home maintenance and adaptation,
- [ ] transportation,
- [ ] assistance with trips out of the home,
- [ ] counselling for coping with stress,
- [ ] education, and
- [ ] physician home visits.

Declining fertility rates in Canada, combined with an increase in the number of women in the labor force has limited the role of women as informal caregivers.

Issues in Home Care

Objectives are often unclear. Earlier hospital discharge is often given as an objective but cannot be important when only 1 to 4 percent of discharged patients are transferred to home care. Delaying admission to hospital is often said to be an objective but if all institutions are full, then the effects of the delay are rather invisible. Encouraging people to stay at home rather than to seek institutionalization is a commonly stated objective which is probably met, although institutional waiting lists still exist. Providing disabled individuals and their caregivers with a better quality of life is one objective that is almost surely routinely met. Other possible objectives include

- [ ] client safety or protection,
- [ ] the preservation of households,
- [ ] reducing the costs of health care by taking advantage of unpaid caregivers,
- [ ] reducing pressure on institutions,
- [ ] humanizing care,
- [ ] allowing individuals to be where they want to be or allowing them to spend disposable income as they wish, and
- [ ] including for the purchase of additional care.

The financial implications of home care are not really known. Studies examining the extent to which home care replaces institutional care tend to ignore the fact that institutions in Canada remain full whether or not home care is available. In this situation, home care is always an add-on cost, although its availability may reduce the demand for construction of new facilities. It also increases medical care costs by reducing hospital lengths of stay and allowing a greater number of surgical and other procedures to be done.

The total potential caseload is still unknown. It does appear that between 1 and 2 percent of the total population will, at any one time, be receiving services at home if there is a reasonable mix of services offered without direct cost to the recipient and without too many rules regarding admission.

There is no clearly preferred organizational approach, and no evidence as to whether home care is best delivered as a separate provincial program (Manitoba), as part of regional public health services (British Columbia and Ontario), as one of the services under the management of a multifunctional regional board (as in selected western Canadian communities), through a network of ambulatory care centres (Quebec), by voluntary agencies (Ontario), or by hospitals (Ontario). Examination might find that organizational charts have little or no bearing on efficiency or anything else. In smaller, one-hospital communities, hospital-based home care can work although it will be probably no better than home care under other sponsorship. In multihospital urban centers, it is administratively more sensible to have a central administration than to have each hospital follow its own patients after discharge.

There is minimal understanding of the extent to which various types of patients benefit from home care. Care, therefore, is often received on the basis of the perceived degree of crisis or on a first come, first served, basis. The cost-effectiveness concept cannot be applied until more is known about the impact of home care on the health status of the clients and other household members.

There is some evidence that delayed termination of home care is common, and that it is most frequent when case managers have caseloads of 100 or more. Regular assessment of the satisfaction and needs of persons receiving home care may not be possible when case managers are responsible for more than 60 to 70 clients.

The New Brunswick extramural hospital program has been widely publicized but appears to offer no special advantages. All services provided in this program have been provided elsewhere. The most successful management strategy in New Brunswick has been *providing home care to some residents of nursing homes who were willing and able to function in the community with this added support*. This allowed the relocation of other patients and residents in the long term care system and the appropriate transfer of long stay patients out of acute care hopsital beds. The waiting for optimal placement was virtually eliminated.

Public
Health
Services

Public health services became a local government responsibility in Britain with the passage of the Elizabethan Poor Laws in the seventeenth century. Concern with disposal of the dead and the operation of poor houses was followed by actions to dispose of sewage, assure clean water supplies, dispose of garbage, and control vermin. By the 1900s, most Canadian provinces had modeled their public health legislation on the *English Public Health Act of 1875*. Earlier activities had been joined by immunization programs and the beginnings of public health nursing. Particular attention was given to the control of communicable diseases and to child and maternal health. The central themes throughout the first half of the twentieth century were public safety, health education, and the use of regulation. The medical officer of health had almost unlimited powers of quarantine, isolation, entry, and closure — powers that have persisted, although with modification.

In recent decades public health agencies have, in all provinces but Quebec, expanded into many areas of counselling and personal care and their role in sanitation has decreased. Garbage disposal and water and sewage treatment are now municipal functions. Food inspection is, at least partly, taken care of by departments of agriculture or food.

In Quebec, public health functions have been transferred to several agencies and departments. Community and personal care services are delivered mostly through CLSCs, the research and planning functions are mostly assigned to the departments of community health in regional hospitals or to the regional councils. The environmental protection functions have been distributed to departments of labor, the environment, and others.

The environmentally-related functions that are the responsibility of public health departments are primarily performed by public health inspectors. Their responsibilities include

☐ the examination of selected aspects of air and water quality,
☐ the control of insects and animals,
☐ the testing of rural water and sewage systems,
☐ food testing,
☐ inspection of eating places and other food premises,
☐ inspection of a variety of public and residential buildings and spaces, and
☐ responding to public complaints.

There is considerable overlap between the duties of public health inspectors, municipal building inspectors, and a broad range of environmental control officers.

Provinces also have quite different approaches to the use of public health personnel in such activities as immunization, family planning, home nursing, sex education, family-life education, pre-natal classes, and the provision of dental care.

For almost a decade, the Council on Community Health Accreditation in Ontario has been accrediting public health agencies. The accreditation process is, unfortunately, a copy of that applied to hospitals. The Council decided at its outset that management was the thing to examine. The examination of outcomes was avoided despite the long history in the public health field of relying heavily on outcome measures.

Many years ago, public health personnel discovered that if water was boiled people did not get cholera or typhoid. No one knew whether the pot was the right size or whether there was a committee to design it *and no one cared*. They were pleased to have no cholera and typhoid. When polio vaccine prevented polio there were very few scholarly papers and no evaluation exercises that concentrated on how the immunization program was organized or whether the person giving the needle (or spoonful) was properly qualified. People were interested only in the effects of the program the reduction in polio. When seat belt legislation and lower speed limits came into being, we looked for changes in highway accidents and deaths and found them. There was no concern over which department wrote the legislation or the qualifications of those who enforced the laws. The Ontario approach to the evaluation of public health units is an immense step backwards. It looks at the bureaucracy rather than the effects.

The exercise of counting visits, listing programs, reading minutes, evaluating the qualifications of staff, and examining organization charts will merely delay the day when evaluators will have time to pay attention to whether priorities have been sensibly set, whether resources are being well used, and whether public health activities are contributing as much as they can to the health status of the people of Ontario. Attention to qualifications, staffing, and organization may lead to a search for more staff and to new organizational structures just because administrative and professional personnel say that changes are in order. The public health industry should ask for more staff and more money only when it can prove that the need to be met or the hazard to be avoided is worth the money to be spent, and that spending more money will appropriately decrease the need or the hazard. Evaluation, therefore, must concentrate on outcomes.

Costs

Public health services cost in the range of $5 to $100 per capita, with the higher costs being associated with extensive personal care programs, especially home care. Most public health services are financed by the province although some municipally operated programs and receive up to one half of their funds from the municipality.

Issues in Public Health Services

☐ Medical officers of health are now primarily planners and administrators but most have little training in either planning or administration.

☐ The historically established authoritarian approach is still sometimes seen. This concept is quite incompatible with the current role of public health personnel in lifestyle change, community development, and the empowerment of individuals and groups.

☐ Although the activities and responsibilities of public health personnel overlap and interact regularly with personnel in a variety of other health and social service programs, there is often limited coordination. Examples of integration or coordination include some community health centers, some multiagency centers (by various names) and the arrangements in Quebec.

☐ The degree of need for public health nurses in the schools as teachers or as caregivers is unclear. Provincial patterns vary considerably.

☐ Should the historical organizational isolation of public health personnel and departments be continued? Quebec has said it should not.

Summary

Community health services face one major obstacle, namely, the issue of financial support. Despite major growth in programs such as home care, there have been equivalent cutbacks in the funding of CHSs in several provinces.

These cutbacks are even more common when one looks at social programs — the housing, income support, recreation, and other services that are crucial to the health of many Canadians.

References

Abel-Smith, B. (1989). The rise and decline of the early HMOs: Some international experiences. *The Milbank Quarterly*, 66 (4), 694-719.

Beland, F. (1985). Who are those most likely to be institutionalized, the elderly who receive comprehensive home care services or those who do not? *Social Science and Medicine* 20 (4), 347-354.

Brosky, G. (1990). HSOs, HMOs, and CHOs: The continuing history of capitation-funded health care. *Canadian Family Physician*, 36, 1402-1406.

Ferguson, G. (1987). The New Brunswick extramural hospital: A Canadian hospital at home. *Journal of Public Health Policy*, 8 (4) 561-570.

Gaumer, G.L. et al. (1986). Impact of the New York long term home health care program. *Medical Care*, 24 (7) 641-653.

Government Reports:

Alberta, (1989). The rainbow report: Our vision for health. Premier's Commission on Future Health Care for Albertans. Final Report. Edmonton, Alberta.

British Columbia, (1991). Closer to Home. Report of the British Columbia Royal Commission on Health Care and Costs. Victoria, British Columbia.

Canada, (1990) Report on Home Care; Report of the Federal/Provincial/Territorial Working Group on Home Care. Ottowa: Health and Welfare Canada.

New Brunswick, (1989). Report of the commission on selected health care programs. Saint John, New Brunswick.

Nova Scotia, (1990). Health strategies for the nineties: Managing better health. Halifax, Nova Scotia: Department of Health.

Ontario, (1990). Health services organization (HSO) information package. Toronto.

Ontario, (1989). Toward a shared direction for health in Ontario: Report of the Ontario health review panel. Toronto.

Ontario, (1989). From vision to action: Report of the health care system committee, Premier's Council on Health Strategy. Toronto.

Quebec, (1990). A reform centred on the citizen. Quebec City, Quebec: Ministry of Health and Social Services.

Kramer, A.M., Shaughnessy, P.W., Bauman, M.K., and Crisler, K.S. (1990). Assessing and assuring quality of home health care. *The Milbank Quarterly*, 68 (3), 413-444.

Mechanic, D. (1991). Changing our health care system. *Medical Care Review*, 48 (3), 247-260.

Muldoon, J. (1991). Publicly financed competition in health care: Legislative issues. *Health Care Management Forum* 5, 39-46.

Newcomer, R. et al. (1990). Awareness and enrollment in the social HMO. *The Gerontologist* 30 (1), 86-93.

Peachy, D., Linton, A. (1988) What you should know about HSOs. *Canadian Medical Association Journal* 138 (4), 352-355.

Ross, M. (1991). Beyond the family: informal support in later life. *Canadian Journal of Public Health*, 82, 79-82.

Shapiro, E. (1986). Implications of demography on the supply and use of nursing home beds, in Review of Demography and its Implications for Economic and Social Policy, Health and Welfare Canada, Ottawa.

Stone, L. and Frenken, H. (1988) Canada's Seniors: Census 1986. Statistics Canada Catalogue, 98-121.

Stewart. M.J. (1990). Access to health care for economically disadvantaged Canadians: A model. *Canadian Journal of Public Health*, 81, 450-455.

Weissert, W.G., Cready, C.M. and Pawelak, J.E. (1988). The past and future of home and community-based long-term care. *The Milbank Quarterly*, 66 (2), 309-388.

CHAPTER 7

Technology, Pharmaceuticals, and Research

Introduction

The public loves miracles. Technology and the industries which prosper from it can now deliver mechanical miracles, and do so with regularity. Technocrats also love the mechanical miracles, and they enthusiastically welcome every new generation of every technological stream.

Within the health field, imaging devices, organ transplantation, and cardiovascular surgery are good examples. X-ray technology was followed by ultrasound, which was followed in turn by computerized axial tomography scans (CAT scan), radioactive scanning, and magnetic resonance imaging (MRI). MRI provides better images in selected circumstances than CAT scans, and these in other circumstances, give better pictures than x-rays. Effects of the better images on patient outcomes are usually not known.

In cardiovascular surgery, angioplasty has allowed coronary arteries to be cleared with lasers. These services are less invasive and less expensive than coronary artery by-pass surgery and are, apparently, just as good in many cases.

Organ transplantation has evolved thanks to advances in tissue matching (now a very sophisticated and machine based process), tissue preservation and transport (which varies from a bucket of ice to life support systems), the ability to conduct long operations on very ill patients (which is possible due to new anesthetic agents and techniques, and advances in intensive care nursing.

Although multinational or global factors dominate when the role of technology is discussed, there are subordinate but still consequential decisions that are under the control of Canada, the provinces, municipalities, the private sector or individual Canadians. We have decided to have seat belts in our cars and, therefore, we have the opportunity to use them. We will probably soon be driving with our lights on at all times (and technology will turn them on and off without our assistance) and we have still to decide whether we wish all cars to have air-bags. Automobiles are usually the major cause of death, of brain and spinal cord injury and of other forms of trauma between infancy and middle life, and it has been estimated that air-bags to complement seat belts would reduce deaths and injuries by 10-50 percent. Canada and Canadians can alter the levels and the nature of factory, household, automobile, and other emissions, but only at economic and social cost. Available technologies in safety, the environment and health care can be used or ignored, and the choice is often ours.

Different choices bring different positive and negative effects. Most choices improve health status in some ways and damage it in others. Policy development is, unfortunately, made difficult by people who want solutions that bring advantages but no disadvantages. We wish our garbage to be disposed of, for instance, but nowhere near where we live. The main point to be made here is that although technology makes options available it is not the villain. If society or individuals make selfish or short sighted choices, the error is entirely theirs.

Technology Assessment

Technologically sophisticated advances have brought benefits, but there is uncertainty as to when benefits are brought, and how large these benefits are. A better picture is not worth anything if it doesn't affect the long term outcome of the patients. If the better picture does bring benefits and it also increases cost, and if the funding is from a fixed public pool, then there is the question of whether the improved outcomes are worth the additional costs.

Technology has, in general, brought great social benefits and has greatly decreased costs of many important components of health care. The current interest in technology assessment appears to arise from several factors.

- The increases in health care costs have been most marked, and most difficult to control, in the tertiary level hospitals, and these are the locations in which expensive technology and high cost cases tend to be aggregated.
- It is conceptually and, in terms of policy, easier to think of controlling inputs than process. There is, at times, a hope that the control of costs will be simple; if the machines are evaluated, the system will then know how many of them are needed and will use them correctly.
- Expensive technology is an easy and impersonal target, and it can be a source of savings.
- Concentrating on such a visible and "safe" target as technology can allow bureaucrats to avoid dealing with, or put off dealing with, other more central problems such as inappropriate professional decisions.

In other words, technology assessment is a needed evaluation but is receiving excessive attention at this moment. It also is being seen as a much more significant source of savings than it will turn out to be, and examination of technology will do little if anything about the inappropriate spending which arises from other, more behavioral, sources.

Improved post-marketing drug surveillance is another form of technology assessment which may become prominent in the near future. It is clear that the long term and rare effects of new drugs cannot always be identified in the clinical trials conducted before the drug is released. It is also clear that there is currently no adequate program in place in Canada to detect the above effects.

This interest in the way technology is assessed and used is quite appropriate, but there may be a tendency to believe assessment is primarily to prevent the introduction of useless or unsafe technologies. The greatest threat is not the existence of unnecessary or intolerably hazardous drugs or equipment, although these should be found and eliminated. The greatest threat to costs and the public lies in the inappropriate use of drugs, equipment, and procedures which are fully legitimate and often essential in appropriate circumstances. There is therefore a need for improvement in the professional decisions which lead to the use of technologies as well as in the assessment of the technologies themselves.

Table 7.1

CT Scanners Per Million Population in Canada, 1990

Alberta	9
New Brunswick	8
Nova Scotia	8
P.E.I.	7
B.C.	7
Quebec	7
Newfoundland	7
Ontario	6
Manitoba	6
Saskatchewan	5

Source: Manitoba Health Report, 1992, p. 61.

An Example of Managing Technology

The total cost of medical imaging has risen in Manitoba from $16 million in 1976, to $41 million in 1982 and $68 million in 1988. Costs include all diagnostics, radiology, nuclear medicine, diagnostic ultrasound, CT scans, and MRI. Manitoba Health reports that of all the MRI's performed in 1989, only 43 percent were appropriate. (1992 Manitoba Health Report, p.61)

The Manitoba Health Report (1992) also notes

"The millions of dollars that are already spent on the application of this technology — and the additional millions that would be required were the government to approve all the requests for additional purchases — are dollars that could be possibly better spent on health services for which there are more efficacious outcomes to patients' needs." (p.62)

This province has set up the Manitoba Imaging Advisory Committee to review some issues such as

☐ the lack of regulatory criteria to protect patients from, and possible adverse dosage impacts from the over-use of imaging technology;

☐ the wide variations in the quality of operations of some imaging equipment; and

☐ the repeated procedures as patients move between institutions.

Manitoba has found no good evidence that the choice of technology or the amount made available has increased risk to the health status of consumers. In addition, as is shown in Table 7.1, variations across provinces are not limited to evidence of greater or lesser health status.

At the national level, a recent comparative study of the availability of medical technology shows the population served by each unit (Table 7.2). There is no evidence in Canada that the health of the population is harmed by the lower number of units when compared to the U.S. level. Note that this is 1988 data and there will be more technology in both Canada and the U.S. now.

Table 7.2

Comparative Availability of Selected Medical Technologies (1988)

	Number of Units	Population Per Unit (in thousands)	Number of Units	Population Per Unit (in thousands)
Open heart surgery	11	2,364	793	307
Cardiac catheterization	31	839	1,234	198
Organ transplantation	14	1,857	319	764
Radiation therapy	31	839	967	252
Extracorporeal shock wave lithotripsy	4	6,500	228	1,069
Magnetic resonance imaging	12	2,167	900	271

Sources: American Hospital Association, Canadian Hospital Association University Hospital, London, Ont., Canadian Association of Radiation Oncology, Canadian Medical Association.

Developed by Robert Cross, Ottawa Citizen.

Research

The Medical Research Council (MRC) will spend $240 million on clinical research in 1992. Almost all of this will be spent on research related to physical health. Mental health, health promotion, primary prevention, improved professional decision making, and the involvement of the patient in clinical decisions will receive little or no support. In other words, the priorities of the MRC have not changed much in the last 20 years, and neither have the family of scientists winning the competition for funds.

The National Health Research Development Fund (NHRDP) will spend about $30 million, mostly in research grants and mostly on projects closer to the clinical focus of the MRC than to the structural, financial, strategic, informational, evaluative, and production questions so central to the future of Canadian health care. The physician/academic community quite easily and continuously captures the NHRDP funds as well as the MRC funds.

Foundations, societies and other private sources will spend $200-300 million on research, most of it clinical research and much of it awarded without rigorous review.

A few years ago it appeared that Canada should concentrate on measuring the value of specific elements of health care. For two reasons this is now not the case. First, the U.S. is now spending $1 billion annually on cost-effectiveness research and a great deal more is being done in Europe. Second, Canada has been slow to make use of information already available.

Canadian research dollars could usefully be directed to learning how to make use of what is known. If the process of change is not mastered we will soon have large amounts of new information (from other countries) but will not know how to amend our health care practices to reflect the new knowledge. Research and development spending is low compared to other industrialized nations. Sweden, Japan, the United States and Germany are the top four investors.

Figure 7.1

Total R&D Expenditures as a Percentage of GDP, Selected Countries 1989 or latest year

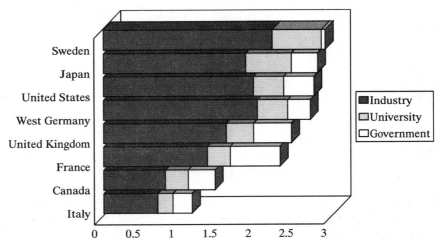

Source: Economic Council of Canada, presentation of Toward 2000 Conference, Ottawa, 1991.

The Drug Industry in Canada

The use of medication is as old as man. The apothecary and his pestle and mortar were early symbols of health care. The pestle and mortar are now largely museum pieces, the apothecary is now a pharmacist, and the pharmacopia has changed. The "magic" of medication, however, is unchanged. Tincture of belladonna, mustard plasters and spirits of camphor have been replaced by tagamet, valium, hydrocortisone and tens of thousands of other names. Arsenic and opium stayed in vogue for hundreds, if not thousands, of years whereas the average medication brought into the market now is barely into the literature before it is obsolete.

Medication in ancient times could usually offer little except psychological benefit and it was often very hazardous. Today the odds are better. Most medication does more good than harm, especially when used wisely, but the volume of inappropriate or questionable drug use in which patient hazard exceeds patient benefit is still high.

Costs

Canadians will swallow, inject, pump, or smear on $7 billion worth of prescription and non-prescription drugs in 1992. Some of this consumption will occur in hospitals or be paid for by a provincial Drug Benefit Plan — a cost that is shared. Many Canadians have a drug plan through their workplace, so the $42.00 average cost of a prescription for a new patented drug doesn't really sting until we add up the cost for 1992 and then look back at the rapid rise in those costs over the past five years.

Table 7.3

**Health Budget Allocated to Drugs in Canada
1980 to 1990**

	1980 percent	1990 percent
Drugs	8.9	14.1
Hospitals	40.9	39.3
Physicians	15.2	16.0
Other Institutions	11.6	10.1
Capital Expenditures	5.4	4.1
Other	18.0	16.4

Source: Science Council of Canada, 1991

Because of the hospitals' use of drugs and because most drugs for seniors are paid for out of the public purse, Canada's health ministers are asking some important questions. How can we make decisions about which drugs to make available, what volumes, for which consumers, and at what cost to society?

These questions are the cornerstone of growing public concern about Bill C-91, currently (in 1992) before the House of Commons. This bill will extend patent protection for brand name drugs and prevent compulsory licensing of these drugs by generic manufacturers. The multinational pharmaceuticals say that this protection is needed to recoup investment in research and development. *Fortune* magazine said in June, 1992, that the **growth** in pharmaceutical earnings will drop from an enviable high of 20 percent to a more modest 15 percent this year. Statistics Canada, Canada's national data bank, reports that return on equity has risen steadily for the past 15 years from 12 percent in 1977 to 27 percent in 1987. That's double the return for all Canadian manufacturing.

Figures 7.1 through 7.5 show the expenditures for prescriptions filled in drugstores, drugs used in hospitals and drug costs for the elderly in the province of Saskatchewan. These figures demonstrate the growth of the drug segment of health care costs in Canada.

Research and development potential in Canada does not have a good track record. Between 1940 and 1975, Canada introduced 3 new drugs, compared to Switzerland's 68, 51 in the United Kingdom, 48 in West Germany, and 622 in the United States. Even with the first round of extended patent protection under Bill C-22 in 1987, few companies operating in Canada have made efforts to develop the size of research and development programs capable of systematic discovery. The regulations of the patent protection law encourage product-related activities, not primary research.

In terms of drug exports, Industry, Science and Technology Canada reports that the 1990 shipment value of drugs in Canada was $4.49 billion. Exports were only 6.6 percent of this total, well below the exports of the U.S. at 32 percent and the European Community at 26 percent.

Drug Price Control

The Drug Prices Review Board, a federal government watchdog, says the cost of drugs is in line with increases in the Consumer Price Index (CPI). Greenshield, a private prepaid, health benefit company disagrees. Greenshield, in a 1992 report, shows that drug prices are rising at more that 11 percent compounded annually — well above the CPI. In 1987 Canada increased the patent protection for prescription drugs and 1988 produced more than 40 percent of the price increases to date. New drugs, especially brand names, have higher prices and little or no competition. Older drugs, many with generic competitors tend to have lower prices.

Figure 7.2

Prescription Drug Sales in Retail Stores (Canada)

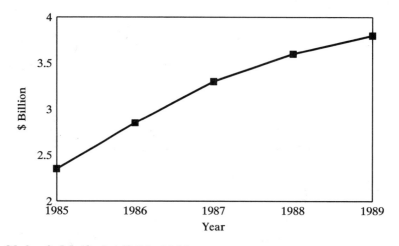

Source: Globe & Mail, April 29, 1992.

Figure 7.3

Estimated Drug Expenditures in Public Hospitals, Canada

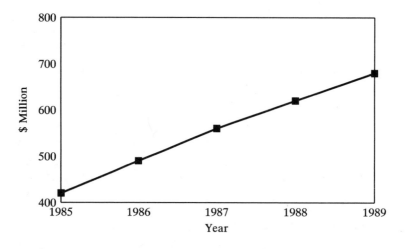

Source: Globe & Mail, April 29, 1992.

Figure 7.4

**Medicines and Aging in Saskatchewan
Drug Plan Beneficiaries**

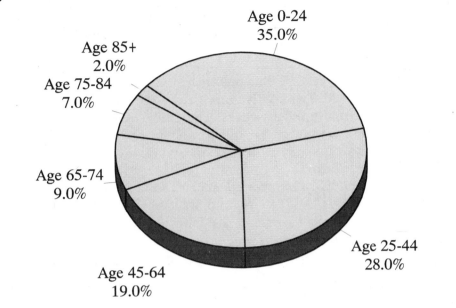

Source: Globe & Mail, May 1, 1992.

Figure 7.5

**Medicines and Aging in Saskatchewan
Cost to Drug Plan**

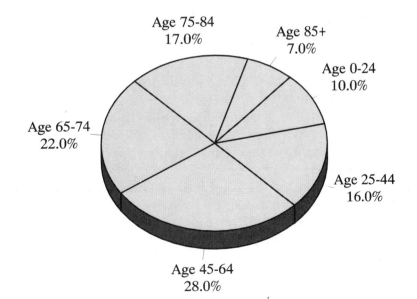

Source: Globe & Mail, May 1, 1992.

In the U.S., the situation is much the same. The U.S. government is trying to constrain price increases on prescription drugs to the level of the Consumer Price Index, but the U.S. already has the highest drug research budget on earth. Efforts at control have begun with threatened curtailment of tax credits to big companies. Discipline from the huge institutions in the U.S. — such as HMOs and mail-order pharmacies — is found in their demands for significant price breaks. The final blow to U.S. pharmaceutical companies is the number of products soon to be available for generic manufacture, a big source of drugs in America.

In 1991, sales in the U.S. pharmaceutical industry were $43.5 billion, up 10.7 percent from 1990. Twenty-five new drugs were approved by the FDA in 1991, an increase from previous years. The 1992 estimates for research and development for new products is $10 billion, about 17 percent of revenues. About three-quarters of this is spent on drug trials and reviews and only one-quarter is spent on original research.

In 1992 and in 1993, a number of generics will come off patent, creating a market opportunity for U.S. generic manufacturers. Until the 1980s generic producers were required to repeat the clinical trials of the original drug company. In 1984, the *Waxman-Hatch Act* cut that requirement and demanded only that the active ingredients of the drug met the same pharmacological standards as the original product.

Notwithstanding the increasing number of generic products, drug prices are expected to rise in the U.S. In 1990, new U.S. federal laws required price discounts for Medicare and Medicaid as for other volume buyers.

The generic drug industry is able, in Canada, to bring some drug prices down. The generic drug can be manufactured at present, either under compulsory licensing from the patent holder during the period of the patent or when the patent runs out. Bill C-91 will extend patent protection to original manufacturers for 20 years if it is passed in late 1992. This bill also contains a proposal to ban compulsory licensing which will conform with GATT rules. Ontario's Minister of Health says this will drive drug prices higher in Canada.

Prescribing and Marketing

Current evidence suggests that Canadians are consuming more drugs than ever, especially the elderly. A 1989 study in Saskatchewan shows that 80 percent of seniors received at least one drug while the most common number of prescriptions for seniors was 18 per year. Figure 7.1 shows the proportion of the population in each age group while Figure 7.2 shows the drug consumption. Note the large consumption by older groups.

A June 1, 1992, study in the *Annals of Internal Medicine* found that ad campaigns help determine how doctors treat their patients. Out of 109 ads reviewed by researchers at UCLA, 100 contained "deficiencies where the FDA (Food and Drug Administration) has established explicit standards for quality." The study found that

- ☐ 92 percent of the ads potentially violated at least one FDA regulation,
- ☐ 50 percent of the ads had little or no educational value, and
- ☐ 59 percent would not lead physicians to proper prescribing.

The United States FDA does not often take administrative action against such ads. In Canada, the Pharmaceutical Advertising Advisory Board must approve, in advance, all advertisements and direct mail to physicians and other health providers. The board is made up of physicians, representatives of medical journals, consumer groups, and the pharmaceutical and advertising industries. The federal drug regulatory agency in Ottawa has an *ex officio* member on the board to ensure that the members carry out their responsibilities properly. There is no cost to the Canadian government because pharmaceutical companies are charged a fee for each advertisement submitted for review. Last year, the board reviewed 1,800 ads, many of them from U.S. drugmakers, nearly all of whom cooperate in Canada's program. Even with this effort, ads routinely offend clauses governing risk, efficacy, support for therapeutic claims, and description of negative features of drugs. Drug companies and drug salesmen (detail men) use an endless supply of gloss, patience, samples and free dinners to aid in the delivery of their messages.

Dr. Joel Lexchin, author of "The Real Pushers," a critique of the Canadian drug industry, says that the Canadian drug industry spends about $10,000 per doctor per year on promotion. This is more than $500 million per year — about twice what drug companies spend on research in Canada.

Pharmacists

Historical Perspective

Traditionally, Canada's pharmacists have worked behind the counter of a drug store or behind the desk of a hospital pharmacy. Our changing economic and political environment is both threatening the traditions of pharmacy and presenting opportunities. How the profession fares will depend upon the survival instincts and adaptability of pharmacists.

Pharmacists and physicians were both seen as reliable sources of drug information, according to a 1991 opinion poll (reported in the May 21, 1991 *Medical Post*). Doctors, however said that they use drug company representatives 66 percent of the time as a source of information. Clearly, there is, and will continue to be, a need for pharmacists to play a significant role in helping patients to manage drugs, especially if more than one physician is involved in the person's care. The Ontario College of Pharmacy says that clinical advice to patients is part of the service paid for by the dispensing fee but as few as 11 percent of consumers actually get advice (Canadian Pharmaceutical Association, 1991). Actually, the dispensing fee as a form of remuneration may act as a deterrent to a pharmacist in the event a patient should receive fewer drugs rather than more.

About 60 to 90 percent of all patients get all their drugs from the same pharmacy, allowing the pharmacist to maintain a complete record of prescriptions and identify potential interactions (Canadian Pharmaceutical Association, 1991). This opportunity to *educate the patient* places a professional obligation on the pharmacist to fulfil this obligation to a much greater degree than they do now. A 1988 Environics survey found that two-thirds of Ontarians believe that doctors prescribe too many drugs to their patients. This public opinion is supported by mounting evidence that many seniors take too many drugs, and as many as 30 percent of hospital admissions of seniors are due to adverse drug reactions that could be prevented by a pharmacist (Dorothy Ley, Chairman, CMA taskforce on Caring for Seniors).

Dispensing

The marketplace for drugs is international. Mail order products from the United States are a great temptation to Canadian consumers, whether they are individuals, institutions or provincial health plans. There will be increasing pressure for original package dispensing that will replace pharmacy preparations as dispensing fees rise above their perceived value to the consumer and to the drug plan. Manufacturers will encourage this practice in order to increase brand name recognition, notwithstanding a potential decrease in service to the consumer. Juggling a commercial enterprise with a health care service will continue to pose conflict for pharmacists.

Billing Governments

Canada's provinces offer a variety of fully and partially paid drug programs for seniors, persons with specific diseases such as cystic fibrosis or AIDS, and persons on welfare. The drug programs will offer fewer products in the future than they do now, and the focus will be on products that are cost-effective. The pharmacist will be obliged to substitute products, and may be required to refuse a product that is not on the drug plan or demand direct payment from the patient. As a result, the pharmacist will be on the firing line between physicians and the government. Politically and economically, provinces cannot allow drug plans to mushroom as they have in the past. Drugs with little or no benefit will be eliminated from the plan. The potentially explosive costs of new biotechnology make it imperative for governments to set guidelines and constraints for consumer access, either directly or through drug benefit plans.

The New "Scrip" Writers

Under current legislative proposals in Ontario, emerging health professions will be able to write a limited number of prescriptions for treatments within their scope of practice. New relationships will need to be developed between pharmacists and the new professions, many of whom will work outside the traditional hospital walls in, for example, community health centers and in home care.

The Rural and Urban Recipe

From an economic and policy perspective, there appear to be two debates in which pharmacists should participate. The first debate is the fee-for-service versus salary versus capitation question which plagues medicine as well. The pharmacist who fills prescriptions for a fee grows rich by filling many, offering little dialogue, and giving little advice. The pharmacist in a commercial enterprise grows rich by selling high profit goods such as cigarettes. The pharmacist on salary in a hospital of health department may not advise enough consumers (or providers) or prevent enough adverse drug reactions to be cost-effective.

The rural pharmacist will work in a very different environment and have many more roles than the urban pharmacist who can become a specialist. The rural pharmacist may receive a part-time salary for managing drug consumption in a long term care facility and for visiting home care patients when their prescriptions need renewal. This pharmacist may also carry many more products in his or her store. The urban pharmacist may belong to a joint venture with a physician group practice and operate a pharmacy full-time.

Post-marketing Surveillance

Monitoring drug use and compliance in post-marketing surveys is another important future role for pharmacists. Clinical trials are generally too small to identify all low incidence events and unusual complications caused by a drug. Since pharmacists have the data on most individual's drug use and have the obligation to advise consumers in return for a dispensing fee, they should also accept the obligation to participate in improving the safety of the products they sell. If not, then government sponsored distribution and monitoring of drugs is the next best alternative.

The Role of Government

The emerging government and academic emphasis of appropriate care may be the factor that changes pharmacy the most. Care at home is preferred by many consumers over care in a hospital. Early discharge, childbirth, palliative care, and chronic care can all be managed at home. The traditional role of the hospital pharmacist may remain if home care is managed by hospitals. If, as present trends suggest, home care will be managed by community centers or public health units, a new role must be developed for pharmacy in the home care team. Nurses are lobbying for regulatory change that will give them the drug management role. They claim, with some justification, that their knowledge of the whole individual including function and health status, gives them the ability to broaden their scope of practice.

The 1987 Golberg Report (page 124) on drug utilization reviews a study showing that pharmacists prescribe more appropriately than physicians in a geriatric facility. If specialist nurses prescribe, is there a role for specialist pharmacists to prescribe? Should physicians refer to pharmacists for prescribing certain categories of drugs such as those for long periods of use or those with potentially harmful side effects or interactions? Should pharmacists always check on the health status of a patient before renewing a prescription?

Changing the focus of health care away from physician dominance and hospital delivery toward new providers and community delivery will change the role of pharmacists. Canada's weak economy (hampered by free trade and the federal Goods and Services Tax) and growing social awareness of the factors that support health have produced a necessary emphasis on appropriate but not heroic care. Pharmacists cannot be excluded from these pressures. If the public is paying a fee for a service it does not get, it won't take long for either professional competition to offer the service or for commercial competition to provide drugs at lower cost because they are prepackaged or by mail order.

Canadians will be better served by their health care system if the knowledgable professionals advise consumers, wherever they choose to be, so that interventions (including drugs) are appropriate and affordable. Pharmacists also have an obligation to participate in the development of public policy so that governments can make informed decisions as they restructure programs to create, support, and renew health.

Drug Benefit Plans

All of Canada's provinces offer some extended drug benefits to some special groups: citizens over 65, diabetics, children with cystic fibrosis, AIDS patients, and others. Not all benefits are similar across provinces. Many working Canadians also have a drug benefit plan through their employer. Some provinces charge deductibles, for example, in Saskatchewan the annual deductible

- ☐ for individuals is $125.00 per year,
- ☐ for a senior family $75.00,
- ☐ for a senior single $50.00.

In Saskatchewan, a diabetic who is a member of a Blue Cross plan is subsidized for up to $300.00 per year for drugs and supplies. In New Brunswick, the Senior's Heath Benefits Program covers part of the cost for vision care, hearing aids, foot care, chiropractic services, prostheses, and prescription drugs. Seniors must pay a premium of $40.00 a year for these benefits.

Public Insurance's Effect on Costs

The effect of universal public drug insurance on prescription drug costs is unclear as is the effect of population aging. Effects of public programs are masked by the widespread coverage of private drug insurance. Costs also vary significantly with the extent to which non prescription items (bandages and aspirin) are covered as long as they are prescribed.

Provinces use three basic methods to control their expenditures on prescription drugs, these are

1. limitating the population who will be given free drugs,
2. limiting the list of drugs and supplies that can be obtained through the drug insurance plans, and
3. controlling price of drugs at the factory gate.

The drug store costs are controlled through mandated prescription fees and/or requirements regarding substitution. In 1984, five provinces had legislation assuring use of low cost suppliers when more than one company supplied the same drug. Substitution was automatic unless the physician specifically ordered, on the prescription, that there should be no substitution.

Provincial formularies list the drugs that will be paid for under provincial drug insurance plans. These formularies can, if wisely and courageously used, both reduce costs and improve patient care. Formularies can identify interchangeable drugs and can set prices for these drugs.

References

Anderson, G.M., Lomas, J. (1989). Regionalization of coronary artery by-pass surgery: Effects on access. *Medical Care*, 27(3):288.

Barkin, M. (1991). Macroethics and microethics: The case of health care. *Canadian Public Administration*, 34(1):30-36.

Brook, R.H., Lohr, K.N. (1986). Will we need to ration effective health care? *Issues in Science and Technology*, 3(1):68.

Evans, R.G. and Stoddart, Greg L. (1990). *Producing Health, Consuming Health Care.* Working Paper Series #90-6. Hamilton: McMaster University, Centre for Health Economics and Policy Analysis.

Evans, R.G. and Stoddart, Greg L. (1986). Medicare at Maturity: Achievements, Lessons and Challenges. Proceedings of the Health Policy Conference on Canada's National Health Care System. Banff: The Banff School of Management.

Fuchs, Victor R. and Garber, Alan M. (1990). The new technology assessment. *The New England Journal of Medicine*, 323(10): 673-677.

Fyke, K., Poole, B. (1991). Doing the right things. *Policy Options*, 12(8):11-12.

Harrison, F., Juzwishin, D., Roger, R. (1989). Quality of care and utilization management: Contemporary tools and strategies. *Health Care Management Forum*, 2(2):18-23.

Linton, A.L. and Naylor, C.D. (1990). Organized medicine and the assessment of technology. *New England Journal of Medicine*, 323(21):1463-1467.

Porter, Michael E. (1991). Canada at the Crossroads: The Reality of a New Competitive Environment. A study prepared for the Business Council on National Issues and the Government of Canada. Ottawa, B.C.N.I.

Science Council of Canada (1991). *Medication and Health Policy: A Research Agenda.* Ottawa: Supply and Services Canada.

Siegel, D.M. (1987). The high cost of medical technology: Getting at the heart of the matter. *Medical Care*, 25(10):979-987.

Singer, P.A., Choudhry, S. (1991). How green is your grass? A comparative analysis of the American and Canadian health care systems. *Humane Med*, 7:47-53.

Wilson, B. (1992). The U.S. pharmaceutical industry: An outlook for 1992 and beyond. *Challenges*, Summer:15.

CHAPTER 8

Mental Health Services

Mental health services in Canada belong to a health service sector that has emerged from complete neglect but that is still struggling to consolidate public acceptance. The age of the large, low-cost, rural, and hidden, institutions in which incarceration was often for life is past, but the stature and the level of financing of mental health care still lag behind those of physical health care.

This section discusses the public and professional perceptions of mental health, the population who have need of mental health services, or whose mental health is at risk and needs protection, and the policies, programs and institutions that comprise the mental health services network.

In 1960, 0.4 percent of Canadians were in mental institutions, and half of them had been institutionalized for more than seven years. By the 1980s, two-thirds of psychiatric admissions lasted less than two weeks, and many of the institutions were either gone or much smaller. These changes have been accompanied by major reassignment of function among institutions and programs. Psychiatric services fall into the same general categories as physical health services — that is, into institutional and noninstitutional, emergency and elective, short term and long term, and preventive, diagnostic, therapeutic, palliative, and rehabilitative categories.

Legislation

The federal *Hospital Insurance and Diagnostic Services Act* (HIDSA) of 1957 specifically excluded cost-sharing for psychiatric services because those services were already being provided at provincial expense. The new *Act* was intended to expand health care access, not to transfer existing provincial expenditures to the federal treasury. Because of this decision, there were, for some time, few major expansions or improvements to psychiatric hospitals — a very fortuitous neglect when one considers how rapidly these institutions lost favor during the late 1960s and 1970s. If psychiatric expenditures had been cost-shared by the federal government, there would probably have been expansion of the supply of these isolated, crowded and soon-to-be-rejected institutions.

The Clients/Users of Mental Health Services and Their Patterns of Ill Health

Inadequate mental health is usually characterized by loss of a sense of reality, by socially unacceptable behavior, or by inability to cope. The clients may be individuals or groups of individuals (usually families). Mental or emotional illness may be associated with psychosis, but the great majority of those who need and use mental health services are not psychotic. Although the definition of good mental health will vary with the values of the beholder, it could be described as a state of mind that allows the individual to develop abilities, pursue goals, meet needs and cope with life's problems without undue stress.

There are four functional categories of people who seek (or might seek) mental health services. Each category requires a somewhat different capability in the health services that deal with it. This functional categorization is non-diagnostic, and is quite different from one based on categories such as cerebral dysfunction, psychosis, mental retardation, personality disorder or social pathology. The four functional categories are.

1. the long term and significantly disabled (for example, the chronic psychotics);
2. the short term seriously disabled (for example, the acute psychotics or those who react severely to situational factors);
3. the distressed (for example, the significantly neurotic or those finding it quite difficult to cope); and
4. the dissatisfied (for example, the bored, alienated, unhappy — neither disabled nor ill).

There is much less need for formal intervention in category four than in three, and the need tends to be less urgent in the last two categories than in the first two. The extent to which formal mental health services are required increases as coping abilities decrease and as the incidence of socially unacceptable behavior increases.

The chronically mentally ill are now seldom permanently institutionalized (as was common a few decades ago), but they tend to be continuously in need of support. Ten to twenty percent of persons receiving provincial disability allowances for medical reasons in Ontario have a psychiatric diagnosis. Another, perhaps larger group are on municipal welfare roles. There is often need for assistance with housing as well as a need for regular counselling, social programs, medication, and professional review. Employment may be possible only in sheltered situations. Household members or other close associates may also benefit from counselling and other forms of support.

Estimates of the prevalence of inadequate mental health usually tend to be between 10 and 30 percent of the general population. Heseltine, in 1983, suggested 25 percent, whereas, in 1978, the Canadian Mental Health Association (CMHA) suggested between 12 and 17 percent. The Ontario study proposed that of the 25 percent of the population with a diagnosable psychiatric condition, at least 90 percent will be seen and handled by nonspecialist services. Most will contact a family physician.

Over half of these will be given a mental health diagnosis such as anxiety or depression. Less than one-tenth of the group with a diagnosable psychiatric condition will be referred for specialist attention. There is, however, little evidence to suggest that this referral rate is either too high or too low.

Of the 1 to 2 percent of the total population with a chronic mental illness requiring ongoing attention, one-third are schizophrenic, one-third have organic brain syndrome, and one-third have other diagnoses. Although 10 to 15 percent of the general population will be hospitalized at least once in their lives with an emotional or mental illness, it is the chronically ill who dominate institutional statistics. Among the 10 to 15 percent of persons who are admitted at least once, common diagnoses include alcoholism, schizophrenia, affective disorders, and neuroses.

Child psychiatry is a rapidly growing specialty, as is **psychogeriatrics**. Major problems in children include hyperactivity, eating disorders, adolescent depression, suicide, and sexual abuse. Two to six percent of young females are raped, 80 percent by males whom they know and who are often members of their families.

Although there does not appear to be an increase in the incidence of psychotic illness, there certainly has been greater notice of non-psychotic emotional problems such as insecurity, anxiety, and depression. An increasing number of users are receiving services from an expanding list of health workers for problems which, in earlier decades, were apparently largely ignored.

Characteristics and Perceptions of Mental Illness

Almost all mental ill health is multifactorial. Only in a minority of cases can one clearly identify a physical cause (in which case the condition can be said to represent physical ill health with mental/emotional symptoms), or clearly associate one event or factor with the emotional problem, as is the case in some reactive depressions. Contributing causes may not all be readily visible and the relative importance of the various (personal and environmental) causes may be even less known. Although this vague relationship between cause and effect can be seen as a deterrent to effective prevention and treatment, it can also be seen as a help. Any number of actions or changes may significantly improve or protect individual mental health.

Public and professional perceptions of the relative importance of mental health and mental health services are best illustrated by a look at a few policies and practices:

- ☐ Only a small percentage of Medical Research Council funds, certainly less than 5 percent and perhaps less than 2 percent, are assigned to mental or psychosocial research.
- ☐ Demands by physicians and by the public for increased funding of acute treatment general hospitals are infinitely more aggressive than demands for increased funding for mental health services.

☐ Child abuse legislation in Ontario makes it a crime to mentally or physically abuse children and requires reporting by health professionals of all cases of suspected abuse. Cases reported, however, are almost exclusively cases of suspected physical abuse.

☐ HWC produced a *Health Hazard Appraisal* exercise in which an individual is asked a number of questions. These questions relate almost entirely to physical health and the only conclusion reached is the predicted life expectancy of the subject. The quality of life and mental health, and the hazards to each, are not considered.

☐ Involuntary retention in psychiatric facilities is now routinely examined by means of a series of mandatory assessments and reviews. These protections did not exist a few decades ago.

☐ Group homes or halfway houses for the physically disabled tend to be more acceptable to residential neighborhoods than those which house alcoholics or the chronically mentally ill.

☐ There is much greater general public support for the idea of community-based care for persons with mental illness than there was a few decades ago.

☐ Mental health services are now seen to have a therapeutic and preventive dimension, whereas, in earlier decades, their primary role was the protection of the public against dangerous lunatics.

☐ Large numbers of individuals with diagnosable mental health problems appear not to be receiving professional help. Failure to receive attention for physical health problems is much less common.

Mental Health Services, Programs, and Facilities

Prevention

Mental health protection can and does occur everywhere. The home and the school environments are probably most important, because the personality of the adult is largely shaped during childhood. However, the environments of our workplaces, communities, recreation sites, and jails are also important in the preservation of reasonable mental health, as are the actions of individuals. Preventive programs that assist children and adults in tolerating the differences of others, and in modifying their own performances so that they are more easily tolerated by others, are likely to be both widely supported and successful.

Caregivers, regardless of the nature of their services, can both promote and damage the mental health of their clients. The way news is delivered, the degree of respect shown for client opinions, the tolerance with which client fear or anger are handled, the patience with which instructions are explained — all affect the self-image and the level of stress of the client.

Health care institutions are a potential threat to the mental health of young children and selected adult populations. For children, the hazardous ages are the infant and preschool years.

Preventive activities include:

- using home care instead of institutional care (some children's hospitals seldom refer children to home care programs);
- encouraging parents to remain with young children as much as possible;
- involving parents in the care of the sick or injured child; and developing institutional procedures that minimize the adaptation needed from the child.

The child is already under stress, and the provision of care should be as nonthreatening as possible. For selected adults, particularly the depressed, demented, and frail elderly, the same general rules apply. Familiar events, surroundings, and faces are generally preferable. New routines, new corridors, and new noises can evoke physical and emotional deterioration which might have been more easily prevented than cured.

One type of low-cost, community-based preventive mental health service deserves mention. Many communities now have one or more centers to which mothers and their infants or preschool children can come. These centers support mothers who are staying at home with their children. These mothers often have inadequate personal support networks, they may not have had experience with small children, and they may be on low and fixed incomes. These centers offer a combination of counselling, peer support, education, short term day care, and emotional support to help the mothers to tolerate the stresses of parenting. The way this successful preventive model must struggle for funding and recognition is another example of our social preference for treating illness rather than preventing it.

The lines between services delivering primary prevention, secondary prevention and therapy are not clear in the world of mental and psychosocial health. **Distress centers** help people remain stable and out of care (a primary prevention role), while, at the same time, advising some people to go elsewhere for help (a diagnostic/secondary prevention role) and also actually being curative for some others (a therapeutic or tertiary prevention role). **Social drop-in centers** for the homeless, the poor, the lonely and the rejected perform the same full spectrum of functions, especially when their range of services includes providing food, socialization, and counselling.

Diagnosis

The diagnosis of mental ill health appears to be made at two levels. Society has a collective opinion as to whether individuals' performances indicate mental illness. When people exhibit socially unacceptable levels of suspicion, intolerance, anger, retaliation, or hysteria, they are apt to be labelled as mentally ill. Society often makes a diagnostic comment through its statements regarding what is acceptable or normal.

At the second level, mental health is evaluated by professionals who, although constrained and influenced by social norms, will also be interested in less visible characteristics. Is the client able to cope? Is he or she a menace to him or herself or to others? Is the intensity of response (for example, to a group home or to an AIDS patient in school) an indication of a more deeply-seated personality defect?

Therapeutic Services, Programs, and Facilities

The Concepts of Mental Health

As with physical illness, treatment of mental illness has, as its desired outcome, either the alleviation of undesirable symptoms or the control of disease. When the diseases are poorly defined, when symptoms cannot be quantified and when the symptoms at some level become "normal," it is not only difficult to know when to start treatment, but is also difficult to know when treatment should be stopped. There is considerable possibility of both over-servicing and under-servicing, although each is difficult to prove. When conditions are the product of many factors, and when improvement can arise from a variety of changes within the individual and the environment, it is also often difficult to know the extent to which improvement is the result of the treatment versus other factors. Despite these uncertainties associated with diagnosis and treatment, there is no doubt about the usefulness of most formal mental health programs and therapies. When the patient can cope moderately well and is able to be tolerated by society, treatment is usually stopped or reduced to a maintenance level.

When the cause of illness is unknown, treatment is less apt to be scientific. The degree of cure or improvement is also difficult to measure, and all of these factors increase the likelihood that there will be disagreement as to the preferred method of treatment.

The therapy for mental illness is quite different from its physical health counterpart. In mental illness, sick role theory usually does not apply. The classical sick role, which often does apply in physical health services, requires that the patient place himself or herself into the hands of the system and passively wait for care or cure. In mental illness, however, the patient and all persons of significance in his or her environment must usually actively contribute to the recovery process and to the maintenance of recovery if outcomes are to be satisfactory. In mental illness, as in other chronic illnesses, improved function is as likely to be found in helping the person adapt to his or her illness as it is in removing a cause.

Mental health treatment in Canada tends to be delivered by multidisciplinary teams within a therapeutic milieu. This is an ecological concept which recognizes environment as part of both illness and recovery. In this ecology, any number of individuals or factors may be an important part of therapy. At any particular time and with respect to a particular patient, the most important team member may be a psychologist, psychiatric nurse, social worker, family member, psychiatrist, nursing assistant, or remedial gymnast. Mental health teams should, ideally, be much less hierarchical than physical health teams, but one can easily find psychiatrists' kingdoms in which a hierarchy definitely exists.

Physical health services and workers tend to say, "Give yourself to me and I will cure you and care for you." Often, this approach works. Mental health services and workers often say, or should say, "Sit down with me and we will try to find a way in which all of us working together can improve the health of those in need of help." To the extent that mental health workers are paternalistic or discourage family and client participation, the system may partially fail. In mental health the "therapeutic milieu" includes the household, the workplace or school, and the social network of those in need of assistance.

The Delivery of Mental Health Services

Inpatient mental health services are provided by psychiatric hospitals and general hospitals with psychiatric units. This care is paid for by provincial governments through the same funding scheme as physical health services.

Psychiatric units in general hospitals, of which there are about 400 in Canada, have replaced isolated psychiatric hospitals as the dominant site of short term, active psychiatric care. The beds in psychiatric wards in general hospitals represent 4 to 5 percent of all acute treatment general hospital beds. Despite the move towards providing care in psychiatric wards in general hospitals, the large psychiatric hospital is still an important source of care which, until 1980, provided twice as many days of care as psychiatric wards in general hospitals. By 1990, these large institutions were downsizing. Psychiatric hospitals and units routinely offer both inpatient and outpatient care, and occasionally operate outreach programs or satellite clinics. Two-thirds of the increase in the number of psychiatric facilities in the last 20 years has been due to the appearance of psychiatric units in general hospitals; the other third has been mostly special treatment centers for children.

Residential care — that is, a living-in arrangement combined with some level of counselling and supervision — is provided in a general category commonly called Homes for Special Care. This category includes homes for the aged, nursing homes, boarding homes, special treatment centers for children, group homes (including homes for ex-psychiatric patients, battered wives and disturbed adolescents) and halfway houses. Mental health assessment and therapy in many forms is available through many nonprofit and a few for-profit agencies. Most large educational institutions and many churches and other agencies offer programs on family-life education, assertiveness training, and life skills — all of which should be seen as part of the mental health services network. A small number of psychiatric facilities (the forensic centers) have the special function of caring for persons who are a major threat to society or themselves.

A mental health services network will be faced with crises as well as less urgent demands, and many communities are not nearly as well prepared for emotional or psychiatric crises as they are for injuries or other physical emergencies.

Current efforts in Canada to develop a good crisis intervention service are based on quick response to housing, multidisciplinary specialized staff, financial aid, and continuous care needs. **Community-based mental health crisis intervention** requires institutional backup, and it must be able to support households as well as individuals. The crisis intervention teams should work closely with the police. Police are often the first to know of the crisis. They are among those who need and welcome good professional back-up. The psychiatric workers will need good police back-up sometimes. Appropriate crisis intervention markedly changes the pattern of institutionalization and frequently shortens length of stay when institutional care is unavoidable.

In the physical health field, we insist on the broadest imaginable level and mix of emergency services being available. Mental health workers regularly work with quite primitive crisis response capability.

Reducing Psychiatric Beds

Canada, at the end of the 1970s, was down to a national figure slightly under 1 (0.8 or 0.9) psychiatric bed per 1000 people. Patient census on any day was down to about 0.7 per 1000 because the institutions were operating at about 80 percent capacity. Besides admissions to psychiatric beds, there is an unknown number of psychiatric and psychosocial admissions to general medical, pediatric, or other beds.

Different provinces have gone through the same trends somewhat differently. In the late 1960s, Quebec had 3.6 psychiatric rated beds per 1,000, the highest number in the country, and many institutions exceeded their rated capacity by 50 to 75 percent. By 1978-79, Quebec had reduced its psychiatric bed supply to 0.6 per 1000 and the patient population in psychiatric institutions had fallen by up to 90 percent. Other provinces had gone through the same deinstitutionalization process, with Saskatchewan being first.

The decrease in facility size and number was associated with a major improvement in all aspects of facility services. More institutions had more and better staff and offered better therapy, improvements which meant marked increases in per diem costs. The move was from warehousing to therapy, from public protection to concern for the recovery and rights of the client. The decrease in beds was also accompanied by a growth in outpatient services. For instance, there was a 300 percent increase in outpatient services in Ontario from 1961-70.

Not all provinces have changed as much as Quebec and Saskatchewan. For example, New Brunswick had, by the end of the 1970s, cut its bed numbers by only about one-half, and the institutions remained full. Preference for one provincial experience over that of some other province will depend on the extent to which provincial policymakers and administrators think people should live in the community and the extent to which community back-up is available to people after discharge.

In Ontario in the period from 1961-76, the daily patient census in psychiatric hospitals fell from 18,000 to 5,000, a fall of 70 percent, while the daily census in psychiatric units in general hospitals rose from 350 to 1,500. In Ontario, from 1965-77, the number of psychiatric patients in homes for special care increased from 1,600 to 7,400. A significant part of the emptying of psychiatric hospitals was accomplished by merely moving the patients to other institutions.

Psychiatric Admissions

Annual admission rates (first admissions and readmissions) in Canada are usually now in the range of 4 to 7 per 1000 (as compared to general hospital admission rates of 100 to 150 admissions per 1000 per year). Average length of stay for the psychiatric patients is several times that of physical health patients, but the great majority of psychiatric admissions are now for less than one month. Admissions to psychiatric facilities are equal to only 2 to 5 percent of admissions to physical care facilities. Age patterns also differ. Ages 20 to 50 are the peak years for psychiatric admissions (at least partly because these are peak years for schizophrenia admissions). Rates for the elderly are 25 to 35 percent lower than the rates for younger adults. Costs of hospital treatment for mental illness in Canada are about one tenth of the costs of the hospital care of physical ailments.

Many mental health programs and institutions, especially the institutions, now have a Patients' Bill of Rights. Ontario psychiatric hospitals now have a formally trained patient advocate on staff whose role is to mediate institution-patient disputes and to assist patients in the protection of their rights.

Community Services

Community-based mental health services provide a broad range of advocacy, education, advice, protection, and therapy. The networks tend to be dominated by nonprofit, low-budget sources of care, few agencies spend over $1 million a year. In 1985, over 300 community mental health programs in Ontario received, in total, less than $50 million of Ministry of Health funds.

Children's mental health services and facilities consist largely of quite expensive and usually residential treatment units, associated with psychiatric hospitals, children's hospitals, or child protection agencies such as the Children's Aid Societies in Ontario.

Addicts are an important subgroup within the users of mental health services. They have a high rate of recidivism, and often have little interest in treatment. Within this category, the alcoholics are almost surely the most numerous, expensive, and socially disruptive group, with prescription drug abusers being their major competitor. Alcoholics and users of illicit drugs are often served through agencies or facilities that serve no other user groups. These include detoxification centers, halfway houses, and Alcoholics Anonymous. Two to five percent of the adult population are alcohol dependent to the point of some interference with social and occupational life.

Detoxification centers provide short term care during recovery from bouts of intoxication. Most centers are of the nonmedical type with no medical staff and minimal nursing and counselling capability. Clients stay 3 to 5 days and are referred to treatment programs if that is their wish. Centers within the medical model are much more expensive and offer few if any proven advantages over the nonmedical model. In the region of Ottawa-Carleton, for example, there are 5 to 6 admissions per 1000 total population per year to detoxification centers — that is, 3,000 to 3,500 per year for a community of 600,000 people.

Addiction recovery programs operate under both for-profit and non-profit auspices. Intensive rehabilitation programs are in such short supply in Canada that almost one-third of those receiving such treatment go to programs in the United States. The largest group of users of these non-Canadian programs are executives aged 35 to 64. A recent Ottawa-Carleton report (on a service area population of approximately 1 million people) proposed a need for 28 more inpatient alcoholic recovery beds and 120 day/evening spaces. One objective was to stop exporting approximately $300,000 a year for services that could just as adequately be provided within the region. Many less intensive alcohol and drug addiction recovery programs exist, often based in group homes or halfway houses. They have variable success rates, none of them very high, but they constitute a personalized and less expensive effort to deal with an endemic and serious disease. A few programs such as Alcoholics Anonymous operate successfully without public financial support.

The importance of **community services for the chronically mentally ill** is easily illustrated. Fifty percent of the patients admitted to the Queen Street Mental Health Centre in downtown Toronto have no fixed addresses. When discharged they will once again have no fixed addresses, and will have an increased likelihood of readmission unless there is an available network of residential, social, and professional support within the community. A 1982 study done in a Whitby, Ontario, psychiatric institution reported that 20 percent of patients were remaining in hospital because suitable community-based support networks were not available.

Sheltered workshops may be described as a form of psychiatric facility. They allow individuals to work in a protective environment where stress is reduced, production standards are different and work can have a therapeutic component. They can be operated by many different sponsors and can serve the intellectually handicapped, the physically handicapped, or the mentally/emotionally handicapped.

Mental Health Manpower

British Columbia, in 1984, proposed that there should be one psychiatrist for every 11,000 people, a figure also proposed by the 1975 Report of the National Committee on Medical Manpower. The figure 11,000 appears to be largely chosen as something modestly below the available number of psychiatrists rather than on the basis of a more objective rationale. Ottawa has twice the provincial concentration of psychiatrists (1 per 3,000 to 5,000 people) and they all are busy. There appears to be no visible ceiling to the capacity of psychiatrists to find patients and provide them with service. In Washington, DC, there is one psychiatrist for every 2000 persons and some parts of California are even better supplied.

If a person feels better when he or she spends an hour a week with a mental health worker for which he or she is spending personal money, then public policy is only marginally affected. In a publicly financed system, however, society is likely to eventually express an opinion regarding how frequently an hour of publicly financed therapy should be available. Psychotherapy and counselling are definitely growth industries, but control should not be pursued unless there is equal attention given to the many types of physical health services that have also expanded, such as many types of surgery and infertility procedures.

Organization and Administration

Integrated, comprehensive networks of mental health services are more the exception than the rule, although high-quality exceptions exist. In most areas, mental health services are provided by an impressive list of uncoordinated and predominantly locally inspired programs. The yellow pages in the Ottawa-

Carleton telephone directory list over 200 sources of mental health assistance, including over 100 providing services exclusively for mental health needs. The Ontario Ministry of Health provides support to over 100 mental health services in the Ottawa-Carleton region. The historical centralization of mental health services in large rural hospitals has been replaced by a wide variety of agencies in which the components are varied and usually quite unplanned. The mix includes agencies specializing in providing health, social, vocational, recreational, housing, income support, and educational services.

A few decades ago, most formal mental health services were part of a psychiatric services branch of a provincial ministry of health. Today, the mental health services network is more complex and less predictable (Figure 8.1). Figure 8.1 is not an organization chart nor is it meant to describe any single province. It merely illustrates many of the components and relationships of mental health services in most provinces.

Institutions which provide only psychiatric services are usually operated by the Ministry of Health, although some are operated by independent boards (examples include the Clarke Institute in Toronto and several institutions in Alberta). When institutions are operated by the Ministry of Health, all personnel, including most psychiatrists, are salaried provincial civil servants. Personnel policies and union affiliations are the same as for other civil servants. The physical plant and its maintenance or replacement may be the responsibility of a provincial department of public works or equivalent.

In Canadian general hospitals, a psychiatric unit together with its associated psychiatric outpatient services make up merely one part of the hospital. They are usually funded out of the hospital global budget and are operated in the same way as any other service unit. Physicians providing psychiatric services within the hospital are paid in the same way as other physicians; as private practitioners on fee-for-service or within some negotiated university contract.

Psychiatric emergency patients often benefit from specialized care. General hospitals whose emergency departments will receive psychiatric emergencies which cannot be immediately referred to an adjacent psychiatric emergency department will almost always have appropriate support in the form of at least a psychiatrist and a psychiatric social worker or equivalent.

Figure 8.1

The Role of Provincial Governments in Mental Health Services

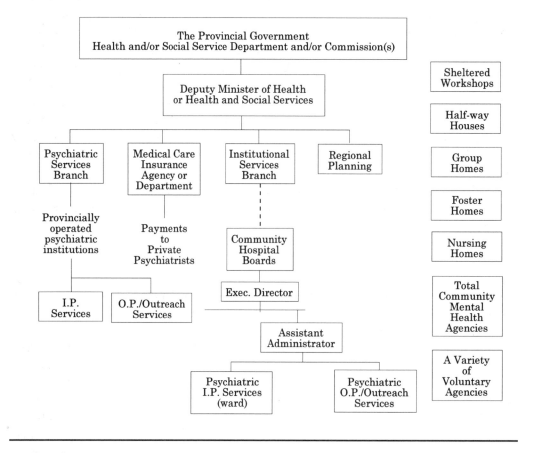

Community-based mental health services are a mixed bag. Private psychiatrists often work alone and, at times, provide services largely to the type of clientele who do not need a multidisciplinary team. These patients might include the worried, the stressed, and members of households in modest conflict. A variety of profit and non-profit agencies provide personal or group counselling, primarily through social workers or psychologists. Most of these cannot bill provincial medical care plans, and income is earned through private insurance, user-pay arrangements, charitable support, or government grants. Other agencies, usually non-profit, operate a variety of residential programs, including group homes and halfway houses. Nursing homes, boarding homes, or homes for special care under a variety of names, are often an important part of the mental health services network because they house many individuals with mental disabilities, including those who have been discharged from psychiatric institutions. In this latter instance, public financing on a per diem basis has replaced public financing through an institutional budget.

Many institutional and noninstitutional mental health programs make regular use of case conferences in which professionals and sometimes the patient and/or the patient's family discuss the diagnosis and develop a treatment plan. As with many committees, these case conferences have two sides.

They are very useful when the complexities of the case require multidisciplinary comment and consensus, but they are expensive. Staff members can spend a good part of their day talking to each other, an activity which significantly reduces the time available to work with clients. One preferred alternative is to use some type of triage in which an intake worker makes a decision regarding the need for case conferencing. Although some patients would miss the benefit attributable to a conference, the patient contact hours per worker would be higher and outcomes perhaps better with a fixed amount of staff.

A few Canadian communities have, at various moments in the past, taken steps towards implementing an integrated, community-wide approach to mental health services. Over 25 years ago in Yorkton, Saskatchewan, it was shown that good, non-institutional mental health services markedly altered the referral of patients to institutions. It was shown that long-term care facilities which routinely referred disturbed, elderly patients to psychiatric facilities could deal quite adequately with these problems on their own if advice and support were available from mental health professionals. Saskatoon initiated a psychiatric home care program over two decades ago which showed how patients could be supported by a multifunctional, community-based agency.

The biggest step forward was made in Vancouver in the mid-1970s with the establishment of a regional service, the Greater Vancouver Mental Health Service, serving several metropolitan municipalities with a combined population of about 500,000 people. This service was created by a special provincial statute and was operated by its own community board. It had close ties with the municipal public health authorities.

This regional service was designed to provide crisis intervention and continuing care for the chronically mentally ill. The short-term ill were considered to be already reasonably adequately served by the private psychiatrists, the wards in general hospitals, and a variety of community agencies. The chronically ill who were repeatedly or permanently hospitalized had no one able to support and treat them in the community. In the Vancouver area, as elsewhere, there were large, isolated psychiatric institutions attempting to reduce census without the necessary coordinated community support in place.

This new service

- [ ] was multidisciplinary,
- [ ] was available 24 hours a day/7 days a week,
- [ ] had close liaison with the police,
- [ ] had good access to institutional care if needed,
- [ ] had temporary noninstitutional housing available, and
- [ ] was willing to provide short term, high-intensity, around-the-clock support if needed.

Service was provided by eight teams with special crisis intervention units, based in the temporary housing. The general teams were led by social workers or psychiatric nurses. All teams included psychologists, psychiatric nurses and psychiatric social workers. Psychiatrists played a consulting role. Several research studies confirmed the benefits and adequacy of the Vancouver approach, but despite international attention, the model has not been duplicated in other Canadian cities. By 1991, this service was available for nearly 1 million residents of the region.

Halifax-Dartmouth decided to take a completely different approach in its search for more rational and adequate community mental health services 10 years ago. The community had no overall plan; there were many agencies, but no way of reducing duplication and plugging gaps. It was decided that better inter-agency communication might be all that was needed. Clients would be more appropriately referred and service adjustments would eliminate gaps. The Minister of Health of Nova Scotia funded the Metropolitan Halifax-Dartmouth Mental Health Planning Board. It involved a great many committees, and a lot of time was spent having professionals talk to each other, but this board has survived successfully for many years.

Besides improving communications, the Halifax-Dartmouth board serves a planning function similar to that of District Health Councils in Ontario. Each year, the Ministry of Health invites the board to rank, in terms of need or importance, all of the proposals for new mental health programs in Halifax-Dartmouth. Recommendations are submitted to the Ministry along with the rationale and criteria used, and these recommendations tend to be accepted by the Ministry.

In Ontario, the District Health Councils have the task of developing plans for regional mental health networks and recommending steps to achieve them. In 1983, the Minister of Health in Ontario proposed that "designated general hospitals with psychiatric units be made the pivot for intramural and extramural community services" within a part of a larger provincial psychiatric hospital. Each community would be the direct responsibility of, and would receive inpatient and outpatient services from, a designated hospital. Services available from this hospital would include crisis intervention and backup services for community-based agencies. Implementation of the plan has, to date, been slow despite the appearance of a new psychiatric facility in Ontario with a broad range of community outreach.

The failure to develop comprehensive/mental health networks in much of Canada provides another illustration of the low status of mental health services. Ontario, in recent years, has introduced a provincial ground ambulance service, a number of central bed registries to assure optimum acceptance of non-psychiatric emergencies, a paramedic program to handle cardiac and other similar emergencies, and a general hospital emergency room categorization scheme. Yet, it was only in 1984 that Toronto received its first community-based psychiatric crisis service in the form of a house with 24-hour staff supported by a 10-bed, short-stay, stabilization unit.

Progress towards comprehensive mental health service networks is steady but painfully slow.

Mental Health in Quebec

In Quebec, the Regional Health and Social Service Councils (CRSSSs) have a broader mandate than District Health Councils (DHCs) in Ontario and can more easily honor their mandate because of the existence of a provincial network of CLSCs. Community mental health needs and services are among the responsibilities of the CLSCs.

When the Castonguay Commission on health services reform was doing its work in Quebec almost 20 years ago, it discovered that the major mental health facilities and programs in Montreal had no well-defined community responsibilities. It was also discovered that most facilities chose not to identify with the 500,000 people in central Montreal. In response to this situation, each institution in the Montreal area was told that it was to be responsible for a portion of the total population. If a client showed up from a particular institution's geographic base, that institution had an obligation to provide care.

Issues and Problems

Salaried psychiatrists. Psychiatry is one of the few medical specialties in which a significant number of physicians providing patient care are on a salary. These psychiatrists are on salary as public servants in provincially operated psychiatric hospitals. They tend to want incomes comparable to psychiatrists on fee-for-service, for whom there are no income ceilings. This situation carries the seeds of continuing dispute. In addition, the continued rapid growth of utilization of psychiatric and other mental health services may emerge as a real or perceived economic problem.

Mental competence. There is continuing difficulty with the concept of mental competence. This has historically been resolved by being arbitrary. The person in question was either fully competent or fully incompetent. The measures of competence tend to relate to socially acceptable conduct or opinion, as well as to the technical ability to understand or decide. Various provinces have, in recent years, increasingly sought compromises which preserve portions of personal autonomy while protecting clients or the public in areas of vulnerability.

In the face of complete or partial mental incompetence, there is a need for the identification of someone else to act on behalf of the incompetent person, and this agent is commonly either a civil servant or a person to whom power of attorney has been given. Newer legislation, such as the 1978 *Alberta Dependent Adults Act*, provides for flexible arrangements for incomplete as well as complete transfers of powers.

The transfer of authority usually creates a situation in which the new guardian can, if he or she wishes, act contrary to the previously expressed wishes of the person involved. This can be seen as ethically unacceptable, and in some provinces the guardian cannot reverse previously clearly stated intentions.

Deinstitutionalization is more a characteristic of the mental health world than of other medical fields. It has, at times, been promoted because institutions are considered to be bad or because community care is thought to be cheaper. Neither reason is acceptable. Institutions are often effective, and community care may only be cheaper if the necessary community-based support services are not offered. It also may be more expensive. Deinstitutionalization does not occur at all when a patient is merely transferred from a psychiatric hospital to a large, highly structured, and often socially unattractive residential facility or to a small room without a supporting social and professional network.

There would probably be no argument with the proposition that some mentally ill individuals are best cared for in institutions. Disagreement, therefore, revolves around who should be cared for in this way, for how long and within what institutional environment.

In considering the extent to which non-institutional care ought to be promoted, it is wise to assume that the environment within psychiatric facilities can be different from that which existed a few decades ago. The traditional psychiatric facility produced institutionalism, a condition characterized by submission, loss of initiative, reduced communication, and personal deterioration. These characteristics included the almost inevitable loss of personal control, loss of privacy and dignity, loss of freedom, lack of social and intellectual opportunities, and emotional (if not physical) brutality.

Institutions do not need to be dominated by the historical model, and most are now significantly better. They show evidence of reduced congestion, more respect for the feelings and wishes of residents, a more personal approach to lifestyles and therapy, and a search for resident improvement. In assisting individuals and families to choose between institutional and community-based care, it is desirable that both of the options be recognized as having good, as well as less desirable, features.

Institutions offer 24-hour support and protection. They can handle unpredictable changes in behavior and can offer a good range of social opportunities. They also tend to impose schedules, reduce privacy, disrupt households, and alter lifestyles. Care in the community varies greatly in the extent to which it assures improved social opportunities and the opportunity for personal decisionmaking. It is usually less able to handle crises. Whether institutional or community-based care should be chosen by or encouraged for a given individual will depend as much on the characteristics of the institution and the community health services network as on the characteristics of the individual. Certainly institutionalized persons are still being released into communities without an adequate system of support services.

Specialization. Some psychiatrists and mental health workers work almost exclusively with the neurotics, acute psychotics, or other patients with shorter-term and more manageable problems. This pre-selection of patients could leave fewer and fewer workers to care for the difficult, more emotionally demanding, and less emotionally rewarding, patients.

Public support. It is difficult to obtain public and bureaucratic support for community mental health programming to a level approximating the degree of public support for physical health programs. As things which engage the public imagination, providing housing, income support, assistance with daily living and help in learning how to socialize are no match for test tube babies and heart transplants.

Stress. Health care providers must consider what stresses people should be taught to adapt to, or be more accepting of, rather than be angry with. How should people be encouraged to respond to unemployment, demotion, divorce, single parenthood, criticism, poverty, discrimination, the possibility of unemployment, spending half of one's disposable income on housing, being unable to afford things, growing old, being disabled, and being institutionalized or deinstitutionalized?

Consent. There will be continued conflict between the sanctity of personal (human) rights and the professional certainty that there are times when therapy must be initiated without the consent of the patient.

Summary

Canada's mental health services are approaching the new World Health Organization's (WHO) definition of health. However, there is still limited public acceptance of the need to consider a wide range of strategies for support of mental health. These include employment, housing, personal security, safe inner cities and clean environments.

References

Austin, C.D. and O'Connor, K. (1989), *Case Management and Program Contexts, in Health Care of the Elderly: An Information Sourcebook*, ed. M.D. Petersen and D.L. White. Beverly Hills, CA: Sage Publications.

Comments on Proposed Amendments to the Patient Act, Consumer & Corporate Affairs Canada, October, 1986.

Kane, L. and Kane, R. (1984). *A Will and a Way — What the United States Can Learn from Canada about Caring for the Elderly*. Columbia University Press.

Health and Welfare Canada (1988). *Mental Health for Canadians: Striking a Balance*, Ottawa: Supply and Services Canada, H39-128.

Haseltine, G.F., (1983) *Towards a Blueprint for Change: A Mental Health Policy and Program Perspective*. (A report produced for the Government of Ontario) Toronto.

Weissart, W.G., Cready, C.M. and Parvelak, J.E. (1988). The Past and Future of Home- and Community-Based Long-Term Care, *The Millbank Quarterly*. Vol. 66 (2):309-388.

CHAPTER 9

Long Term Care Services

The Evolution of Long Term Care in Canada

M uch of the evolution of long term care (LTC) merely reflects the larger events in society. Elitism, for example, has given ground to universality, and human worth now has dimensions other than productivity. Three evolutionary phases are easily described.

The first phase was characterized by social disinterest. Families cared for their disabled members as well as they could. Public assistance for the indigent portion of this unproductive population was limited to isolated and low-cost institutional warehousing. Charitable (usually religious) institutions were the only other option. In phase one, the objectives of government, to the extent that it was involved through funding or legislation, was to keep costs down and keep the disabled and the indigent elderly out of sight. The institutionalized persons were treated as inmates and frequently referred to as inmates.

The second phase was firmly in place by the 1960s. It brought benevolent paternalism characterized by family, professional, and societal protection and dominance of "the less fortunate." Patronizing institutions and professionals using the medical model became surrogate parents, regardless of the mental competence of the dependent persons. The concept of second childhood became enshrined in our processes of assessment, placement, and care. Professionals evaluated the patient, decided the appropriate location for care, and then planned its delivery. The role of the user in decisionmaking was minimal.

In the early stages of this period of benevolent paternalism, the LTC institutions copied the hospital model through the use of regular schedules, professional control, uniformed staff, prohibition of alcohol, and limited visiting. As phase two has matured, serious efforts have been made to make institutions more stimulating, flexible, personal, and pleasant — more home-like — and to recognize client individuality. Many institutional professionals, administrators, and many families, however, still believe that institutionalized adults, regardless of their mental competence, need someone to make sure that they do nothing foolish. The LTC client who was earlier treated as if he or she were in kindergarten is now treated like an adolescent.

The objectives of phase two, at least the latter part of it, could be described as follows.

☐ To protect life by providing a safe physical environment and regular medical supervision by paying attention to nutrition, by encouraging exercise if possible, and by demanding compliance with professional decisions when thought necessary.

☐ To improve quality of life by humanizing institutions and by offering greater opportunity for resident decision making.

When the two major objectives come into conflict, the policy makers, administrators, and caregivers, unfortunately, still often opt for protection of length of life over protection of quality of life, although the trend is towards client choice.

Paternalistic phase two is steadily and peacefully merging into phase three. In the third phase of LTC evolution, the dependent adult is treated as an adult rather than a child. This phase is dominated by the idea that adult status is not compromised by physical dependency. The extent to which this latest phase has arrived, how its full arrival can be hastened, and the implications of its arrival are questions now open for discussion.

Definition of Terms

Long term care (LTC) and **chronic care** cannot be precisely defined. Most people would agree that facilities such as nursing homes and chronic hospitals provide LTC, and that persons in these facilities are receiving LTC, but agreement then begins to weaken.

A person with a long term illness such as asthma, psoriasis, hypertension, or diabetes, who is receiving regular and multidisciplinary services but is leading an active and normal life, is not considered to be receiving LTC. Similarly, a person with a chronic disability such as an amputated finger or foot, a moderate hearing loss, a speech impediment, or absence of vision in one eye is not considered to be someone who needs LTC. Continuing care in psychiatric facilities is also not considered to be part of long term care. If, however, psychiatric patients are cared for in a nursing home, then the patients will, by virtue of their location, be categorized as LTC patients even if not physically disabled or dependent. It is clear that, through custom and evolution, we consider the term "long term care" to have a strong institutional connotation even though it can be delivered in the community. A person is considered to be a candidate for LTC only if quite physically dependent with little or no possibility of future physical independence.

Distinctions between psychiatric and nonpsychiatric patients are unclear and changing although institutional classifications remain relatively unchanged. Persons with long term brain dysfunction arising from physical disease or injury, whether accidents, Alzheimers, or toxic agents, are increasingly likely to be cared for in LTC facilities and programs. At one time, these persons were admitted to psychiatric facilities. Persons with quite similar handicaps arising from psychiatric disorders are more likely to be cared for in the mental health services network (unless there is also major physical disability, in which case care may come from outside of the psychiatric network). Terminology has become convenient for statisticians, institutional operators, and those who pay bills, but is often of minimal use to planners and makes little sense to users.

It is useful to distinguish between disability and handicap while recognizing that some people use them synonymously. An amputated hand or emotional instability is a **disability**. A **handicap** is the effect of a disability. For example, handicaps associated with the loss of a hand may include inability to play most musical instruments, to open a door, or to be a laborer, while those associated with emotional instability restrict one's employment opportunities and endanger personal relationships. Disabilities and handicaps can be minor or major, temporary or permanent. Many disabilities, even quite severe ones, produce few if any handicaps, and sometimes the biggest handicaps flow not from the disability but from the way others see it. A paraplegic or a blind person, for instance, may not be thought to be capable of managing a job. In some instances there are major handicaps and no disability, as when a stabilized epileptic is refused employment.

Two final definitional comments may add clarity. First, **senior citizens** and **long term care** are not synonymous. The majority of the persons receiving LTC are elderly, but more than 90 percent of elderly Canadians are not in LTC. The LTC network responds to dependency (handicap), usually a physical dependency, in persons of all ages. Secondly, **geriatrics** is that branch of medicine which treats problems peculiar to old age. **Gerontology** is the clinical, biological, sociological, and historical study of aging.

Current Structure of Long Term Care

All contemporary LTC has one or more of the following goals or objectives, but never all of them:

- ☐ to prolong life and maintain health,
- ☐ to improve the quality of life of the LTC recipient,
- ☐ to support household caregivers and protect their quality of life,
- ☐ to reduce agency or program cost,
- ☐ to reduce total system cost,
- ☐ to reduce departmental cost,
- ☐ to reduce user and household cost,
- ☐ to protect acute treatment hospital beds from "bed-blockers,"
- ☐ to make a profit, and
- ☐ to be cost-effective compared to other sources of similar care.

Factors Affecting the Size of the LTC System

The size of the LTC system is a product of the number of people receiving care and the volume of care delivered per person. The number of persons receiving care in the total network, or any part of it, is controlled by the same general categories of determinants that apply to all health services:

☐ by factors which lead the user and the system to feel that entry is appropriate,

☐ by factors which determine the volume of care to be delivered, and

☐ by factors which affect how long the user remains in the system.

Some interpretations and considerations, however, are quite specific to LTC.

As stated earlier, many of the people in LTC, especially in LTC institutions, are there for life. Until a few years ago discharge for other than acute illness or injury was rare. For those institutionalized persons who will not be discharged into the community, length of institutionalization is determined entirely by how long they live.

The entry of an individual into LTC, and the mix of services delivered, is determined partly by type and degree of measurable disability/dependency, partly by societal perceptions of dependency, and partly by the volume of LTC resources available for purchase with private or public money. Diagnoses are almost completely irrelevant, and age is of only slightly more significance. Inability to walk, feed oneself, or think clearly requires approximately the same group of services whether the person in need is 25 or 85 years of age. Some changes in need arise from different interests in such things as education, employment, sex, marriage, and children, but many needs are the same regardless of age.

Principles That Should Govern the Organization and Delivery of LTC

The following 13 principles are emerging in the Canadian LTC network to reflect support of patient and personal rights.

1. The place where a person gets his or her mail and is enumerated to vote should be considered his or her home.

2. The mentally competent but significantly physically dependent population has the same rights, privileges, and responsibilities as the less dependent population, including the right to make decisions and choices. For example:

    ☐ This population should be able to use disposable income to increase the levels of or quantities of care received, to improve the nature of their accommodation, or to be catered to in whatever ways they can afford. This is already the case with respect to paying for private or semi-private institutional accommodation but the choices should and can be much broader.

    ☐ They should personally choose those with whom they share private living space. No person should, for prolonged periods, be forced to share his or her home or bedroom with one or more strangers whom he or she did not choose. (This practice is not considered to be desirable even in a jail.)

    ☐ Dependent adults should be as much in charge of their lives and lifestyle choices as the rest of us. Personal preferences should be honored to roughly the same extent that the rest of us have the opportunity to have our personal preferences honored. Choice should be possible with respect to sexual activity or orientation, private consumption of alcohol, use of addicting substances, refusal to comply with professional advice, privacy, social contact, employment, travel, and how and where to spend leisure time.

☐ They have the same responsibility as do the rest of us to be considerate, thoughtful, respectful, and positive, and to refrain from demanding or expecting more care or attention than is appropriate.

☐ They have the right to a reasonable level of health care, usually without reduction in quality or quantity merely because they are elderly or disabled.

3. All adults have the right to be considered mentally competent until proven otherwise, and the determination of mental competence should rely on *legal* criteria, process, and decisions rather than on medical ones. LTC practices and personnel frequently appear to assume mental incompetence in the elderly or the disabled when there is no evidence for the assumption.

4. Partial loss of, or limited development of, mental competence should not prevent client choice and control in areas in which adequate competence exists. A person may be unable to find his or her way home from shopping but may, at the same time, recognize surroundings, have a good recollection of the past, and remember the financial details of his or her life.

5. Persons with even very limited cognition (perceiving, thinking, remembering) should be given adequate and respectful care. The question of how much care to provide to persons with permanent absence of cognitive skills is an ethical issue on which current consensus is unlikely. It needs active discussion.

6. Family and social networks represent more than a vital part of the psychosocial environment of the disabled; they are major sources of care. Preserving households and outside social contacts reduces the loss associated with disability and reduces the need for and cost of outside care.

7. Because we wish to give the disabled choices with respect to where they live, who they live with, and what risks they take, it is incumbent on planners and policy makers to be certain that these choices exist if they can be made available at reasonable cost.

8. Image is important and self-image reflects social image. If society sees dependency as synonymous with inferiority, then dependent persons will see themselves as inferior. Society must, therefore, promote and support the concept of equality.

9. When the primary objective is the protection of and elevation of quality of life, an institution or care provider must allocate available resources

in such a way that highest priority is given to meeting the needs that are seen by the consumer as most important.

10. Prevention of illness and support of health is relevant to all age groups.

11. New LTC accommodations should be designed and operated as adapted housing and not as modified hospitals.

12. Society has the right to decide what volume of resources will be made available at public expense to a particular group of persons or to any one person. Being physically dependent should not markedly reduce one's mental independence but it also should not allow the user to demand residential or other options that are deemed by society to be unnecessary or overly extravagant.

13. Persons requiring long term support should be able to exercise significant control over how they choose to use whatever resources society chooses to assign to them. This is the principle within which some other social support programs now operate, to some extent. Our financial support systems, our ambulatory health system and our educational systems are examples.

Besides the above principles that should govern the planning and delivery of care, there are at least two different perceptions within which we can plan and provide LTC. One of these leads to the proposition that regardless of the extent to which noninstitutional options are improved, there will always be a large number of persons, including many mentally competent persons, who must be housed in institutions. This assumption underlies Canada's continued construction of LTC facilities. Another concept, significantly different from the first, proposes that LTC services of virtually any degree of complexity and volume can be delivered to people living in personal, rather than institutional, accommodations. The only significant provision associated with the second concept is that, for some clients, this personal accommodation may need to be specially constructed if adequate service is to be provided at acceptable cost.

Deciding which concept is correct is fortunately quite simple. Endless experiences and examples have shown that the immobile, the incontinent, the visually impaired, those who need respiratory assistance, those who cannot feed or dress themselves, and those who are frail, medically unstable, or in need of regular injections or dressings or other procedures, can all be cared for either in institutions or outside of them. The assumption that institutionalization is the only credible option in the face of major physical dependency is, therefore, invalid.

Not all persons seeking to help the elderly have put forward principles similar to those just proposed. A White House Conference on Aging in the early 1980s, for example, adopted the following set of rights for the elderly.

☐ To have self-esteem in an agist and sexist society.
☐ To have adequate economic support to cover needs for food, shelter, clothes, and health care.
☐ To have adequate health care and to be treated with respect, as an

individual whose life is valuable, by sensitive health care providers.

☐ To have access to honest legal and financial advice and consumer protection.

☐ To have a positive representation in the media.

☐ To be free from fear of crime, isolation, poverty, and abandonment.

☐ To be seen as a unique individual who is productive, attractive, intelligent, and interesting.

☐ To express sexuality in whatever manner is preferred.

☐ To be free from society's stigma of incompleteness which is applied to a woman who is alone.

☐ To have employment opportunities when work is wanted, and to receive fair wages.

☐ To have worthwhile volunteer opportunities available.

☐ To choose alternate lifestyles and living arrangements.

☐ To maintain optimum control over one's life and possessions.

☐ To be given the opportunity to continue to grow intellectually, spiritually, and socially.

☐ To avoid dependence on others, to speak for oneself, and to learn to serve oneself.

The principles in this list are of importance to all persons, not just the elderly or the disabled. To write rules such as these merely strengthens the incorrect supposition that the rights and responsibilities of the elderly are fundamentally different from those of the rest of the population. The acceptance of the elderly as a "normal" part of the population is best accomplished by acceptance of the general proposal that the disabled have the same rights and responsibilities as the less disabled and that age does not alter those rights and responsibilities.

The Elderly and the Future Elderly

Because most dependent persons are elderly, and because planners and society are inordinately preoccupied with the aging of the population, the elderly, as a population, will be examined before looking at the dependent population of all ages.

In 1986, approximately 11 percent of Canadians (2.7 million) were 65 years of age or older. If projected life expectancies, fertility rates, and immigration volumes materialize this percentage will increase over the next 40 to 50 years to 22 to 25 percent. Our population is aging partly because people are living longer but mostly because our fertility and birth rates since about 1970 have been low. From 1950-70, birth rates and immigration rates were quite high. Beyond 2035-40, the elderly as a percentage of the total population will, unless predictions are in error, fall to current European levels of 15 to 19 percent.

Until 1972, there had always been more males than females in the total Canadian population, but females had always dominated the older age groups. Projections suggest that in 35 to 40 years there will be 3 females for every male among 80-year-olds.

Life expectancy at birth is now about 73 years for males and 82 years for females in Canada. The gap between the sexes steadily widened after female life expectancy passed that of males early in the twentieth century. Since 1985, however, the gap has remained relatively constant. Perhaps changes in female lifestyles (using tobacco more, taking on male occupations) or an improvement in male lifestyles (less smoking) are at work.

The fact that females live longer than males partly explains why there are more widows than widowers (part of the explanation also lies in the fact that husbands tend to be older than wives) but does not directly or fully explain why there are more females in LTC. The major cause of this is the fact that females not only live longer but they also have, on average, twice as many years of major dependency, a difference that is apparently more sex-related than age-related.

One very impressive feature of our elderly population is not that 4 percent at age 65 or 35 percent at age 85 are in institutions, but that 96 percent at age 65 and 65 percent at age 85 *are not*. Aging does not lead to automatic dependency, as is sometimes portrayed. It is, however, commonly associated with certain changes.

☐ Senses deteriorate (sight, smell, touch, adaptation to dark).
☐ Reflexes are slower.
☐ Vital organ functions become less adequate.
☐ Recovery time is slower.
☐ Height goes down, posture changes, joints deteriorate.
☐ Wrinkles and grey hair appear and there is less subcutaneous fat.

There are a number of other perceptions of aging that are, however, myth rather than fact.

☐ That old age is a disease.
☐ That all elderly people suffer the "regular" bad effects of aging.
☐ That the elderly cannot be creative or innovative.
☐ That sexual interests disappear.
☐ That memory and other mental abilities automatically become poorer.
☐ That the elderly cannot do a day's work.
☐ That the elderly cannot learn new skills or change their values.
☐ That old age brings tranquillity.
☐ That there is usually fear of death.

Various authors have shown that judgement, vocabulary, comprehension, problem solving skills, and concentration can increase up to a very advanced age.

Will Our Aging Population Overwhelm Us?

Many analysts speak of a crisis of national bankruptcy, of pension plan bankruptcy, of no institutional space for acute care, of thousands of LTC beds needed, and of doddering elderly everywhere with no one to care for them. These predictions are so widespread and so often overstated that the assumptions on which they are founded need to be examined.

Certainly the population is aging. Barring some major global catastrophe, a surge in birth rates, or massive immigration, the number of older people in Canada will almost certainly increase in both an absolute and a relative sense until 45 to 60 years from now, at which point both absolute and relative numbers are likely to fall.

Dependency ratios are a common basis for propositions that we will be short of caregivers and unable to afford the burden of an enlarged elderly population. The most commonly used dependency ratio refers to the ratio of workers (age 20 to 64) to nonworkers (age 0 to 19 plus those 65 years and older).

In 1901 there were 99 dependent children (0 to 19) and older persons (65 and over) for every 100 persons in the working ages (20 to 64) in Canada. Ten of the 99 were older persons and 89 were 0 to 19 years of age. By 1981, these figures were 16 and 56 respectively for a total of 72, and in 2031, the year with the highest projected dependent population, the estimate is that the figures will be 33 elderly and 47 children for a total of 80. Dependency ratios do not present a frightening picture. As currently calculated, they should be ignored. They understate the size of the dependent population by ignoring

- the 1 to 2 percent of those 18 to 65 who are permanently incapacitated and dependent,
- the 1 to 2 percent of those 18 to 65 who are in school,
- the 8 to 12 percent of the workforce who are unemployed, and
- others such as single parents who are on welfare or other social assistance.

The dependent population is overstated primarily by assuming that all those 65 and over are dependent. Five to ten percent of this population are working and many others are living primarily on savings and pensions accumulated during their working years. In addition, many of those over 65 and not working are fully able to work. If Canada reaches the point where workers are needed and/or we merely want to make the dependency ratio look better we can gradually change the entry age of the "elderly." In association with a change in the age at which one becomes elderly, we could change the point of onset of the automatic old age pension. There could be a phased extension to age 70, and we could encourage the 65 to 69 age group to remain at work if workers are needed.

The high costs of inappropriate use of health institutions is one contributing factor. Many Canadians whose health could be supported at home, for example, are in hospital at a much greater cost. Provinces such as Manitoba are working to place the dependent population in more appropriate settings (Table 9.1).

Table 9.1

Per Diem Operating Cost of Manitoba Services 1991-92

Service	Cost
Teaching Hospital	$775.00
Community Hospital	410.00
Personal Care Home	60.27
Home Care	16.75
Support Service to Seniors	0.51

Source: Quality Health for Manitobans, the Action Plan, May 1992, Government of Manitoba.

More sophisticated calculations incorporating all or various dependent and independent populations could be made to allow us to more rationally discuss dependency ratios of the future. Unfortunately, we do not fully understand the probable impact of technological change, but it will surely eliminate many jobs, worsening the dependency ratios more rapidly than the aging population.

What about the proposals that we will need to build hundreds of LTC beds per year for the next 50 years, or that the onslaught of the elderly will completely fill our acute care beds? The former contention is easier to deal with than the latter. Our predicted LTC institutional needs become unreasonable when we note that Britain, Denmark, and others have only 50 to 70 percent as many LTC beds per 1000 people over 65 as we have, that a variety of Canadian governments and regional planning agencies are committed to controlling institutionalization, and that there are excellent alternatives to institutions that are cheaper and more suited to the LTC objectives and philosophies of today.

If we used LTC institutions as sparingly as other countries, our current supply could be adequate until our elderly population reached 18 percent of the total population, around the year 2010. If we keep building at our present rate we may, by the year 2000, have enough LTC beds to last until 2035, after which we may have empty beds as the percentage of elderly falls.

Users of LTC Who Are Physically Dependent but Mentally Competent

The prevalence of major physical dependency increases with age, but there is a physically dependent population in all age groups. Physically dependent persons who are mentally competent are, in many respects, similar to the remainder of the population.

☐ They have varied lifestyles, personalities, expectations, likes, dislikes, and prejudices. They are not homogeneous. Systems designed to serve them, therefore, need to be pluralistic rather than monolithic, and within the limitations of practical constraints each person in need should be able to have his or her needs met in a way that is consistent with his/her values and preferences.

☐ The majority of them are living at home.

☐ Maslow's Hierarchy of Needs is valid. Some attention must be given to food, shelter, and safety before giving attention to such things as affection, self-esteem, human contact, and peer approval.

☐ The health and social needs of women differ from those of men.

☐ There are varying degrees of need and want for emotional support, social contact, privacy, and the opportunity to be productive or useful.

☐ Different people have quite different perceptions of what is most important for a good quality of life.

☐ Almost everyone has an address and, therefore, a home.

☐ Almost everyone has his or her own relatively unique network of family, friends, confidantes, and advisors. However, this physically dependent but mentally competent population is, in other ways, quite different from the less physically dependent population.

☐ Because they are more dependent, they are more vulnerable. They are easier to coerce, constrain, exploit, or abuse.

☐ They are older.

☐ They respond differently to illness and injury.
1. Recovery time is much longer. The termination of an acute illness is often not followed quickly by a return to the former level of activity or capability. Even short periods of inactivity can produce long term sequelae.
2. Acute illness or new disability is frequently masked by the chronic disabilities or illness.
3. They are frequently slow to report illness or change in status. Regular screening or continued surveillance of high-risk populations can, therefore, be of great importance.

☐ The disabled, especially the elderly disabled, sometimes adapt poorly to new environments and may be confused by them. Relocation or major changes in the living environment should therefore be accompanied by appropriate resident involvement, information, and comment where appropriate.

☐ They tend to have multiple diagnoses and disabilities so assessments must be thorough.

☐ Social and economic services are increasingly important to independence. In a relative sense, therefore, health services become less important.

In the face of the limitations imposed on the dependent person, three things determine how well the individual will adapt or survive. These are his or her inherent ego strength, the severity and duration of the stress, and the support system available. The LTC services network can do almost nothing regarding the first, can affect the second, and is largely responsible for the third.

Long term dependency, by definition, means a loss of some independence; it means loss of control over some parts of one's life. **Paternalism**, by definition, places limits on the range of decision-making of the child or anyone treated like a child. When paternalistic attitudes and practices are imposed on physically or psychiatrically disabled and dependent persons who have a significant degree of mental competence, these persons are forced to deal with a double threat to their sense of control.

Power and Quality of Life

Power is vital to all people. Everyone wishes to control something. How much control is expected, and over how many things, varies immensely from person to person. The required sense of power/control can, for some people, be centered in what appear to others to be quite trivial events, opportunities, or objects. Words such as status, prestige, and self-image are central to the concept of power and how each person preserves his or her self-image or status is usually fully known only to him or her.

Prolonged loss of power, especially if the loss is seen by the client as permanent, produces anxieties, insecurity, and depression. If this is sustained, it will lead to confusion and serious mental deterioration. LTC administrators and caregivers must, if they value the quality of life of their clients, develop attitudes, skills, and practices which decrease the client's sense of powerlessness, in particular the feelings of powerlessness arising from

- ☐ loss of control over self or environment,
- ☐ lack of understanding of what is happening and of the future,
- ☐ loss of abilities and income,
- ☐ loss of social contacts, and
- ☐ controls and barriers set up by administration, such as imposed schedules and routines, which cannot be overcome.

When assertiveness fails and optimism goes, the next state is apt to be aggressiveness and depression. Restoration of control can be in the intellectual, emotional, or physical domain. Several strategies are available

- ☐ **Involve the user in decision making and respect her or his choices** whenever the making of those choices is consistent with individual rights.
- ☐ **Provide information.** Knowledge is more likely to increase than decrease security.
- ☐ **Create trust that preferences and choices will be accepted without retaliation or ostracism.** Remember that the dependent are vulnerable and are not likely to exercise control if they sense that the family or caregiver also wants control.
- ☐ **Help families and staff to acquire the skills and attitudes that will allow the dependent person to have control.**
- ☐ **Modify the environment.** Remove physical barriers and provide devices to allow performance of tasks without outside help.
- ☐ **Help the individual to set attainable goals.**

In offering people the opportunity to exercise control, it must be remembered that how much control a person chooses to exercise is for him or her to decide, and some people do not wish to make many decisions. New opportunities for control may also, at times, lead to behavior which is considered unacceptable or undesirable. This result is most likely to occur when control has been absent for a long time (as is the case after long term institutionalization) or is thought not to be sincerely offered (when the user may be testing the system).

The Mentally Incompetent Users of LTC

Institutional care has been described as an unnecessary and undesirable interference with the rights and life of mentally competent but physically dependent adults, unless being institutionalized is their preference. There are, unfortunately, a growing number of adults who are permanently unable to exercise choice.

Classification of this **mentally incompetent** population is hazardous but it can be described as a mix of the severely brain-damaged, the severely mentally retarded, the severely psychiatrically disabled, and those with advanced dementia. The brain-damaged include accident victims (mostly injured in motor vehicle accidents), victims of prolonged anoxia (as after cardiac arrest), some post-stroke patients, and severe organic brain syndrome patients (often the result of chronic alcoholism).

The **moderately or severely demented** are mostly persons with Alzheimers disease. In early decades many were housed in chronic psychiatric facilities, but most are now either in LTC facilities or being cared for at home. There is considerable disagreement regarding the extent to which home care, day care, and other services can allow this severely cognitively impaired population to stay at home. The wishes, capabilities, and emotional survival of the family caregivers deserve major consideration when creating care plans. Caring for a severely brain-damaged individual has been described as a living funeral. The caregivers often receive no rewards for their emotionally exhausting services.

Many LTC facilities in Canada do not accept demented individuals, especially if the dementia is accompanied by aggression, noise, or other unacceptable intrusion into the lives of other residents. Segregation of the seriously disruptive is recommended, although there is disagreement with regard to the degree of disorientation and disruption that merits segregation.

Staff who care for the **severely cognitively impaired** are subject to burnout with associated insensitivity, depression, absenteeism, and transfer. They need access to counselling, education, and periods of relief. They benefit from knowledgeable and interested senior administrators, and criticism should be tempered with appreciation and by awareness of the difficulty of their jobs. It is difficult to be eternally patient, kind, and loving to individuals who either do not respond or who respond with anger or abuse.

There is much written about the benefits to the demented of freedom to move about and to be outside in pleasant surroundings. Reality therapy or other behavior modification therapies can be helpful and there is a need for humane and rehabilitative surroundings. All of these are desirable, but all are sharply limited in their effects. This population must be worked with to be understood. Cost-effectiveness questions will be difficult to answer.

The **mobile brain-damaged** may progress to immobility and vegetation. In an age of scarce resources, society needs to seriously and calmly search for a definition of life as well as death. How many unresponsive adults should be diapered, tube fed, regularly turned, and routinely medically treated, and for how many months or years should such treatment be offered?

Long Term Care Services in Canada

LTC services and their delivery are fundamentally different from acute care. **Acute (short term) care** can usually concentrate on diagnosis, therapy, and rehabilitation. **Chronic care** should always give major attention to long term preservation of the quality of life of the individual. Chronic care is always delivered in a person's home, even when that person is living in one of the beds in a public ward in a LTC institution. Chronic care can be immensely supported by (and also delivered by) friends, family, and strangers. Most neighborhoods also have these sources of care. Bureaucratic and professionally dominated systems should seek to use and sustain, rather than exclude, this massive potential source of help and human warmth which is of much less importance during episodes of acute care.

LTC is obviously more sustained than acute (short term) care. Everyone would agree that a few weeks of illness or recovery from injury usually would be and should be cared for within the acute care system. There would also be agreement that multidisciplinary care over a number of years to a significantly dependent person is LTC, but the grey area between these two examples is large. It is, of course, common for patients to intermittently receive care in the acute care facilities and programs while more permanently receiving LTC.

Society appears to have responded to the needs of the dependent of all ages through a cycle in which economic assistance was provided first, health care and housing were offered next, and individualized quality of care items such as recreation, independence (autonomy) and leisure-time opportunities were made available last. This sequence exemplifies the breadth of the network that serves dependent persons.

Income Maintenance

There is minimal direct financial assistance routinely available to families caring for children requiring LTC, but low-income, permanently dependent adults qualify for disability-based support payments usually financed and administered by a provincial government. Special groups such as pensioned war veterans or persons injured at work have other income. Elderly persons, including the disabled elderly, have a number of potential federal, provincial, and private sources of income. Private pension payments are available primarily to persons who had stable employment with an employer who had an associated private pension plan. A variety of devices are also available to the elderly to protect their incomes, including reduced travel fares, extra income tax deductions, reduced recreation and entertainment admission fees, special shopping discounts, reduced tuition fees, municipal tax exemptions, and home maintenance or renovation assistance.

Although age 65 should be of no importance in itself, it has acquired significance by virtue of its selection as the age at which retirement occurs and private and public pension payments usually begin. Its relevance here is that income maintenance has an important bearing on the need for LTC.

Transportation

Most larger urban communities and some individual facilities and programs now have special buses or bus systems to respond to the local transportation needs of the handicapped. Costs per passenger are higher than those of regular transit systems, and service is usually less developed. User fees may or may not apply, depending on municipal and provincial policy.

Recreation and Social Activities

Most of these services are offered by churches and other private non-profit agencies, but municipalities increasingly offer special recreation programs through public facilities. Unfortunately, many private facilities, including churches, are not very accessible to the mobility- impaired. Recreation and social functions are also within the scope of day care centers, day hospitals, and senior citizen centers.

Residential Options

All types of LTC institutions are considered to be residential options. These include chronic hospitals (which include auxiliary hospitals, chronic care units in acute treatment hospitals, and palliative care units), and intermediate care facilities such as nursing homes and homes for special care, homes for the aged, hospices, and geriatric assessment units. Other residential (domiciliary) options include boarding homes, hostels, halfway houses, group homes, foster homes, and sheltered housing.

Long term care institutions are not usually thought of as homes but they should be. The *Ontario Nursing Homes Act* contains the phrase,". . . a nursing home is primarily the home of its residents. . ." Despite this acknowledgement, the resident is admitted, as to a hospital, is obliged to ask others for permission to go out for an evening or weekend, may be charged exorbitant fees for a private room without the protection of rent control, may live in a multibed room with strangers, has no lock on the door and no right to restrict staff entry, and cannot usually be in charge of his or her own medication regardless of mental competency. There are usually few things that will remind the resident that he or she is "at home."

The *Ontario Nursing Homes Act* also states that residents must be consulted on and involved in the planning of any program affecting their lifestyles. This is a strange burden for the nursing home administration to bear considering that the *Act* itself demands regular and continuous actions that affect lifestyle but over which neither the resident nor the nursing homes have any control. The *Act* includes a patients' Bill of Rights dealing with such things as privacy and freedom to associate, things that the institutional environment and the operating regulations have already almost destroyed.

Community LTC services can be categorized in many ways, and this list is arbitrary.

- **Services delivered to an individual at home**. These may be provided by agencies able to deliver a broad spectrum of multidisciplinary services or by agencies which specialize in only one type of assistance such as homemaking, public health nursing, meals on wheels, telephone monitoring, or emergency reporting systems. Agencies may deliver care to many types of users or may be user-specific as with palliative care.
- **Services outside the home**. These include legal aid, wheels to meals, social centers, respite care, sheltered workshops, day care, and day hospitals.

Among the community LTC services, day care, day hospitals, palliative care and placement coordination services have been selected as typical of Canadian services.

Day Care and Day Hospitals (Geriatric Day Care and Geriatric Day Hospitals)

Day care and day hospitals are discussed together because their separation may be more clear in theory than practice. Both programs receive clients 1 to 5 days a week (usually 2 to 3 days a week) for 5 to 6 hours a day. The day hospitals offer a more extensive range of professional services (physicians, nurses, physiotherapy, occupational therapy, social work, and perhaps others), give greater emphasis to rehabilitation and are twice as expensive per day ($80 to 100 vs $40 to 50). All usually provide a noon meal; they may or may not provide transportation.

The line between clients who significantly benefit from regular professional evaluation and therapy and those who require only social and recreational services and/or non-professional supervision is unclear. It seems likely that day hospitals regularly provide more expensive care than is appropriate.

Palliative Care (PC)

PC is more an attitude and a philosophy than a single program or institution. PC programs arose because of the inability or unwillingness of caregivers and health care institutions to respond appropriately to the needs of the terminally ill.

The ideal palliative care program is both community based and institutionally based. The institutions may be part of the acute care or LTC network or they may be special purpose free-standing palliative care institutions usually called hospices. Whatever the form of the institution, the PC team should be able to follow the patient into the community as well as be involved in institutional care.

PC in hospitals is sometimes delivered by teams who go to the patients on any ward and is sometimes delivered on wards used only for the terminally ill. Some PC programs use the same personnel to provide support at home and in hospital, an attractive arrangement. Most programs deal primarily with persons dying with cancer and a few deal exclusively with cancer patients. Most PC patients are persons whose death will be painful and/or whose death is considered untimely. The PC services respond to the stress suffered by the family as well as by the patient and some programs stay in touch with families during the period after their family loss.

PC is not cheap and is not promoted as being a means of reducing cost. Investigative, surgical, and therapeutic costs tend to be significantly lower, as is hospital use, but total nursing and social service costs rise. The objective is to replace technological and cure-oriented personnel with a calm, caring, and supportive team.

The palliative care and modern hospice concepts are usually credited to Dr. Cecily Saunders in England who was a pioneer in the field. In the past decade the movement has expanded quickly in Canada. In 1987, the Palliative Care Foundation of Canada, (established in 1981) reported that about 300 palliative care programs were operating across the country: 42 percent were entirely hospital-based, 24 percent were operating only in the community and 34 percent operated both in the hospital and in the community. Despite the increase in the number of programs, they serve less than 5 percent of all dying patients and perhaps 10 percent of patients dying with cancer.

Assessment and Placement Services

The use of regionally or provincially **standardized assessment practices** is necessary if selection of the volume and the types of care that should be delivered to each LTC patient at public expense is to be equitable. Common assessment forms and personnel reduce the likelihood of institutional or practitioner manipulation of who is eligible for various levels of publicly financed services. They also reduce the ability of institutions to manipulate in the interest of getting long stay patients out of acute care beds.

Central control, or at least influence, over placement is crucial if the needs of patients, as seen by them, are to be reasonably matched with the capabilities of various programs and institutions and if individuals in the community and in acute care hospitals are to have relatively equal access to all LTC spaces. It reduces the likelihood that there will be informal arrangements between LTC and acute care facilities, arrangements designed to serve the institutions rather than the individuals involved. Central assessment and placement can also assure consideration of utilization of noninstitutional options when possible, although many regional agencies have been undesirably institutionally oriented. Standardized procedures should be designed to provide ample opportunity for users to examine placement and treatment options and decide which they prefer.

The Role of Acute Treatment Hospitals in LTC

Acute treatment hospitals will continue to have a major role in the provision of LTC. A number of years ago, Quebec hospitals were told to designate 10 percent of acute beds as chronic beds and to make the necessary program adaptations. In Ontario, available LTC beds in chronic hospitals, nursing homes, and homes for the aged are given first to qualified applicants living in the community. Those receiving care in another institution are admitted next. This policy assures people at home that they will be admitted reasonably quickly if conditions worsen. It is hoped that this assurance will encourage dependent persons to stay in the community as long as possible. Acute treatment hospitals should accept their responsibility for the care of many LTC patients and should develop special programs for them.

Foster Homes, Home Sharing, and Granny Flats

These are not designed for persons with significant degrees of dependency. Each is attractive to some persons and households.

Foster homes usually offer room and board and minimal personal care or supervision. It is quite reasonable, however, for foster homes to care for individuals with more severe dependency. Payment should vary with the level of care required.

Home sharing matches the homeless with persons who have extra space. It can offer advantages to both parties in the form of income, social contact, or assistance of many kinds.

Granny flats are small residences in the yards or homes of family caregivers. The older generation in rural societies has, for years, shared a home with younger generations. The biggest hazards to this program are bureaucrats who write unreasonably complex rules and who demand unreasonable standards, and neighborhoods which are more concerned about property values or street esthetics than about helping families support and be close to elderly or dependent members who wish a home of their own.

Sheltered Housing

This term refers to a variety of architectural and service arrangements in which a number of domiciliary units are supported by on-site staff. The support staff can be limited to basic assistance, or it can consist of three shifts of full-time workers able to offer levels of care comparable to those available in LTC facilities. As many as 5 percent of the elderly in the United Kingdom live in sheltered housing.

In Canada, this arrangement is routinely available only for the young physically disabled. Quadriplegics in special housing may require up to six hours of personal care a day. This care may include being turned through the night, being helped in and out of bed, being dressed for school or work, and being fed. This need for a large volume of care does not prevent the disabled from being tenants in the fullest sense rather than institutional residents. The care is delivered as home care rather than as institutional care and costs compare favorably. This model merits major consideration as another residential option for the disabled elderly.

Services with the Primary Objectives of Prolonging Life and Maintaining Physical Health

Prolonging life has often been considered the prime objective of LTC. Compassion and client involvement in decisionmaking become expendable in the face of the fear that clients might, for example, fall and be hurt.

Most LTC services at least indirectly protect life or maintain physical health, but a few of these services have no other primary objective. Some disabled, for example, now carry devices through which they can call for assistance if it is needed. Others live in apartments with communication or alarm mechanisms that will, in an emergency, alert neighbors or staff who will then visit. Programs such as Postal Alert or those offering a daily telephone call are designed to prevent prolonged failure to get help. The telephone monitoring services are usually conducted by the elderly themselves, sometimes by residents in LTC institutions.

Services with the Primary Objective of Protection and Elevation of Quality of Life

Having a decent home and enough money to remain there comfortably and safely are probably more important to most people than a comprehensive network of community-based health and social services, but as dependency increases, the latter eventually are needed. One cannot predict which programs and services will protect or elevate quality of life for a specific person. This objective is, however, usually thought to be served by those things that allow people to stay in their own homes if they wish, that help to preserve households, and that encourage user decision making with respect to such things as accommodation, privacy, and social activities.

The protection of quality of life is not assured by the mere availability of a full range of services. It also requires planners who vigorously seek to provide viable choices, and caregivers and advisors (professionals, family members, and friends) who will sincerely support whatever option the client chooses. The concept of viable options can refer to levels of privacy, volumes of social contact or physical activity, types of recreation or entertainment, degrees of decision making or degrees of risk or safety, among other things.

Services Which Can Make it Possible for a User to Remain at Home

These services fall into four main categories.

1. Services which make the physical environment more tolerable or manageable.

    ☐ **Home maintenance activities** such as the removal and installation of storm windows.

    ☐ **Home adaptations** such as the installation of ramps, grab bars in the bathroom, or better lighting.

    ☐ **Improved security and emergency alarm systems**. These were listed earlier as services that protect life but for that part of the population for whom a feeling of security/safety is essential to peace of mind, these services also improve quality of life and eliminate one of the reasons for leaving one's own home.

2. Services which provide basic householder functions.

    ☐ **Meals on wheels**. These services, most of which are run by voluntary organizations, usually pick up meals from a hospital or LTC facility and sell them at cost to persons unable to prepare meals. There is usually one delivery per day, five days a week, of a hot lunch and cold supper. Drivers are often volunteers.

    ☐ **Wheels to meals**. Drivers, once again usually volunteers, deliver isolated individuals to central dining locations. This service provides social opportunities as well as nutritional support.

    ☐ **Homemaker services**. This service provides assistance with cooking, cleaning, laundry, and perhaps some counselling and socializing. Homemakers are available with or without public subsidy and subsidy, when available, may be with or without means testing. The homemakers may have almost no training or be graduates from 3 to 6 month homemaking courses. The services are available from profit and non-profit agencies although the great majority are provided by staff of non-profit agencies.

3. Services which deliver personal care such as assistance with bathing, toileting, or transferring. These services are usually delivered by semiskilled personnel.

4. Professional services offered through several administrative arrangements and several kinds of personnel.

☐ **Nurse visits to the home**. Most programs limit attendance to 1 to 2 visits per day maximum and 1 to 3 visits per week as an average, although for palliative care or short term problems more frequent visits may be available.

☐ **Home visits** by physicians, physiotherapists, speech therapists, nutritionists, clinical nurse specialists, and other professionals. Physicians' home visits appear to be more appreciated than needed. Their availability, or lack of availability, does not appear to be a factor in whether or not patients stay in their own homes versus being admitted to an institution. Physician visits are most likely to be needed for prescribing medication, giving advice, assessing the patient, carrying out procedures, or counselling.

☐ In some provinces, certain senior citizen buildings have an in-house medical office with regular attendance of a variety of health care professionals but with the public health nurse being the central caregiver. Office and apartment visits are available during normal working hours.

☐ Twenty-four-hour staff adjacent to disabled persons in private residential units. This is a variation on home care. It is provided through several different noninstitutional models in which the residents are tenants rather than "admitted" patients. The apartments and group homes may be owned and operated for profit or they may be nonprofit. There may or may not be a central dining room. They may or may not accept disabled persons with families. The staff may be all nonprofessional or a mix of professional and nonprofessional. Costs vary with the extent to which services are provided. When the residents pay all costs the rent and services may cost $2,000 per month or more for a very modest level of assistance.

Services Which Preserve Households

When a household requires levels or types of care that cannot be delivered through existing programs or by other members of the household the person in need will either not get the care or will lose the pleasures of staying with friends and/or family. Of the service arrangements listed earlier, only the option of 24-hour immediate availability of adequate volumes and types of care, delivered to residential units of the needed size, can preserve households in the face of almost all situations of dependency. Other arrangements can meet intermediate levels of dependency.

In speaking of the preservation of households, one must remember that the dependent person is only one of the individuals to be considered. Other household members also face financial, career, and personal challenges. The LTC network must consciously identify and work to meet these challenges if the household is to be preserved and the quality of life of all household members protected. Additional stress may be placed on women (as traditional caregivers) if they also work outside the home.

Stress to the household caregiver(s) arises from

☐ the dependent person's wandering, aggression, and incontinence,

- ☐ the additional expense,
- ☐ the destruction of the quality of the caregiver's personal life,
- ☐ the inability to obtain short term relief, and
- ☐ fear of injury or illness.

Supporting the household caregivers would seem to be logical both to reduce these stresses and in the interest of cost control through continued involvement of no-cost providers. Unfortunately the system has, in the past, often failed to welcome or to support family caregivers. Fifteen years ago in Ontario, a family with a developmentally handicapped or autistic child, for example, either provided care without system support or admitted the child to an institution. The caregivers were isolated and exploited. In recent years several devices have been used to support household caregivers.

☐ **Financial aid**.
1. In British Columbia, funds are provided by government to families who care for their severely retarded children at home. The amount to be paid is determined by a voluntary agency (The Living Society) acting as an assessor, counsellor and quality control vehicle (within Ministry guidelines). Financial aid can be used to hire help, to enable the family caregiver to stay at home or to meet various direct and indirect costs such as drugs, equipment, and laundry.
2. A number of states in the United States provide tax incentives. At best these are not very effective and are of no value to households that pay no tax.
3. When the dependent person is mentally competent, the required extra money can be given to him or her to purchase required services. This practice is followed in some European countries.

☐ Legislated or voluntary **sabbaticals from work** without penalty and with job protection.

☐ **Training and education** regarding caregiving skills, understanding the situation and coping with stress.

☐ **Respite care programs** which provide household caregivers with relief for a few hours, days, or weeks. The need may be scheduled, so as to allow vacations, or unexpected, as when the caregiver becomes ill. Relief may be obtained by bringing another person into the home or by taking the dependent person to another location. Generally speaking, the term "respite care" is not meant to include short term relief such as that provided by a homemaker or a day care or day hospital unit, although the benefits are similar to those associated with longer term separation of regular caregiver and care recipient.

Respite care arrangements are currently not adequate. Most accommodation is in the form of one bed in a home for the aged or nursing home. It may not always be available, and it usually is poorly publicized. Too often, there are rules that limit access to not less than one week and not more then 2 to 4 weeks per year. There is minimal availability of regular weekend relief.

Administrators do not tend to welcome personalized arrangements. Just as there is little effort to help institutionalized persons to regularly spend time with family, there is not much imagination applied to the question of how to help dependent persons stay at home for 50, 40, or 30 weeks of the year, or for 4, 5, or 6 days a week. The household is routinely expected to adapt to bureaucratic rigidities, instead of the system adapting to household problems and constraints. The same attitudes are seen in day care programs that serve a major relief function but are useful only to those caregivers who can adapt to 9:30 to 3:30 service.

For selected persons, in particular those who are confused or acutely distressed by new caregivers and surroundings, consideration should be given to respite care in which the alternate caregivers are persons who are known and who will provide care in familiar surroundings.

In summary, the services that most directly preserve households include all those which either protect the household caregivers from financial, emotional and/or physical burnout or which provide care at home of a type that cannot be provided by the household caregiver.

Services Which Promote User Control

Any service which allows anyone to be independent in any respect obviously increases that individual's opportunities for control. Examples of such services or might be a seeing eye dog, a ramp, a telephone adaptation for the hearing impaired, an electric wheelchair, or additional disposable income. Conversely, anything which prevents a person from exercising independence reduces that individual's opportunity for control. Such barriers to independence include institutional regulations regarding pets, plants, visitors, outside visiting, or how one may spend available wealth.

In general, it is assumed that all of those services which allow a person to stay out of an institution also increase the opportunity for user control. This assumption, however, is not always correct. The private living arrangements of many dependent persons may be isolated, not physically adapted, and generally more restrictive than the environment of an institution committed to resident decision making.

The Financing of LTC

Acute care in Canada is almost routinely financed through global budgets or fee-for-service. The financing of LTC, however, has no standard pattern.

Some degree of care at home, at least to the level of public health nursing, is publicly funded in all provinces. Beyond this level of service there is a mixture of public/private financing in the Atlantic provinces, with those who request additional services usually being means tested. In six provinces, additional levels of care at home are universal and publicly funded.

Long term care institutions are partly or entirely publicly funded through either a global budget, a per diem rate, or, as with municipally owned Homes for the Aged in Ontario, an initial budget plus assured coverage of operating deficits. Institutions such as chronic hospitals in Ontario, which care for the most severely disabled, are funded through a global budget in exactly the same way as an acute care hospital. In some other provinces payment is via a fixed and standardized per diem rate. Alberta and British Columbia have led the way in establishing standard assessment procedures and standard payments for persons at a particular level of care. Payments do not vary on the basis of the ownership of the institutions; rates are the same for profit and nonprofit institutions.

In all provinces, most clients/residents pay $300 to 600 per month toward the cost of care. The payment is usually set so that it can be met by the old age supplement while leaving a $50 to 100 per month comfort allowance. Residents also pay for semi-private and private accommodation in most institutions. A private room in Ontario in a chronic hospital can cost over $600 a month. This outrageous fee for the privilege of being alone in a small room represents the only residential rental payment in Ontario to which rent control does not apply. (Several years ago the Ontario government removed the ceiling from preferred accommodation rates and gave 100 percent of that revenue to the institutions. Many hospitals, both acute and chronic, immediately sharply increased their rates.)

LTC can also be financed by making funds available to the users or their guardians or agents.

Summary

Many questions have been raised. Should we consider the elderly to be the same as the rest of us but older? The answer is, very definitely, yes. Do we believe the disabled population should have the same opportunities as the rest of us to the extent feasible? Once again, the answer is definitely yes, and this answer rules out all paternalistic professional control that reduces the opportunity for a disabled person to make decisions.

Existing LTC institutions and some of the legislation which governs them are incompatible with the principles enshrined in the literature, the political speeches, and the mission statements of the institutions themselves. Social intent is good but adaptation of professionals and institutions is slow to the point of being a barrier to progress. Never have such a large group of users been so in need of advocates.

References

Hendrick, S.C., Inui, T.S. (1986). The effectiveness of cost of home care: An information synthesis. *Health Services Research*, 20(60): 851-880.

Lane, D. et. al (1985). Forecasting demand for long term care services. *Health Services Research*, 20(4): 435-460.

McDaniel, Susan A. (1986) *Canada's Aging Population*, Toronto: Butterworth.

Thornton, C., Dunstan, S.M., Kemper, P. (1988). The evaluation of the National Long Term Care Demonstration: The effect of channeling on health and long term care costs. *Health Services Research*, 23(1): 129-142.

CHAPTER 10

Emerging Health Professions, Dental Services, and Emergency Services

H istory, technology, economics, politics, and geography have helped to determine Canada's present mix of health workers. Florence Nightingale created the generalist nurses that are still graduating from nursing schools today. Nurse anesthetists established their competence 50 years ago but they could not survive in Canada in the face of the organized and male power of physicians who wished to control the discipline. Respiratory Technologists appeared for uncertain reasons; nurses could have absorbed this new component of patient care if they had been interested or the cylinders of gas had been lighter. The need to provide care to small isolated northern settlements led to the special training of nurse practitioners. In the south, however, the physicians again exercised their power and relegated the nurse to limited functions in even more limited locations. In Saskatchewan, economics led to the creation of a childrens' dental program dependent on the dental therapist; politics in a later era gave the program back to the more expensive, but more politically favored, privately practicing dentist. A scarcity of trained laboratory technologists at the time of the introduction of mass cervical screening (Pap smears) led to the use of job specific technicians to do the work. Yet, despite a similar shortage of physiotherapists and the proven adequacy of physiotherapy aides, we have very few aide training programs because physiotherapists do not approve.

There has been a rather random pattern in the appearance of new kinds of health providers who work in association with physicians or dentists. Orthopedic technicians who repair or apply casts were welcomed by the interns and surgeons who previously put on the casts. Dental hygienists are routinely employed to perform examinations and preventive functions formerly performed by dentists. However, at the same time, physicians are objecting to the appearance of midwives, and dentists have opposed expanded roles and freedoms for denturists. The mixture of acceptances and rejection is a practical one. New workers, or new roles for existing workers, are usually welcomed if they will reduce physician/dentist work without loss of physician/dentist fee-for-service income. If there is a threat to income the new workers or new roles tend to be opposed.

The question of the future role of the registered nursing assistant (RNA) is a matter of importance. Nursing associations have proposed that no one but a registered nurse (RN) should provide direct nursing care, a proposal with conceptual, economic, and social consequences. Conceptually, we should defend the idea of high volume work being done, when possible, by the least skilled person who can do it adequately. We should promote the idea of assigning skilled persons to the level of work for which they are prepared. Financially, we should want to keep the lower cost RNA, and socially we should resist changes which reduce the employment opportunities for semi-skilled, often middle-aged and usually female, workers. This battle is far from over although some active treatment hospitals have already reduced their employment of RNAs.

The male-female mix of health care workers is also changing. Canadian health administration schools have many more female than male graduates and females are approaching or have reached parity in many medical schools.

Education of Health Workers

Health worker training in Canada is usually partly academic and partly practical. The academic portion leading to a degree or diploma is usually provided by an educational center which is within the jurisdiction of a department of education. The academic program usually includes practical training as well as academic material but the academic experience is also commonly supplemented by a quite separate and often mandatory period of apprenticeship after graduation. Within these general specifications there is considerable variation.

A registered nurse (RN), for instance, may be a graduate of a 2 or 3 year community college program or a 3 or 4 year baccalaureate program but no postdiploma or post-baccalaureate apprenticeship is required for professional licensure. During the baccalaureate program the student may usually, at her or his choice, concentrate on one field of nursing such as public health, psychiatry, pediatrics, or geriatrics. Besides the academic exam, the graduate nurse may need to pass a provincial exam to be eligible for provincial licensure or certification.

The one year postgraduate certificate programs which were formerly common in public health nursing and psychiatric nursing, for instance, have now been largely abandoned due to increased attention to these nursing fields within the academic nursing programs. Prior to the 1960s, nursing education was usually based in a general hospital where psychiatric and public health nursing experience were often not available. There is, unfortunately, considerable evidence that the new graduate nurse is not adequately prepared for many of the tasks that will be assigned, including work in the operating room, the emergency room, and the intensive care units. This is a significant problem considering the fact that 80 percent of all nurses are employed in hospitals and that there are only a few large scale post RN programs offering specialized clinical training.

The great majority of new nurses continue to be graduates of non-baccalaureate programs, but the Canadian Nurses Association (CNA), with the support of provincial nursing associations, has announced its wish that all nurses should, by the year 2000, be graduates of a baccalaureate program. This objective, which seems reasonable in light of the stature of nurses and the responsibility given to them, can be met as long as there is

- ☐ early planning for expansion of university nursing faculties and other resources,
- ☐ acceptance of the need to lower the current admission standards of university nursing programs, and
- ☐ a willingness to utilize less expensive personnel where reasonable patient outcomes can be achieved.

Most of the necessary faculty should be available in the existing community college programs, but faculty with the academic credentials usually required will be in short supply.

There appear to be no insurmountable financial, cultural, conceptual, or logistical problems associated with the change to baccalaureate training for nurses. The major financial hazard lies in increasing training costs because university education is longer and more expensive per year than community college training. The pay differential between a baccalaureate and non-baccalaureate nurse is small and nurse pay scales are already commensurate with or better than those associated with other baccalaureate graduates. Employment costs should, therefore, change very little. Nevertheless, despite the apparent feasibility and appropriateness of the CNA proposal there has been little hospital or governmental support for the idea of converting to the baccalaureate model.

Governments, health care institutions (including hospitals), and the public are not particularly concerned about how competence is acquired or who approves it, they merely wish it to be there. Nursing leaders who strongly push an expansion of clinical masters degrees in nursing would do their profession a service if they chose instead to concentrate on the development of a multitude of hospital-based post baccalaureate nurse specialist programs. This is the pattern which produced the internationally renowned British midwife and the neurosurgical nurses trained at the Montreal Neurological Institute. The current practice is for nurse graduates to acquire special skills while on the job and, although this undoubtedly results in good competence after several years in the same clinical setting, it would be of benefit to all if the special skills could be more thoroughly acquired through supervised and formal post RN programs taken before attempting to provide sophisticated nursing care.

Dental Services

Providers of dental care still look after teeth and gums but dental occupations and patterns of morbidity, financing, and organization have, in the past 20 years, undergone significant change.

Manpower

The dental model, in which the dentist is the only one who can prescribe, has been modified. It is now common for a denturologist (Quebec), a denture therapist, a denturist, or a similar dental worker by some other name to legally fit, produce, and sell a denture or partial denture or to repair a denture, with little or no contact with a dentist. In Saskatchewan for almost 15 years, dental therapists (originally called dental nurses) filled, extracted, and capped the teeth of children without on-site supervision by a dentist.

The range of dental specialization has increased and now includes

- orthodontics,
- dental (oral and maxillofacial) surgery,
- public health dentistry,
- pedodontics (children),
- periodontics (care of gums),
- endodontics (care of roots of teeth),
- prosthodontics (the production and use of prostheses), and
- oral pathology.

Orthodontists are the largest specialty group followed by dental surgeons.

In addition to increasing specialization by dentists, there has been aggressive entry of many unspecialized general dentists into some of the specialty fields. Whether all specialties, especially pediatric dentistry and endodontics, can survive in the face of this trend remains to be seen.

Dental hygienists, whose role is primarily patient education and the cleaning and assessing of teeth, continue to work under the immediate direction of dentists. In provinces such as British Columbia, hygienists are lobbying for some independent practice, including such activities as cleaning teeth for residents in long term care. Dental assistants, who may or may not have formal training, provide chairside assistance to dentists. Canada has one dentist per 2,000-2,200 population with regional variations of from 1 per 1,500 (British Columbia) to 1 per 4,400 (Newfoundland).

After peaking in 1983, dental school enrollment in Canada has been steady at about 450 entering students per year. Dental school enrollment in the United States fell 23 percent from 1978 to 1985 and the trend is likely to occur in Canada. The supply of dental assistants and dental hygienists continues to increase. They work primarily in dentists' offices on salary and are sources of assistance and additional income for the dentist.

There is general acceptance that both Canada and the United States have a current oversupply of dentists. Whether a condition of oversupply continues will depend on such diverse factors as

- whether the current middle-aged population, who use dental care quite regularly, will continue to do so when they are elderly,
- whether the capitation approach to financing increases with its associated need for fewer dentists,
- whether the use of auxiliaries, whose adequacy was confirmed in the Saskatchewan dental program, will be controlled or allowed to grow, and
- whether or not research, by virologists or immunologists for example, will develop vaccines or new therapies to control periodontal disease.

The greatest growth in dentistry has been in the field of aesthetics. Orthodontists were, at one time, interested in a good fit of upper and lower teeth. Now both they and their patients wish a perfect appearance as well as a perfect bite. Braces are now chic and crooked or darkened teeth are passé. There has also been a marked increase in dental involvement in therapy of the temporomandibular joint.

There is now also an increasing sense that teeth are to be saved at all costs. A lost tooth or a removable denture represent dental failure. Root canals and implants have increased. One area of probable growth in dental services is in long term care institutions, many of which now operate with minimal consideration of the dental needs of residents.

The Saskatchewan Children's Dental Program

No discussion of Canadian dental care would be complete without a description of the creation and partial destruction of the children's dental care plan in Saskatchewan.

In 1968, with federal assistance, a three-year pilot program of dental care for children 3 to 12 years of age was put in place in the town of Oxbow, Saskatchewan. Teams of one dentist, two dental nurses, and three dental assistants provided the care. The nurses extracted deciduous (baby) teeth and placed fillings in deciduous and permanent teeth. On the strength of the success of this trial, which drew extensively on the dental nurse program in New Zealand, plans were made to introduce a province-wide children's dental program.

Training of the necessary staff was provided through a specially created community college program. The *Saskatchewan Dental Nurses Act* was passed (1973) authorizing the dental nurses to do selected dental work. In 1974, with the graduation of the first class of the new dental workers, the program was begun. In 1974, services were offered only to children born in 1968. The program was expanded at a rate consistent with the expanding supply of dental nurses until all children over the age of 3 were enrolled. Over 400 permanent clinics were established in schools throughout the province. Enrollment was voluntary but over 85 percent of eligible non-native children were enrolled. Less than half of eligible native children enrolled.

In 1976, three outside dental specialists evaluated more than 2000 fillings and 97 steel crowns in 410 children. They did not know whether the work had been done by dentists or by dental nurses and work was classified as unacceptable, adequate, or superior. The work of the nurses was considerably better than that of the dentists.

Table 10.1

Quality of Dental Work in 410 Saskatchewan Children by Type of Provider — 1976

	Dentist	Dental Nurse
Superior	16.5	47.4
Adequate	62.4	48.6
Unacceptable	21.1	3.7

Source: Annual Reports, Saskatchewan Health Dental Plan.

Costs per child fell steadily for the first 6 to 8 years and then climbed in keeping with inflation. The condition of the teeth of the children improved markedly, at least partly because of the large educational component of the program.

The initial dental team in the Oxbow trial had one dentist and five auxiliary workers. By the early 1980s the team ratio had become one dentist and approximately twenty auxiliaries. (In usual dental practice the team is one dentist to two or three auxiliary workers.)

This program is one of the truly excellent cases of how new health programs should be introduced. The new program was tested and shown to be feasible, a program was created to train necessary staff, the necessary legislation was written to allow the new staff to provide dental care and there was preservation of a consultative role for dentists with a steady trend toward transfer of work to less expensive personnel. The services emphasized prevention as well as treatment. The program was expanded at a rate consistent with the production of new personnel so that jobs were available for the new graduates and so that those promised services were able to get them. Moreover, the quality of the dental work was evaluated by outside, extremely credible dentist evaluators (members of dental school faculty). There was a regular and startling (sometimes 50 percent) annual reduction in the dental pathology in the children seen and costs per child fell steadily throughout all of the early years of the program.

The unique features of the Saskatchewan dental plan are now largely dismantled. The dental nurses (who were officially renamed dental therapists) are largely unemployed and dental care has been returned to dentists on a fee-for-service basis with limited provincial financial responsibility. Political debts and orientations, plus the wish to reduce public expenditures even when private costs for the same or fewer benefits would be higher, have eliminated an administrative and service model that should have swept the country.

The Dental Health of Canadians

In Ontario between 1972 and 1986, there was a 51 percent reduction in caries in 5-year-olds and a 53 percent reduction in 13-year-olds. The percentage of these children with no caries rose from 42 to 66 percent for 5-year-olds and from 8 percent to 31 percent for 13-year-olds. The decline has been greatest in communities with fluoridated water but has occurred everywhere. Other factors at work include fluoride toothpaste, fluoride mouth rinses, the addition of vitamin D and other nutritional requirements to milk and other products, and better oral hygiene. Preventive activities in dental offices, including cleaning and use of topical fluorides and of sealants, also contribute, as does a higher level of treatment of existing caries. There is a possibility that the widespread use of antibiotics may also be a factor. Improvement does not appear to be due to changes in dietary habits, in particular in our consumption of sugar.

Despite these improvements, there are still great inequities in accessibility and utilization of dental services. Eighty percent of the caries that are identified exist in 20 percent of the children. Improvements in the dental health of children will be reflected in the health of future adults.

Dental Care Costs, Payment, and Financing

Dentist earnings have, for a number of years, stayed close to 5 percent of each dollar spent on Canadian health care. Although almost all dentists are paid on a fee-for-service basis there has, in recent years, been an increase in the number of prepaid dental insurance programs in which dentist payment is by patient year or family year, that is, by capitation. The plans are often operated by insurance companies which wish to have more predictable costs. They are attractive to dentists because there is an assured supply of patients and a guaranteed income in a highly competitive market. Dental associations are vigorously opposed to these new plans on the grounds that patients will be underserviced. There has not been equal concern about the probability that fee-for-service is associated with the provision of unnecessary care. The capitation approach has been shown to cut costs per patient per year by approximately 40 percent. Employer/employee sponsored dental plans have grown rapidly since the early 1970s with about one third of the Canadian population, now enrolled (coverage is highest in Ontario).

Other Health Services

Response to Physical Emergencies

Physical emergencies occur everywhere: at home, at work, at play, at school, and in the hospital. Major components of the emergency response system include

- a communications network,
- case finding mechanisms,
- on-site first aid,
- on-site professional care,
- transportation arrangements,
- care in hospital emergency departments (ED) or rooms (ER), and
- disaster planning.

The Area-Wide Approach to Emergency Care

There was a time when every hospital had an emergency department and serious emergency cases were spread among them all. Specialization and referrals were uncommon. Evidence has now proved that high quality emergency care requires a different model. In Russia, some hospitals are dedicated fully to trauma care. British experts believe that a population of approximately one million is the proper base for one highly sophisticated trauma center with a full range of specialized services available 24 hours a day, 7 days a week. The armies of the world are masters of triage, and triage plus a hierarchical and integrated network of care centers has immensely improved recovery rates.

Emergency services are a stand-by network. They never know when difficult obstetrical, cardiac, infectious, or traumatic cases may arrive. They must be ready for head injuries, eye injuries, chest injuries, burns, respiratory difficulties, and severe blood loss, and each of these requires its own mix of specialized services. It is economically unreasonable to maintain the highest level of stand-by capability in any institution at which very few complex cases arrive per month or per year. It is also impossible to maintain the clinical skills of the medical, nursing, and other staff unless there is a reasonably steady arrival of cases requiring those special skills.

Canada has been very slow to plan and allocate resources for its emergency care, although some progress has been made. In many smaller urban centers, for example, only one of the two or three hospitals is now operating an emergency room, and global planning in large metropolitan centers is beginning.

In the early 1980s, Ontario proposed that all hospital emergency departments be placed in one of four categories — comprehensive, (of which the most sophisticated would be called a trauma center), major, general, and basic. Staffing, budgeting, and hours of operation would correspond to the category assigned. This categorization, which is still in its earliest stages of implementation, will help clients and ambulance personnel know where to go and it will provide better care at less cost. In time, if the categorization is implemented, only a few urban hospitals will operate a 24-hour emergency service, with most other hospitals and some free-standing health care units operating a less comprehensive service for 10-to-18 hours a day. The volume of minor emergencies during the night hours is low enough to be handled by the stand-by staff in the higher level emergency centers.

Sudbury, Ontario, is an example of a city with fully integrated hospital emergency care. Sudbury General has 24-hour emergency coverage, Sudbury Memorial closes its emergency at midnight, and Sudbury Laurentian has no emergency department at all. In Toronto, three hospitals have been designated as trauma centers — Sunnybrook, St. Michaels, and The Hospital for Sick Children. Wellesley Hospital has the only burn center in Toronto.

The major fear of the population when a reduction in the number of 24-hour emergency departments is suggested is that people will suffer or die because of the additional travelling time. There is no doubt that occasional headlines will arise when someone dies en-route to an urban emergency department when another hospital would have been closer, but there will be many more people who will be saved because they arrive at a better-equipped and better-staffed emergency department. The number who are harmed by a few more minutes of travel will be even less if patients are transported in well-equipped and well-staffed ambulances, and the quality of these vehicles and staff is constantly improving. The person who dies while travelling a bit farther will usually be someone who would have died anyway. The principle of centralization of 24-hour emergency services is much less applicable to rural areas, but even here patients would often be better served by travelling farther in a good ambulance to a better-equipped and better-staffed emergency department.

Reducing the functions of emergency departments will be most firmly resisted by medical staff. Many medical practitioners expect some of their patients to be admitted through the emergency department, and rerouting of emergency patients to another hospital will transfer those patients to the caseloads of physicians who are on staff at the other hospital. The clinical realignments will be quite major in some communities. For example, in greater Ottawa, with less than a million people, there are 6 emergency units staffed 24 hours a day, and many other cities show the same oversupply.

Hospital emergency departments designed to handle major emergencies should expect to have periods without much to do. At other times there will be too much to do. The more one tries to make sure the staff are always busy, the less prepared the department will be for new major emergencies.

Central Monitoring

When several or many emergency departments are operating, as is the case in all major urban centers, there is no good way of predicting which departments will be under excessive pressure at any given hour. The unexpected arrival of an unmanageable volume of patients, or a back-up in the ER of patients waiting for transfer to wards with no empty beds has, in the past, led to some hospitals declaring their emergency departments temporarily closed. This closure has, at times, occurred without knowledge of whether other hospitals were any better able to handle the emergencies being turned away.

Several major centers (Hamilton, Toronto) now have a centralized monitoring service constantly aware of the availability of beds in all hospitals and of the volume of patients awaiting care in all emergency departments. This central office advises ambulances and others of the best place to go, and it can determine whether or not it is reasonable for a particular emergency department to be temporarily closed to additional cases. The central monitoring (often referred to as a central bed registry), plus ER classification, will allow ERs to act more like a coordinated network.

Emergency departments with over 40,000 visits per year should have a permanent formal referral arrangement through which selected patients can be referred to an ambulatory care unit during high volume hours. Toronto General Hospital has made such referrals since 1986. Many patients who come to ERs are better cared for in a normal office setting, where routine examinations and counselling are the service best delivered, than in an ER where heroic measures and early referral are the norm. Referral can, after triage, transfer many patients to a hospital outpatient department, a community health center or some other site of office-based care. These offices are much more appropriate for the immediate care and the follow-up of the kinds of emotional, social, and medical problems that are common among ER patients.

ERs and Routine Ambulatory Care

Seventy-five to ninety percent of patients who come to emergency departments have problems that are not life threatening, which can be dealt with in a relatively ordinary office, treatment room, or minor surgery, and whose treatment can be safely deferred for a few minutes or hours.

A small percentage of patients have a major illness or injury which, after examination and minimal stabilization, leads to rapid transfer to an intensive care unit, a coronary care unit, or an inpatient ward (assuming that a bed is available). A very small group require major, immediate, and sometimes quite sustained, multidisciplinary attention in the emergency room.

The volume of patients in the first group (the 75 to 90 percent) is on the basis of previous experience fairly predictable for any good-sized emergency department. Volumes vary with time of day, day of week, season of year, and specific local events or conditions. The second two categories of patients arrive quite randomly, although higher volumes can be expected on selected evenings such as Saturdays, in certain weather conditions, or on selected long weekends. These seriously ill or injured persons are the ones who require the major standby capability that characterizes a high quality trauma center.

ERs are a major source of routine medical care, receiving 0.5 to 1 visit per person per year. There is considerable disagreement over whether or not most of these users are receiving care in the right place. Certainly many could be cared for at home (though few doctors make house calls), or in an office (though offices are more often closed than open), but do these facts mean that the visit is inappropriate? Providers of care are often critical of persons who come to the ER with a rash, a headache, or a sore back, especially when the problem has been present for some time or appears to be minor. These persons are often referred to as abusers of the system; that is, they are thought of as persons who are taking advantage of the service and should somehow be discouraged.

Patients who are seen as abusers of emergency services also include the inebriated, the neurotic, the terminally ill, the chronically ill, the socially detached or maladjusted, and those who drop in on the way home from a party for advice about a chronic complaint because they do not want to take time off from work. All but the last group are persons to whom emergency services should be offered without complaint. Emergency assistance should be available through social work staff, mental health staff, and formal referral arrangements. To be hungry, cold, confused, or drunk can be as hazardous as having pneumonia or a protruded intervertebral disc.

The terminally ill are especially stressful for caregivers as well as family. The family is frightened and may become angry when hospital admission is refused. The family is emotionally unsupported in the face of an impending family death and they would like some help. Emergency physicians, on the other hand, may feel that acute treatment hospital services are not needed and may not be appropriate. Referral to a palliative care team should be routine, but palliative care backup is not always available.

The chronically ill can be equally difficult. These include patients with problems such as panic syndrome, chronic asthma, muscular dystrophy, or chronic obstructive lung disease. Good links with social work staff and home support systems will reduce the user/institutional conflict arising from unwillingness to admit.

It is easy to be quite critical of "callous" emergency room staff but, in the face of quite precise and necessary criteria for hospital admission, these caregivers must regularly play the role of gatekeepers. Their decisions cannot always be acceptable to everyone, nor will they always be right, but most of them do as well as the rest of us would.

The discussion of when individuals are abusing emergency departments is not worth much effort, since no good devices have been found to keep patients away. Long waiting times aggravate everyone and bring unreasonable inconvenience, discomfort, and sometimes hazard. Triage and the use of an affiliated ambulatory care unit can improve efficiency and quality and can protect the stand-by capability needed in major ERs.

Special Communication Problems

All medical care, including emergency care, must be delivered to the deaf, the aphasic, the mentally retarded, the emotionally disturbed, and those who speak languages other than those most commonly in use. Some hospitals, such as The Hospital for Sick Children in Toronto, have a vast army of volunteer interpreters. All major emergency departments should be prepared for patients speaking any of the languages used fairly commonly in their community, and all should have personnel trained in the handling of persons with other communication problems.

Disaster Response

The emergency department in even a sophisticated trauma center is hard pressed to handle 5 to 10 serious injuries that arrive simultaneously. Occasionally, however, a community is faced with hundreds of casualties or with the need to evacuate hospitals and/or neighborhoods; how does it cope? It usually copes best if it has a carefully described disaster plan that has been regularly tested.

The basic components of a disaster plan are as follows.

☐ A pre-established authority structure which disregards existing physician and administrator prerogatives. Someone must be in overall command and specified persons must be in charge of specific tasks such as triage, identifying hospital patients who are to go home or be moved to other facilities, arranging patient transfer, providing information and traffic control, and calling in off-duty staff. The most senior administrative personnel should operate from a central command post well away from the disaster and the ER.

☐ A pre-established role for, and cooperation among, the police, the fire department, the ambulance system, the ham radio operators and other adjacent institutions, and possibly the armed forces, the Red Cross and other such groups, all of whom may be essential in various situations.

☐ A central casualty distribution plan to ensure that those in need, when picked up from their place of injury, are delivered to the place most able to care for them in terms of special competence and/or available space. Without this dispatch arrangement, all casualties may show up in one place. Minor emergencies should go to some established first-aid post quite geographically separate from the hospitals so that hospitals can receive only the seriously injured or ill.

☐ A communications network to handle outside enquiries (families, friends, the press) and ensure the continued availability of contact between all participants in the disaster response.

☐ A pre-established plan for each of the functions listed.

The effects of smaller disasters can be handled within the region; examples might be a fire requiring evacuation of one institution, or a structural collapse or other event whose casualties require less than 15 to 25 percent of locally available beds. In other situations, all local institutions may be out of action, as in Mississauga in 1979 when three hospitals, six nursing homes and a quarter of a million people were evacuated because of an overturned railroad car leaking chlorine. One thousand hospital patients were transferred either home (42 percent) or to one of over a dozen hospitals outside Mississauga. Only 2 to 3 percent of the LTC patients were able to go home. The remainder went to outside LTC institutions or to emergency accommodation. The move involved 160 ambulances and other vehicles and took 19 hours, and there had been no disaster.

A tornado in Barrie, Ontario, in May, 1985, demonstrated the chaos that accompanies a disaster when 8 were killed, 160 injured, hundreds of homes and other buildings destroyed, and major disruption of communication, transportation, and electrical systems occurred. Emergency housing, the allocation, feeding, and sheltering of hundreds of emergency workers, the unmanageable volume of enquiries and the documentation of the dead, injured, and displaced were only reasonably well done. Follow-up counselling, especially of children, was needed for many months to overcome feelings of panic whenever high winds or similar sounds brought back memories of the tornado. Another less expected need in the recovery period was protection of the victims from unscrupulous builders and exploitive prices.

On July 31, 1987, the Edmonton area was hit with lightning storms and a series of tornados. Lightning knocked out the ambulance dispatch tower, the telephone answering service (controlling all physician pagers) and many of the city's telephones. The tornado produced over 25 deaths and many hospital admissions. The vulnerability of a disaster plan to the loss of communication networks was vividly illustrated. No one knew what was going on.

The Mississauga, Edmonton, and Barrie experiences were modest challenges compared to the Halifax explosion of World War 1 or the more recent disasters at Bhopal, India, or Chernobyl in the former Soviet Union. We can benefit from planning for those large scale disasters that are more common than we think.

Mobilizing the System for the Usual Small Scale Emergency

The first step in the emergency care sequence is knowing that an emergency exists. In most cases this need for emergency care is immediately reported by the victim, co-workers, family members, bystanders, or others. The report is made to the police, fire department, ambulance system, or health care worker or facility. Many Canadian communities now have a special, easily remembered and toll free telephone number, usually 911, providing direct contact with the emergency network. Not only is the call simpler to make but the message is received by a center, usually the police, the fire department, or an ambulance dispatch office, that can respond immediately and that is in radio contact with all resources.

Sometimes the call for help is more automatic. High-risk patients may carry monitoring devices that will call for help when it is needed. The postmen play a role through their Postal Alert program (in which the postman alerts authorities when mail has not been picked up), as do the many programs in which a high risk person is phoned daily at a prearranged time. If there is no answer an investigation begins. Some of these programs are staffed by residents of LTC institutions.

Ambulance Services

Uncoordinated, user-pay, and privately operated ambulance services are now uncommon in Canada. They had the disadvantages of being financially hazardous to the operators (many clients were uninsured and did not pay), duplicated services (people in need often called several ambulances and only the first one there had a fare), somewhat unreliable (all companies might decide this was a good call to ignore), and of variable quality.

These unsatisfactory features have been steadily reduced or eliminated by regional or provincial organization, regional dispatch systems, and co-insurance plus provincial financing. Central dispatch systems for ambulances arrived about 20 years after they were firmly established in the taxi industry but technology is now being effectively used to ensure high quality contact between ambulances, the police, the fire department and the major hospitals.

Ambulance utilization is in the range of 50 to 150 trips per 1,000 population per year, of which up to 30 percent may be for scheduled services such as interhospital transport or taking patients home for the weekend. These trips may appear to be the inappropriate use of expensive staff and equipment, but they are an economical use if the expensive stand-by team would otherwise be idle. Besides the usual well-equipped ambulances there are now more super ambulances able to provide sophisticated life support during transportation.

For a number of years ambulance costs in Canada rose rapidly, but as of about 1982, as ambulance systems in a number of provinces matured, costs have stabilized. Data on ambulance cost is limited because Quebec does not report separately for this sector. The data also reflect the total expenditures of federal and provincial governments and workers' compensation boards. Surface vehicles equipped with life support and air services are included in Table 10.1.

Table 10.1

Change in Ambulance Cost, Canada 1975-1987

Year	Cost in Millions	Cost Per Person
1975	$ 92.7	$ 4.08
1978	149.1	6.33
1979	159.1	6.69
1980	176.2	7.32
1981	186.0	7.64
1982	201.0	8.17
1983	216.7	8.74
1984	243.7	9.75
1985	284.0	11.28
1986	313.1	12.34
1987	321.8	12.55

Source: National Health Expenditures in Canada 1971-1987, 1990, p.38-40.

In Ontario the total emergency services network cost $165-to-170 million in 1987-88, or about $20 per capita. These costs cover air transport, 640 ambulances (1:13,000 population) a small number of special support units and critical care transport units (for inter institutional transfer of stabilized patients), over 200 first response/administrative vehicles, regional dispatch centers and central administration. In 1987-88, about one million ambulance calls were made, or 120 calls per 1000 population.

Ambulance services have no national pattern. The degree of public financing and of provincial organization is extremely varied. All Ontario ambulance services operate under the *Ambulance Act*, and all are fully or primarily financed provincially. Nine area ambulance services are administered directly under the Ministry of Health, 5 (including that of Metro Toronto) are municipally managed, 66 are hospital operated, primarily in smaller communities with one hospital, 65 are privately owned and operated and 32 remote areas are served by volunteer services. Metro Toronto is unique in that Metro is reimbursed by the Ministry of Health for only about 65 percent of its costs and the system is operated by the regional government.

The characteristics of a good emergency transportation system include providing prompt response and having competent staff, modern equipment, good communication with physicians in hospitals, and a knowledge of the best destination for a particular patient. Improvements have, in the past decade, occurred in all respects, primarily because of increased public planning and financing. A province-wide, provincially operated and financed air ambulance service was started in Saskatchewan almost 40 years ago and all provinces offer some air evacuation assistance. The Canadian Coast Guard provides rescue services in marine emergencies.

Field health care personnel in the armies of the world have always been well trained, but the caliber of staff in Canadian ambulances has only recently begun to reflect the best features of military experience. Most provinces now use ambulance personnel with community college or university training. In Ontario, for example, they have at least one year of training. Basic ambulance attendant training may be followed by trauma training and by training in advanced cardiopulmonary life support skills.

In 1984, Ontario began training paramedics who must take a one-year course on top of lower level attendant training. As these graduates become available they are joining the ambulance network. They are trained in advanced life support (ALS) including the use of laryngoscopes, intubation, defibrillation, physical assessment, cardiac monitoring and use of drugs. One area under constant review is the range of judgments that can be made and acted upon without referral to a hospital. In light of the amount of training and the regular field experience of these personnel, it will be in everyone's interest if they are left to exercise considerable judgment as to when to contact a physician for advice or authorization.

The upgrading of emergency care personnel has occurred in hospital emergency departments as well as in ambulances. The practice of rotating a large number of physicians through the emergency department of the hospital has now been discontinued in most larger cities although it is still common in smaller centers. Emergency departments are now staffed primarily by full-time physicians, often with special training in emergency medicine. The staff may also be made up of hospital residents in training or physicians earning extra money while they develop a practice.

In most provinces, the physicians who work in hospital emergency departments are paid by fee-for-service, although use of this method of payment has made the low volume night shift unpopular. In some provinces such as Manitoba, the physicians in at least some emergency departments are salaried. In 1987, the Manitoba salaries of $50-60,000 could not compete with incomes offered elsewhere, including those available to emergency physicians on fee-for-service in the same province. Some emergency departments were temporarily closed for lack of medical staff. By 1990, remuneration of emergency physicians was competitive with other specialties.

Walk-in clinics, an exploding phenomenon in Canadian cities, are a new competitor for hospital emergency departments. Provincial governments have expressed concern over the add-on cost, lack of continuity of care and the possible encouragement of unnecessary utilization and the impact of these clinics on the per unit costs of hospital emergency departments where stand-by capability must be maintained.

A new type of "hospital without beds" is also being added to the emergency care spectrum. These facilities

☐ offer diagnostic services,

☐ usually integrate health and social services,

☐ may offer day care or other quasi-institutional services,

☐ may offer general medical care,

☐ may offer outpatient surgical services,

☐ usually offer 15 to 18 hours a day of minor emergency care, and

☐ may have a 1 to 2 bed holding unit for emergency stabilization before transfer.

The role of the public in emergency care is long established through such organizations as St. John Ambulance. The role of the public in cardiopulmonary resuscitation (CPR) is more controversial. In Seattle, one in five adults has CPR training, compared to one in eighty in Toronto.

Some information services are important to emergency care. Poison information centers tell mothers and other caregivers what to do. Telecommunication networks advise caregivers in isolated communities as to the most appropriate treatment and/or referral of patients, sometimes after transmittal of x-rays or other images for review by the central specialists. Patient registries and computerized patient medical histories will increasingly be valuable to a physician or other caregiver faced with a seriously injured person.

A 1986 survey of the Ontario public showed that only 59 percent rated emergency hospital care as "good" or "excellent," far below the 82 percent accorded hospital services overall. Waiting times, waiting areas and staff attitudes are cited as unacceptable. However, because Canadians have access to so many sources of emergency care, the conditions and waiting times are far less onerous than those in American public hospitals.

References

HWC (1983). *Pre Hospital Emergency Care Services; Report of the Subcommittee on Special Services in Hospitals*, Health Services and Promotion Branch, Ottowa: HWC.

Ontario (1986). *Directions for the Development of Emergency Health Services in Ontario*, Toronto: Ontario Ministry of Health.

Swimmer, G. (1991). *The Final Report of the Emergency Medical Services Review*, Toronto: Government of Ontario.

CHAPTER 11

The Health of Canadians

What Is Health

Protection and improvement of the health of Canadians are the most basic objectives of Canadian health services. To discuss these objectives, we need to know something about the extent to which Canadians are currently healthy, and why. To determine this, we must have some understanding of what we mean by health.

If an elderly person has a terminal illness but is looking forward to tomorrow and is content and relaxed today, to what extent is that person unhealthy? If a star teenage athlete in excellent physical health commits suicide, was he or she healthy? If a severely physically disabled person is optimistic, has a job, accepts responsibility well, and is anxious to contribute to the quality of life of his or her friends, to what extent is that person healthy?

Health will be considered to be, first of all, a reasonably optimistic and contented state of mind. This definition is preferred because state of mind is usually the major determinant of quality of life, and an acceptable quality of life is what makes life worth living. The greatest threats to the health of Canadians are, therefore, not necessarily those things which end our lives or interfere with our physical perfection. They are those things which ruin the quality of life. To concentrate on preserving life can be discouraging because, in the end, everyone must die. Concentrating on preserving the quality of life is, however, very apt to be rewarding because quality of life can almost always be improved. None of this is meant to suggest that the preservation of life and of physical health is unimportant. Poor physical health can seriously damage the quality of life.

If the protection and improvement of state of mind, or quality of life, are the primary objectives of health services, then these services will be delivered with enthusiasm and purpose even if a life is near its end (although the nature of the services may significantly change at that time). Because quality of life is subjective, health workers cannot protect or improve it until they know what things are important to each patient. Services can then be offered in ways that are compatible with, and supportive of, the priorities of the patient.

Recently the World Health Organization (WHO) European Region has defined health as a resource for everyday living, and as the extent to which an individual or group is able to realize aspirations and satisfy needs while also changing with, or coping with, the environment. Others have defined health as physical and mental well-being, as freedom from disease, pain or defect, as normal physical and mental functioning, or as a perception of the world and of oneself in it. Health care professionals tend to think of it as the absence of physical abnormalities.

Mental health and **emotional health** can be used synonymously but there is also, at times, a degree of difference. Mental health carries a more psychiatric connotation. Mental ill health, therefore, tends to be associated with institutional care and inability to function in society. Emotional ill health, on the other hand, may be seen as the depression, anxiety, or panic that happens to "normal" people. It can be perceived to be "normal" and not "psychiatric" even though mental health workers and programs may be involved in counselling or support. Some chronic mental disorders such as schizophrenia or manic-depressive states may be the product of a systemic and physical factor, but for the moment they continue to be classified as mental rather than physical disorders. Emotional disorders are predominantly a reaction to some situation, like bereavement, unemployment, failure, loss of independence, lack of social-ization, or continuing insecurity.

Intellectual health is not a commonly used term. Presumably, it is used to refer to the extent to which a person is able to use his or her inherent intellectual abilities. **Social health** is a collective term applying to populations rather than individuals. Social pathology exists when too many members of a population have undesirable characteristics such as fear or anxiety. Social health, as well as individual health, is threatened by such things as unemployment, war or the threat of war, starvation, or natural disaster.

The Blurred Margin Between Sickness and Health

Not only do we have trouble with the word health, the definitions of disease and illness are also unclear. Because health services are created to respond to ill health or injury, our network of health services will change as our concept of ill health changes. Not everyone considers all of the following situations to represent ill health, and not everyone wishes the health system to respond to all of these situations. Nevertheless, each of the following seven types of situations can be seen as disease or illness.

1. Situations in which subjective symptoms/complaints are consistent with objective observations, for example, sore throat due to tonsillitis, sore foot due to a broken bone, itchiness with a rash.
2. Situations characterized by an asymptomatic biomedical abnormality, for example, high blood pressure.
3. Situations with no physical abnormalities, but with symptoms which are consistent with history, lifestyle or environment, for example, chronic cough in a smoker.
4. Situations with no physical abnormalities, but with observable behavior patterns or described thought patterns that are outside of the norm.
5. Situations in which concerns or complaints cannot be explained after subjective and objective investigation; for example, headache, itchiness, insomnia.

6. Situations in which the patient sees nothing wrong and the biomedical exam indicates no abnormality, but in which society sees the patient as sufficiently deviant to be considered abnormal or unacceptable; for example, homosexuality, compulsive behavior.
7. Situations in which the patient or the patient's agent wishes action but others may consider action to be unnecessary; for example, cosmetic surgery, abortion, sterilization, mild interpersonal conflict.

There is no clear line between health and ill health, normal and abnormal, the point where no external support or care is needed, and the point where it is justified. When is a laceration large enough to deserve medical attention? When does unusual behavior become deviant and socially unacceptable? When has anxiety or pain exceeded the levels that ought to be tolerated without attention? There is ample room for the great debates that surround the use of emergency rooms, the abuse of medicare and the overservicing or underservicing of patients. What is called disease or illness obviously changes with the perceptions of the victims, caregivers, observers, or policy makers involved. There can be disagreement as to whether or not disease or sickness exists. Sometimes disease is perceived to be the biomedically demonstrable condition, whereas illness is considered to be what the patient experiences.

The Indicators of Health Status

When deciding whether or not a particular individual is "healthy," what indicators should be used? Would blood pressure, cardiac reserve, respiratory function, and vision be measured, or would degree of self-confidence, level of job satisfaction, ability to cope with stress, and ability to love be on the list? Emphasis on the first set of indicators would require a health bio-technocrat to do the appropriate tests, while emphasis on the second set of indicators requires the tools and uncertainties of the social scientist. The first set of indicators suggests a primary interest in physical health and the preservation of life and the second set suggests a primary interest in the quality of life. Either set of indicators could be used in the determination of "health."

Indicators of health status can be found in data describing populations or individuals. To assure oneself of a balanced view of health status, one must choose indicators of mental, physical, psychosocial, spiritual, and economic health. These indicators should represent behavioral, psychological, social, and physical (physiological) functioning, and may include measures of attitude and perception. Figure 11.1, for example, uses homicide as a measure of social health, infant mortality reflects physical health and life expectancy effects both economic and physical health. In the examination of health status, especially in the areas of attitude, perception, and behavior, it is necessary to look for and measure positive attributes (optimism, emotional stability, contentment) as well as negative attributes (depression, emotional instability, insecurity). Psychosocial well-being is, even more than is physical health, the presence of positive characteristics, not just the absence of negative or pathological characteristics.

Figure 11.1

Selected Quality-of-Life Indicators, Canada and U.S.

Jurisdiction	Homicides*	Infant Mortality**	Life Expectancy
Ontario	2.0	7.2	75.5
Quebec	2.4	7.1	75.0
New York	12.5	10.7	73.7
Michigan	10.8	10.7	73.7
Ohio	5.4	9.3	73.5
Illinois	8.6	11.6	73.4

* Per 100,000 population 1988.
** Per 1,000 live births 1987.

Sources: Statistics Canada, 1992, Statistical Abstract of the United States, 1992, Canadian World Almanac, 1992.

The determination of health status is more difficult when health is understood to include a great deal more than physical health. Deciding on the degree of happiness, optimism or enthusiasm that is present is more difficult than measuring the function of kidneys and the pituitary gland and deciding whether they are normal. Unreasonable expectations and asbestos fibers are both threats to health, but the former are more difficult to measure and prevent.

Selection of Standards

What is "good" health or "bad" health or "average" health? When is a person "normal?" Our psyche is not expected to survive in the face of endless negative strokes or emotional deprivation, but it should be able to tolerate the normal stresses of work and world. Legs are not expected to be speedier than the fastest bullet, but healthy legs on healthy people should be able to climb a few flights of stairs. Therefore, the first general rule when describing health status is that standards tend to be set to be consistent with the frailties and typical performance of a human being of the appropriate age and sex. "Good," "normal," or "acceptable" health tends to be defined in terms of what healthy peers can do.

Nowhere is this perception more confirmed than in our discussion of disability. The fact that none of us can run 60 miles in an hour is not seen as a disability, but to have 20/200 eyesight or to be unable to lift a cup of tea is a disability.

Reports on Health Status

The 1978-79 Canada Health Survey (CHS) conducted by Statistics Canada involved 40,000 individuals. It consisted of questionnaires and personal health examinations and was designed to answer three questions:

1. Who is exposed to the risk of future illness?
2. What is the current health status of the population?
3. What is the impact of illness?

The findings said a great deal about the health status of Canadians.

☐ Almost one-half of respondents said they had no health problems. Therefore, over half reported that they had at least one health problem.

☐ One-half of those with a health problem considered it too minor or too controlled to need attention.

☐ Almost one-half reported using some form of medication (pills or ointments, for example), in the average two-day period. One quarter of those taking medications reported no associated health problems.

☐ Low-income families experienced greater levels of emotional disorders, heart disease, and chronic respiratory disease than high-income families. Generally young, less educated male Canadians were most likely to endanger future health through current lifestyle.

☐ There are 200,000 persons with definitely dangerous blood pressure elevation.

☐ There are 2.6 million persons with blood pressure elevation which probably should be lowered.

☐ Three million individuals have excessive blood cholesterol levels.

☐ One-quarter of women over 65 take three or more kinds of drugs.

☐ Only about one-third of Canadians get enough exercise.

☐ The prevalence of various categories of health problems is quite different when one looks at population survey data as opposed to health services data. Limb and joint diseases and skin conditions are much more prominent in the client-generated data.

☐ Acute respiratory infections and injuries (trauma) are the major causes of disability days (which average 15.7 per year per person).

☐ High blood pressure, skin conditions, and mental disorders are the conditions most commonly associated with the use of drugs.

☐ The general prevalence of disease and disability showed little overall change in the 27 years between the Canada Sickness Survey of 1951-52 and the 1978-79 Canada Health Survey, but the physical health of children markedly increased.

☐ Many population groups are relatively unhappy; for example, women, teenagers, the elderly, the widowed, divorced and separated, low income, and those in poor health are the most likely to be depressed.

Causes of Death and Premature Death

Mortality data are still often used as measures of the healthiness of a population. Mortality data tell us what appears to have caused us to die. They do not tell us much about how healthy we are. About 200,000 Canadians die annually. Of these, about one-half die from diseases of the circulatory system. Within this category the biggest killer is coronary artery disease. Another 20 to 25 percent of deaths are caused by cancer. Deaths from cancer are increasing (Figure 11.2) likely because the population is aging (Figure 11.3), but also from increasing environmental causes.

Figure 11.2

Causes of Death

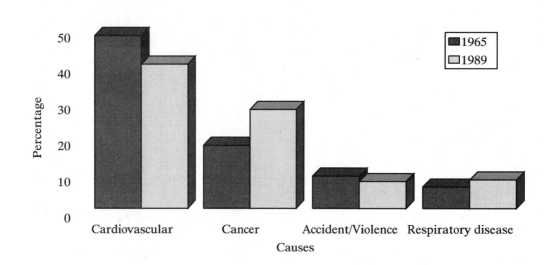

Source: Statistics Canada

Figure 11.3

Percentar

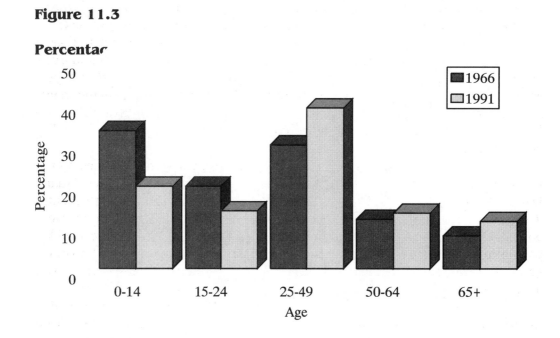

Source: Statistics Canada

A different picture emerges if one counts the extent to which different hazards shorten life as well as end it. This approach gives added emphasis to deaths that are premature. This is done by adding up the years lost when an individual dies prematurely. A death at age 45 represents about 30 years of life lost, whereas a death at 70 years is only 5 to 6 years away from the average life expectancy. Using this approach of "potential years if life lost" the big two (cancer and circulatory disease) are joined, and sometimes surpassed by, the effects of injuries. Accidents and suicide are the big killers in children and young adults and every death represents the loss of 45 to 75 years of potential life.

The five greatest contributors to loss of potential years of life of males are coronary heart disease, car accidents, suicide, lung cancer, and perinatal mortality. This is the order of importance of these causes of premature deaths in most parts of Canada, although in the Yukon and the North West Territories suicide is number one. This information is critical when considering how to improve the health of Canadians and how to avoid premature deaths. The first four of the five conditions respond better to prevention than treatment and the fifth is partially the result of avoidable factors. The picture for females is essentially the same with the exception that breast cancer is usually in the top five. (McCann, 1988).

Activity and Life Expectancy

Canadian women outlive men by about seven years, but they pay for it through more years of restricted functional abilities. A recent study in Quebec reported a male life expectancy of 70 years, with 60 years of healthfulness, versus a female life expectancy of 78 years, with 61 years of healthfulness.

The Canadian Health and Disability Survey (CHDS) conducted as a supplement to the Canadian Labour Force Surveys of October 1983 and June 1984 was based on almost 65,800 households representing over 126,000 persons. Nineteen screening questions determined mobility, agility, seeing, hearing, speaking, and mental handicap. All persons who reported disability were followed up with a personal interview that examined the effect of the disability on the person's life.

Among persons 15 years of age or older, 12.8 percent were identified by the CHDS as disabled, slightly less than the 14.3 percent identified in the Canada Health Survey (CHS) of 1978-79 (the CHS figure includes those with mental disabilities while the CHDS does not). Thirty-seven percent of disabled adults were 65 and over. In this 65 plus age group, 39 percent reported disability. The disabled population varied little by sex. Over one-third of the population with less than ninth grade education reported disability, compared to 10.5 percent of those who have all or part of high school and 5 percent of those with a university degree.

Among the 13 percent of the population 15 and over who reported a functional deficit (which was interpreted to be synonymous with a disability), 65 percent had problems with mobility, 54 percent with agility, 26 percent with hearing, 13 percent with seeing, 5 percent with speaking, and 8 percent with other deficits. Three percent of the total population were reported to have a mental handicap. This low figure may be partially a product of the bias of the questions towards physical disability. Among the 13 percent disabled, 37 percent had more than one functional deficit and 14 percent had more than two. These figures represent 4 percent and 2 percent, respectively, of the total population 15 years of age and over.

In 1981 The Canada Fitness Survey (CFS), with a base of 12,000 households and 24,000 people, was carried out "to provide basic information on the fitness levels and lifestyles of Canadians." It is sometimes difficult to know the exact relationship between lifestyle and health, but the CFS did tell us a great deal about things that we *think* significantly affect our future health.

Physical fitness and its associated programs will, for many people, reduce morbidity and mortality. For other persons morbidity and mortality will be increased, but the net effect of physical activity is very positive. It seems likely that most persons who participate regularly in recreational physical fitness activities find them enjoyable and emotionally rewarding as well as physically useful. It is quite possible that fitness activities are more important as sources of improved quality of life than of lengthened life. There are apparently few studies which compare the effects of fitness programs on people who enjoy them with the effects on persons in the same programs who do not enjoy them.

The CFS indicates that two populations with high morbidity and mortality statistics, the over-40 and the socioeconomically disadvantaged, have the lowest involvement in fitness programs and are the least physically fit.

Benefits of physical fitness (and therefore of the activities which bring fitness) include having the energy needed to enjoy other aspects of life. Energy is especially needed in advancing years when an undesirably sedentary lifestyle reduces one's ability to take part in a variety of pleasant activities such as sports, sex, work, and travel. These activities also reduce hazardous body changes such as osteoporosis. Physical activity also reduces tension (the tranquilizer effect) and can be a socialization device.

Use of drugs can be considered a measure of health status. A study titled "Alcohol and Drug Use Among Ontario Adults in 1984," and "Changes since 1982" reported

☐ the number of alcohol abstainers went down to 15 percent but the number of heavy drinkers also fell,

☐ the number of marijuana users did not change but use was less frequent,

☐ there were 9.3 percent using tranquillizers (no change), and

☐ Seven point one percent of 18 to 29 year olds had used cocaine at least once (one-third of the United States utilization rate).

Physical illness can have major impact on the emotional health of both patients and their families. Spouses of ostomy patients exhibit earlier and higher levels of stress than the patients themselves, especially early in the diagnosis/treatment cycle. Later in the cycle, as recovery is slower than expected, the patient copes less well than his or her spouse, and at later stages many household caregivers show signs of emotional burnout.

The Canadian Health Promotion Survey (1985) reported on over 11,000 households, approximately 1000 from each of the provinces and the Yukon/ Northwest Territories. An adult contact person was identified in each household. The response rate was over 80 percent, with most nonresponses being due to unanswered calls or household representatives not available for an interview. The survey method missed households without a phone and persons institutionalized in hospitals or chronic care institutions.

During the survey, health knowledge, attitudes, beliefs, and behavior were explored. The objective was to find out "what Canadians think, feel and know about health" rather than to collect information about physical health status or lifestyles. Questions examined

- perceptions of personal health,
- what people were doing or intended to do to protect or improve health, and
- the social and health environment in which the individual lived.

The survey made a good effort to escape from the preoccupation with physical health that characterized earlier federal health promotion and health survey activity. The escape was not complete, however, and the report of the survey reflects some confusion. When people were asked about their state of health, a great many of them replied in terms of only their physical health. The majority of key indicators chosen — for example, limitation of activity — are entirely indicators of physical health. Other parts of the survey asked questions about quality of life. Inconsistencies between the respondents' perceptions of physical health and quality of life should have been both expected and understood.

Sixty-one percent of Canadians rated their health as good or excellent. Forty-two percent reported they were very happy and 54 percent reported they were pretty happy. Happy people reported better health than unhappy people.

Hypertension can be thought of as a threat to health or as ill health. Elevated blood pressure increases the risk of vascular disease with increased risk of illness or death from stroke, heart attacks, heart failure, and kidney failure. It has been estimated that 5 to 20 percent of the adult population has hypertension, that one-half to two-thirds of those affected are unaware of it. Half of the cases found are not being adequately treated. Because the cause of hypertension is usually unknown, prevention is not feasible. Treatment, however, can be highly successful and can reduce the long term risks.

Health Status of Children and Adolescents

The concerns of individuals are a part of their health status, and these concerns vary greatly between age groups. A survey by the Children's Hospital of Eastern Ontario, in 1984, of 1,000 teenagers (73 percent response rate) revealed the following concerns. The percent of respondents who had these concerns is in brackets.

- Acne (47 percent)
- Academic difficulties (36 percent)
- Menstrual problems (33 percent of females)
- Family problems (32 percent)
- Nervous and emotional problems (26 percent — 33 percent for females and 17 percent for males)
- "Too fat" (26 percent, again 2:1 female dominance)
- Birth control (females 13 percent, males 5 percent)
- Drugs, alcohol and venereal disease (2 percent)

With respect to lifestyle features, teenagers revealed the following.

- ☐ 36 percent of females and 13 percent of males smoked regularly
- ☐ 15 percent used recreational drugs
- ☐ 49 percent used alcohol at least occasionally
- ☐ 25 percent of females and 18 percent of males reported sexual experience

In 1984-85 the Canada Health Attitudes and Behaviors Survey of over 30,000 children 9, 12, and 15 years old reported lifestyles and feelings that are considered to indicate a less than optimal health status. Twenty to thirty percent of the children reported difficulty sleeping because of worrying, and among 15-year-olds 30 percent used alcohol at least twice a month. Twenty-five percent were smokers and 20 percent reported use of cannabis. Sugars and fats dominated diets and activity levels were often very low. Television was more popular than exercise. Children with higher activity levels reported less depression, a happier home life and a more optimistic attitude to life.

The Ontario Child Health Survey of 1983, which was based on a sample of over 3000 children, reported on the psychiatric health of children aged 4 to 16 and on their use of mental health services. It documented two types of psychiatric behavior primarily affecting the child; neuroses such as sadness, tension, self-harm, somatization disorders with physical symptoms but no apparent physical disease, and psychiatric problems with major impact on the environment, like hyperactivity and socially unacceptable conduct such as stealing, violence and bullying (Figure 11.4).

Thirteen to twenty-two percent of females and males in each of the age groups were identified as having a psychiatric diagnosis. Diagnostic decisions were based on information from parents and teachers (for the 4 to 11 year olds) and parents and the youths themselves (for the 12 to 16 year olds). It was the norm for information from the two sources to present completely different pictures of the child. Psychiatric diagnoses were somewhat more common among urban children than rural children (perhaps because there are more psychiatrists in urban centers).

Figure 11.4

Prevalence of Psychiatric Disorders in Children in Ontario

Ages	Somatization or Neurosis (Internalizing Disorders)		Hyperactivity or Socially Unacceptable Behavior (Externalizing Disorders)		Both Types of Disorders	
	F	M	F	M	F	M
4-11	9.2	6.7	2.7	8.1	1.3	3.6
12-16	15.7	3.9	2.5	11.0	3.5	3.7

Source: The Ontario Child Health Survey, 1983

Infant Mortality

Infant mortality is almost entirely due to three major factors, these being crib death (Sudden Infant Death Syndrome or SIDS), congenital abnormalities, and prematurity. The infant mortality rate for Canada has now fallen to below 8 deaths per 1000 live births.

Figure 11.5

Infant Mortality Rates Among Selected Nations Per 1000 Live Births

	1980-82	1983-85	1986-87
Canada	9.8	8.3	7.6
United States	12.2	10.9	10.1
Japan	7.2	6.0	5.3
Germany	9.8	8.8	8.2
United Kingdom	11.5	10.1	9.4

Source: WHO Geneva 1991.

Native Health

The health status of our native population is a disgrace to the nation. Suicide levels in the 15-24 age group are six times the national average. Violence is the cause of 35 percent of all deaths (15 percent is considered very high in any population). Inuit women have lung cancer rates 15 to 30 times greater than that of other Canadians. Some native communities have a high incidence of diabetes. In Alberta in 1982, 23 percent of native deaths were alcohol-related. This is from two to six times the national average (depending on what national figure you accept).

In 1985 the infant mortality rate for native peoples was 50-60 percent above the national rate. In the post-neonatal period the mortality rate for Canada in general was 3.1 per 1000 while for natives it was 12.2 per 1000, four times greater. Native health care is not delivered through provincial systems, rather through a cumbersome federal department. There are now significant pressures for native control of health care with pilot projects showing lower infant mortality and better child and adult health.

Trends

Gains in life expectancy, which have occurred at all ages, included a significant reduction in premature deaths of males, 35 to 64 years. Longevity gains in all ages have been, to a significant extent, due to a reduction in deaths from cardiovascular disease and motor vehicle accidents (MVA). From the late 1960s to 1983, age standardized mortality rates from cardiovascular disease declined between 15 and 30 percent.

Following a peak in 1973, death rates from MVA had, by 1983, fallen from 40 percent to 60 percent in different age groups and sexes, but the decline was major in all age groups and for both sexes. The pattern is similar when examined in terms of mortality and injury rates per billion kilometers driven.

Cancer mortality rates, excluding lung cancer, have fallen 5 percent for males and 12 percent for females in the last 15 to 20 years. Lung cancer mortality rates have, at best, stabilized for males while rising sharply for females. The rates for breast cancer remain stable while death rates from cervical cancer have fallen 50 percent (1950-80). Female lung cancer deaths will very soon exceed deaths due to breast cancer. The rate of deaths from stroke continue to fall steadily, a trend established 15 to 20 years ago.

Figure 11.6

Life Expectancy of Canadians at Birth 1931-1989

	Males	Females	Both Sexes
1931	60.0	62.1	61.6
1941	63.0	66.3	64.6
1951	66.3	70.8	68.6
1961	68.3	74.2	71.3
1971 (70-72)	69.3	76.4	72.9
1981 (80-82)	71.9	79.0	74.9
1989	73.7	80.6	77.6

Source: Official Canadian Life Tables in Progress in Health Status of Canadians, HWC, 1992.

Age standardized mortality rates per 100,000 population for Canadian males in 1982 were 70 percent higher than those for females. Recent data suggests the gap between the sexes is falling. This is partly because males are living longer but also because female age-standardized mortality rates are rising.

Maternal mortality has declined from over 100 per 100,000 live births (0.1 percent) in 1951 to 6.2 per 100,000 (0.006 percent) in 1981, a drop of 94 percent. In 1981 there were only 23 maternal deaths in Canada.

Disability rates are almost surely increasing, at least in the elderly, although the terminology in the relevant surveys is not consistent and the amount of increase is uncertain. Only part of our increased longevity will be disability-free years. From the Canada Sickness Survey (CSS) in 1951 to the Canada Health Survey in 1978-79, the percentage of the elderly with disabilities rose from less than 30 percent to more than 40 percent. Dementia, predominantly Alzheimers disease, is now a major factor in all long term care, affecting 1 percent of the population at age 65 and 20 percent at age 80.

The most common less serious and short-term health problems reported in the 1951 and 1978-79 surveys changed from trauma, digestive disorders and headache to limb and joint disorders, and allergies.

End stage renal disease, in which kidney function can no longer sustain life, continues to occur, but the availability of dialysis and kidney transplants has changed the outlook from one of certain death to one of either a normal life or a life dependent on modern technology. Transplants are the preferred treatment in economic and human terms, but despite a steady increase in the number of kidneys available, the waiting list is long. The number of persons on dialysis in Canada rose from 2,300 to 2,800 between 1981 and 1985. Home dialysis is becoming less popular in most provinces, with fewer than one-quarter of patients now being treated at home.

Health status and the threats to it are not static. Ulcerative colitis was, a decade or two ago, far more common in children and adolescents than Crohns disease (regional ileitis). Crohns disease is now 10 times as common as ulcerative colitis. Other diseases have also become more common. Anorexia nervosa, for example, has risen predominantly in women and hepatitis B has increased in the general population.

AIDS in Canada

Acquired immune deficiency syndrome (AIDS) is the new and terrifying element in Canada's spectrum of epidemics. In June 1987 the British Columbia government reported that in 18 months of testing for the human immunodeficiency virus (HIV, formerly referred to as HTLV2), over 8 percent of 14,000 samples had tested positive. With the number of tests per month rising sharply, the percentage of positives was unchanged. Later, in 1987, New York City estimated that 50,000 New York City females in their reproductive years were carrying the virus. Canada is not experiencing epidemic growth in the number of new cases reported.

Figure 11.7

Reported AIDS Cases as of January 1991

Country	Up to 1986	1987	1988	1989	1990	Total
Canada	1,236	865	961	1,026	339	4,427
United States	39,125	26,551	31,787	34,601	22,727	154,791
Japan	25	34	31	92	112	294
Germany	1,083	1,036	1,250	1,406	725	5,500
United Kingdom	802	631	790	833	828	3,884

Source: WHO, Geneva, 1991.

Health Status Data

Information on the health status of Canadians is available from the following sources.

Vital statistics (in particular, death certificates). Mortality statistics expressed as rates (per 1,000 or per 100,000) and using the same diagnostic codes (for example, The International Statistical Classification of Disease and Injury, ICDA) are one of the most commonly used measures of health and disease.

Special studies. Many community or regional special studies (needs studies, impact studies, marketing studies), report on some aspect of health status, but their findings are often of questionable quality and usually of only local or regional interest. Many of these reports — as well as many individualized questionnaires, wellness checks, or hazard appraisals — suffer from a lack of attention to psychosocial or emotional content. The national studies of greatest consequence have already been summarized earlier in this chapter.

Registries. All provinces participate in The Canadian National Cancer Incidence Reporting System, but they supply data with varying completeness and accuracy. This registry illustrates the simplicity of the registry concept, the complexity of its implementation and the fact that data can be collected for years and used very little. This registry has almost 20 years of quite well-standardized data, although some provinces, such as Ontario, joined only recently. The implementation of mandatory reporting, or use of reliable sources such as death certificates, can increase the availability of cancer data. Saskatchewan uses a slightly different approach to assure the reporting of cancer. Physicians are not paid for cancer care unless the patient is registered with the Saskatchewan Cancer Commission.

The Canadian National Institute for the Blind (CNIB) maintains a registry of the blind population in Canada. The registry contains only persons voluntarily registered with them but the material is well coded and available for use.

A Canadian Renal Failure Registry, maintained by Health and Welfare Canada (HWC) and the Kidney Foundation of Canada, records the pattern, treatment, and outcomes of end stage renal disease.

Most disease or disability registries are provincial. For example, the British Columbia Health Surveillance Registry is a group of separate registries covering congenital anomalies, genetic defects, and several chronic disabilities. It began in 1952 and has undergone several metamorphoses. The Manitoba Infant Deafness Risk Register documents infants at risk of hearing damage. These infants are routinely registered and are followed by regional hearing centers and the Provincial Office of Hearing Conservation. An Ontario Crippled Children's Central Care Registry is maintained by the Easter Seal Society. As with many voluntary registries, the information is not sufficiently complete to provide total incidence or prevalence of handicapping conditions.

Difficulties With Data

In discussing the state of the nation's health we should appreciate some of the factors which decrease our ability to reach fully accurate conclusions. Provincial reporting is not always standardized; for example, the provincial lists of notifiable diseases vary. In August 1984, AIDS was a reportable disease only in Ontario, Saskatchewan, Alberta, and British Columbia, while all provinces reported in 1992. In addition, not all cases of disease are reported even when there is mandatory notification. The more often sexually transmitted diseases (STD) are treated in private offices, the more they will be underreported. In addition, the less importance a practitioner attaches to a condition, the more it will tend to be underreported (for example, rubella). Reporting may increase if a condition acquires notoriety, as with the 60 percent increase in reported cases of herpes virus infections in Canada between 1978 and 1983. This increase is probably more a factor of better reporting than it is of increased prevalence of the condition.

Diagnostic and disability reporting are each subject to error. The usefulness of hospital and ambulatory care diagnostic information is limited by the rather random way in which primary diagnosis is sometimes selected in multiproblem patients and by the regular underreporting of alcoholism, psychiatric conditions, and suicide. In the reporting of disability there is a tendency for each study or region to develop its own definition of major or minor disability, or its own categorization of mobility or other handicaps. Comparison is, therefore, often difficult.

One's definition of abnormality will, as already mentioned, sharply influence data describing it. What is a normal blood pressure? Certainly clinicians cannot fully agree. What amount of variation in the cervical cells of a pap smear should be accepted as normal, and when should these changes be called questionable or abnormal? How much distortion should there be in the spine of a child before it is called scoliosis? What pattern of carbohydrate metabolism should exist before a patient is called diabetic or prediabetic? What personality characteristics merit use of the term personality disorder or panic state? The degree of disagreement over what is normal is quite astonishing, even when dealing with tangibles such as x-rays or EKGs, and this disagreement can markedly weaken the comparability or equivalence of data.

Because discussion of health status tends to be comparative among communities and populations, it is necessary to adjust data so that selected differences in the populations can be taken into account. Examples of important differences would be age, sex, or socioeconomic status. The need for standardization of data is easily demonstrated.

Cause and Effect

Unfortunately, even when health status or changes in health status are adequately documented, it is not always easy to identify the causes of inadequate health. For example, the number of deaths from heart attacks (the age standardized mortality rate for ischemic heart disease) has fallen 5 to 30 percent in most industrialized countries, including Canada, in the past 15 to 20 years. The extent to which the decline was due to a decrease in cigarette smoking, reduced consumption of polyunsaturated fats, better exercise patterns, better detection and control of hypertension, better treatment of heart attacks when they occur, or some other factors, is not fully known. We do know, on the basis of major studies which have followed large populations over many years, such as the Framingham studies, that the reduction in cigarette smoking is certainly one of the major factors.

Selected kinds of ill health are now effectively avoided or reduced. Whether we are more healthy as a nation than we were two or three decades ago is unknown, but many indicators, especially those related to physical health, indicate improvement. If a healthy state of mind is considered to be the most dominant characteristic of a healthy person, then we do not know for certain whether we are becoming more healthy, because we have not been collecting the necessary information about expectations, optimism, happiness, peace of mind, and contentment. Using mortality rates as one index of health, Canada stands high in world rankings. Though it falls behind a few countries such as Japan and Sweden, it comes ahead of the United States, Britain, and France.

Lifestyle Choices

An HWC survey in 1982 showed that 22 percent of Canadian teenagers smoke daily, with the percentage increasing from 8 percent at 12 to 14 years to 39 percent among 18 to 19 year-olds. Females were more apt to be daily smokers (24 percent vs. 21 percent of males), but were less likely to smoke a pack a day or more. A high percentage of smokers and nonsmokers were aware of the hazards of smoking.

Smoking is being attacked by means of legislation, social pressure, pressure at work, warning labels, and higher prices. However, about 35 percent of males 15 and over and 32 percent of females in the same age group continue to smoke. A combination of chronic cough, impaired taste, discoloured teeth and furniture, $1,000 to $2,000 (Canadian) of direct cost, and 38,000 smoking-related deaths per year has not stopped 35 percent of adult Canadians from smoking.

A second addiction reinforces the importance of lifestyle as a determinant of health. About 65 percent of adult Canadians use alcohol at least once a month. About 10 percent of these will have some alcohol-related disability, over half a million are alcohol dependent, and at least 100,000 have a disabling dependency. Thirty percent of suicides, 50 percent of homicides, over half of our automobile fatalities and perhaps 10 percent (15-18,000) of our total annual deaths are alcohol-related. Besides causing these deaths, alcohol is a factor in 50 percent of divorces and 50 percent of welfare families, and although tax revenues from alcohol sales now exceed five billion dollars, the social costs may be twice as high. Although the taxes on alcohol appear substantial, there was, in the period from 1962 to 1982, almost a 50 percent reduction in the cost of a liter of liquor (or the equivalent amount of alcohol from wine or beer) if the cost is expressed as a percentage of personal disposable income. In the same period there was a 30 percent increase in consumption per person.

Alcohol and tobacco are not the only lifestyle activities of consequence to mental and physical health. There is danger in physical inactivity, inappropriate diets, obesity, abuse of narcotics, unsafe use of all forms of transport, and abuse of prescription drugs.

Heredity/Biology

Our genetic pool is a major determinant of physical health status, but it is a factor we can usually do nothing about. Genetics as a medical science deals with over 3000 conditions such as Tay-Sachs disease, sickle-cell anemia, hemophilia, and phenylketonuria, all of which are deviations from what is called normal. It should also be remembered that our genetic pool is the primary determinant of lifespan, of the capacity of our kidneys and livers to handle toxins, of the pattern of osteoporosis, of the structural inadequacies of our knees, shoulders, and backs, and of the adequacy of our immune system. The question of the extent to which emotional/mental health is genetically rather than environmentally determined is largely unknown, but our genetic pool is definitely a factor in a few specific psychiatric conditions.

Public Policy as a Determinant of Health

The decisions made by governments and governing bodies affect our safety, our opportunities, and the mix and character of our social and economic institutions — all of which affect our health. These decisions are the product of the knowledge and the values of the decisionmakers and of the pressures acting upon them. Decisions and policies can be seen as products of social and economic environments and can be discussed under those headings, but it can also be argued that public policies ought to be considered as a separate factor affecting health.

Summary

In any discussion of health in Canada we should remember that increasing our material standard of living may not increase our level of health proportionately. At the moment we measure national success in terms of GNP or balance of payments. We should also be developing measures of group tolerance, capacity for compassion, willingness to share, and willingness to oppose our drift to increased economic centralization. Good health is difficult to maintain in individuals who must act and live in patterns, and in communities shaped by forces beyond their control.

This chapter has argued that the total health of Canadians is influenced heavily by those factors that strengthen and promote such things as mental health, security, nondestructive lifestyles, safer workplaces, and a healthier environment.

The actions taken to improve health have changed over time. The first big advances in health status were due to socioeconomic and public health measures which included

☐ improvements in housing and water supply,
☐ the preservation of food,
☐ the pasteurization of milk,
☐ sewage control,
☐ garbage disposal, and
☐ control of communicable disease.

These were followed by an acceleration of scientific and technological progress, by the prevention and cure of infectious diseases and by a greater understanding of mental health problems and endemic chronic diseases. Associated with the onslaught of chronic diseases was the need for new treatment and prevention strategies but especially for new attitudes toward the relative importance of state of mind as opposed to state of body.

A third phase of health protection is related to the burgeoning volume of social and environmental pathology. We are still adapting to these and are not, as yet, skillful at dealing with them or at recognizing how and why they develop.

The major determinants of health are, today as always, outside of the purview and mandate of the health system. They include the level of employment, the quality of interpersonal interaction, the quality of our social and physical environments, and the safety of our workplace. At this point in time, we often ignore major threats to health while lavishly supporting selected health services whose impact on health is much smaller than we believe.

References

Ableson, J., et al. (1983). *Perspectives on Health*. Ottawa: Statistics Canada.

Balram, C. (1989). Impact of Chronic Diseases on the Health of Canadians. *Chronic Diseases in Canada*. May issue.

Canada (1987, October). Booze, Pills and Dope, Reducing Substance Abuse in Canada. Ottawa: Standing Committee on National Health and Welfare, Government of Canada.

Canadian Institute of Child Health (1984). *The Silent Epidemic: Childhood Injuries*. The Canadian Institute of Child Health.

Department of National Health and Welfare and the Dominion Bureau of Statistics (1960). Illness and Health Care in Canada: A Report of the 1950-51 Canada Sickness Survey. Ottawa: Department of National Health and Welfare and the Dominion Bureau of Statistics.

HWC (1984). Alcohol in Canada. A National Perspective, Second Edition. Ottawa: Health and Welfare Canada.

HWC (1984-85). Canada Health Attitudes & Behavior Survey. Ottawa: Health and Welfare Canada.

HWC (1986). Canadian Health & Disability Survey 1983-84. Ottawa: Health and Welfare Canada.

HWC (1987). *Chronic Diseases in Canada*. June issue.

HWC and Supply and Services Canada (1987). The Active Health Report—Perspectives on Canada's Health Promotion Survey 1985. Ottawa: Health and Welfare Canada and Supply and Services Canada.

Lapierre, L. (1984). *Canadian Women: Profile of their Health*. Ottawa: Statistics Canada.

McCann, C. (1988). Potential Years of Life Lost, Canada 1982-1986. *Chronic Diseases in Canada*. 9:98-100.

National Council of Welfare (1985). Poverty Profile. Ottawa: National Council of Welfare, Ministry of Supply and Services.

National Council of Welfare (1987, April). Progress Against Poverty. Ottawa: National Council of Welfare, Ministry of Supply and Services.

Statistics Canada (1981). The Health of Canadians—The Report of the 1978-79 Canada Health Survey. Ottawa: Statistics Canada.

Statistics Canada (1983). The Canada Fitness Surveys, 1976 and 1981. Ottawa: Statistics Canada.

Statistics Canada (1992). Causes of Death. Ottawa: Statistics Canada.

Wingle, D.J. and Mao, Y. (1980). *Mortality by Income Level in Urban Canada*. Ottawa: Health and Welfare Canada.

CHAPTER 12

Ethical Issues, Cost Control, and Evaluation

T his chapter is not about the biomedical ethics of treatment decisions. Rather, it is focused on the broader issues of rationing, evaluation, and public choice. Within the area of public choice are emerging trends in Canada such as living will legislation, the empowerment of new health professions, different forms of health care organization, and community control of health services for the native people of Canada's First Nations.

Ethical dilemmas occur often in health care, as in many other aspects of life. Constrained resources make many of these dilemmas more pressing. The practice of ethics is primarily an orderly way of gathering evidence, knowing the legal precedents, exploring principles, and determining the consequences of choices. It also requires the making of a judgment in which the intention is to do good, not evil.

The Canadian View of Social Justice

There are three competing interests in health care delivery in Canada: society at large, patients, and providers. Demands for resource allocation by these groups will require resolution in order to achieve justice for the common good. Fairness and equity must occur among persons or groups. One cannot benefit more than another.

To see this kind of macro-justice in operation in Canada, one needs only to look at the advocacy or lobbying activities of each group as it attempts to influence spending. A hospital may try to encourage society to spend more on health promotion or increase funding to health care generally, knowing that some of this spending will trickle down to them, or several patient advocacy groups may join together to lobby for increased funding for the elderly or for persons with AIDS.

One of the best U.S. examples of the hospital and macro-justice is the example of the Board of the Massachusetts General Hospital in Boston thinking in the ethics mode. In 1980, trustees debated the issue of heart transplants, paying attention to "the effects of the procedure on the allocation of costly and limited resources" (*New England Journal of Medicine,* vol. 302, no. 19, p. 1087-88). They elected not to proceed with such a program.

Dr. Alexander Leaf, Chief of Medical Services at the Massachusetts General Hospital commented (*NEJM* ibid, p. 1088): "If one considers that the medical profession has historically been fostered and supported to serve a societal need and not to supply physicians with a privileged status, one can find little argument with the course that MGH trustees thoughtfully and responsibly followed."

At the micro level of justice, the hospital promises to be fair to patients and residents currently in the system and to those who may enter in the future. For example, a hospital needs fair criteria or equitable standards for admission. A hospital is responsible for fair allocation of such services as palliative care and diagnostic services.

The third kind of justice is an intermediate or mezzo justice and can be applied to staff, management, and health professionals who work within the organization. Issues at this level include which physicians get privileges and for which procedures, and which groups have renovations to their working space. Commonly asked questions are, "Should fewer RNs be hired so more assistants can be employed?" or, "Should union or non-union contractors be used to deliver a hospital-based service?"

The overall question is about allocation of resources. To answer it, decision makers, whether managers, trustees, or governments, must know the facts, the options available, and the basic ethical norms underlying their mission statement.

Toward Fully Informed Consent

The consumer age is said to be characterized by a wish for the ability to make choices for oneself, and this has been shown to apply to many lifestyle choices. The extent to which the change has altered health care, and altered the wish of patients to exert greater control over clinical decisions, is unclear, but certainly many users of health care wish to understand what is going on.

People are more likely to support reduced spending on health care if they believe they can receive all of the health care they really need with less spending. If they become convinced that less health care is just as good as the amount being delivered now, they will know that some of what they got before should not have been provided. They will also know that some of the professionals who provided the care made inappropriate decisions.

What will this do to the patient-provider relationship, in particular, that of doctor-patient? Will people believe that their physician is routinely correct, but that other physicians should be more careful? Or will an increasing number of patients, and advocates of patients, be increasingly skeptical of the advice they receive?

The mystery of medical care will decrease as diagnostic and therapeutic alternatives are described to patients and as the risks associated with care are more fully discussed. Many patients will continue to wish all decisions to be made by their physician or other health care professionals, but many others will decide, or have already decided, that professional advice should not be accepted without question.

Discussions of the adequacy of professional decisions will also expose the extent to which medicine is not an exact science. The mythology of modern medicine has produced a sense that physicians always know what to do, what to prescribe, when someone will die, how much everyone should weigh, and so on. Many patients will not like to know that there are often options, and that there is often no way of being at all certain of which option will produce the best outcome.

The rights of the patient have been established.
Patients now have:

- ☐ the right to be told, in language they can understand, about the medical care alternatives available to them,
- ☐ the right to have the benefits and the hazards of each health care option explained to them in language they can understand,
- ☐ the right to select the treatment option that will be used,
- ☐ the right to refuse treatment, regardless of the consequences of the refusal. If a caregiver is aware of a previously stated objection to a specific treatment or procedure this statement must be honored (for example, as expressed in a card refusing blood transfusions or in a medical directive refusing resuscitation).

Health care professionals may, in situations in which the patient cannot comment, provide emergency life saving care unless this is contrary to the known instructions of the patient. Provision of any other care or investigation without consent is assault.

Hospitals have led the way in requiring consent and refining the process through which consent is confirmed, but the rules apply in all locations.

Older health care professionals remember the time when patients were told very little. The physician might have announced, "Your gall bladder needs to come out and I've booked you into the hospital next week," and that was that (although the date of admission might be negotiable). The law always gave the patient the right to refuse care, but the sanity of the patient was though to be questionable if medical advice was not accepted.

Now, not only may patients wish to know more, but both the regulations of the medical societies and the law require that patients be informed of the health care options that are available as well as the implications of the options. The precedent-setting case in Canada was *Reibel vs Hughes*, a case in which the patient was not informed of the risks of the procedure, became hemiplegic as a result of surgery, and successfully sued his physician.

In a similar trend, the protection of the rights of the mentally ill and those presumed to be mentally ill have been strengthened. Appeal processes are available, mandatory reviews are routine and, in some provinces, salaried advocates review the cases of persons being detained without their consent. In some provinces these processes are said to have protected the rights of the patient to the point where treatment and assessment are difficult or impossible.

Perhaps only one fundamental right is still not available to Canadians, namely, the right to buy hospital and physician services in Canada with their own money if that is their wish. The services of hospitals and physicians remain perhaps the only completely legal product which is produced in Canada but cannot (with a few exceptions such as a cataract clinic in Calgary) be bought by Canadians with their own money.

Hospital Ethics

In Canadian law, a hospital is a corporate person. The hospital makes decisions on such issues as whether to respect a patient as a person, fulfill contractual obligations, provide certain types of services, and give equal pay for work of equal value. In addition to being a corporate person, the hospital is also a registered charity that serves the needs of a particular community, even if the community is as large as a province. This service mandate is reflected in the mission statement of the hospital, and here the ethical agency of the board of the hospital becomes important. Thus, the hospital makes a promise to provide a service in a specific way to certain consumers for a predetermined amount of resources. In detail, these promises can be grouped into three categories: competency, meeting social expectations, and ethical norms.

1. **Competency.** The hospital will demonstrate the scientific foundation of clinical care, education and research.
2. **Social expectations.** The hospital will not break the law, nor will it neglect government regulations governing financing, contracting, and professional conduct. This is essentially a legal dimension of ethical conduct.
3. **Ethical norms.** The hospital will not harm a resident or patient. In fact, there should be benefit attached to a hospital stay. The ethical norms of health care facilities will be met. For example, respect for individuality, informed consent, privacy and confidentiality will be upheld. The hospital will also be fair in determining access to services.

Evaluation of Health Care

Many devices are used to evaluate health care institutions and workers. Formal qualifications are demanded and re-licensing is routine.

Colleges of nursing and medicine investigate complaints. In some instances, there is recurrent testing of competence (such as the Ontario College of Physicians and Surgeons Peer Evaluation Program) or a requirement for proof of involvement in continuing education (the College of Family Practitioners of Canada). There are accreditation programs (hospitals, long term care institutions, and public heath agencies) and, within the accreditation surveys, a variety of audits of the quality of medical and nursing care. Quality assurance programs are now present in most hospitals, and many of these programs are now changing to total quality management programs.

Despite what may seem to be an impressive array of evaluation activities, evaluations of the total system — or of major components — are inadequate. There is only a general understanding of the importance of most procedures done and prescriptions written. When even long-standing procedures are scientifically and validly evaluated, 15 to 20 percent of them are found to be, at best, of no value to patients, and at worst, to actually harm them. Another group of procedures were found to be less useful than they were formerly thought to be. Many decisions to question these procedures in Canadian medicine occur when American studies identify limited value in such procedures.

Evaluation cannot be considered to be reasonably complete until we know two things. First, how much do various health care activities protect or improve the health status of an individual or a community? Second, how much does each activity cost? When society has this information, it will be able to more rationally decide what to do with the resources that are available (always remembering that culture, values and the need to finance other social activities will also influence what we decide to buy). Evaluation is therefore bound by ethical norms, and the implementation of program changes will be bound by ethical principles or codes of ethics.

Moving Toward a New Ethics of Care in Native Health

Heated debate has surrounded both the issue of native self-government in Canada and the desire of the First Nations to control their own health services. Many groups still have no treaty, and land claims have never been settled. Some success in autonomy over health care is now evident in groups such as the Nisga, who live along the Nass River in British Columbia. The Nisga have a Valley Health Board that employs 42 staff, including two doctors and four nurses, to provide care to 2,500 people in four villages. The Health Board was developed by the Nisga Tribal Council in collaboration with the Medical Services Branch of Health and Welfare Canada (the former provider) and the B.C. Ministry of Health (the new partner). The funding is provided 70 percent federally and 30 percent provincially.

Because the valley is isolated, a helicopter pad has been installed for emergency airlift. Services at the center include x-ray, laboratory, a fully equipped emergency room, and a connecting ground ambulance service to a hospital 90 kilometers away in Terrace. Other services include a drop-in center for teens, two pre- and post-natal classes, alcohol and drug counselling, and two nursing stations in outlying villages. The center works towards integrating modern medicine with traditional healing in Nisga culture.

The Ethics of Constraint

Controlling the cost of health care is part of the distributive justice practiced in Canada. It is the limiting of the resource consumption by health care so that social spending for other valued goods and services can occur. This process exists for the wider social good, which must balance the redistribution of resources to patients, hospitals, and providers.

The capping of budgets, which is the most common regulatory tool for the control of expenditures (a global budget is one form of "cap"), is quick and easy. It was, and is, a rational policy choice if health care professionals will routinely make good spending choices and when it is believed that professionals know which choices are best. Programs which are not capped are a threat to cost control, including, for example, private laboratories, drug insurance programs, and fee-for-service practitioners.

Capping is everywhere in health care. The budgets of Ministries of Health are capped (overruns are not acceptable to Cabinets). The budgets of each sector within the Ministry have their budgets capped. In some provinces the total spending on physicians' services is capped; payments to individual professionals can also be capped, as are total physician payments in Quebec and Ontario.

Actions To Constrain Cost

There are two ways to improve constrained spending:

1. lower production costs (ie., be more efficient, produce the same service but at less cost per unit of service); and
2. buy only those products (services) which bring significant benefits per dollar spent. The desirable combination is to buy only the most beneficial services, at the lowest possible cost per unit of services.

The administrators and evaluators of health care have, for several decades, been concentrating on lower unit costs. The lowering of unit costs can occur through a change of location, a change of process, the elimination of some elements within the unit cost, the use of less expensive personnel, and the use of lower cost generic drugs, etc.

Use of outpatient surgery to replace inpatient surgery and the centralization of services such as obstetrics or pediatrics to achieve economies of scale are examples of lowering cost through a change of location. Shortening the length of hospital stay or the reduction of unnecessary laboratory tests are examples of elimination of items which formerly added to the total unit cost. Group purchasing is a new way to perform the same tasks, as in the lowering of energy costs.

None of the examples described is designed to change the mix of patients served. Most of them are not designed to change the mix of services provided to patients who enter the system.

Many information systems have been developed to allow better measurement of cost and better comparison of costs. Provinces routinely compare the cost of various elements of care in one hospital with the cost of the same service elsewhere.

The same attention and energy has not been applied to alteration of the services that are delivered. Evidence of inappropriate health care has been accumulating for some time, but efforts to reduce the inappropriate care are spotty. The efforts that have been made have been mostly in teaching hospitals and include limited access to selected drugs and services, routine review of selected kinds of services and a requirement for predelivery justification of selected care.

Ethics and Legislation

There are expanding amounts of literature and increasing public pressure for individual autonomy over treatment choices. In response, several provinces in Canada have initiated living will legislation, or, in legal terms, advance medical directives. These usually consist of two parts; an instructional directive and a proxy directive or durable power of attorney. The first gives health providers a patient's wishes regarding life-sustaining treatments. The second designates someone to make decisions on one's behalf. In Nova Scotia and Quebec, this proxy is identified by statute.

In Canada, living wills began to influence care choices following the Karen Ann Quinlan case in the United States in 1976. Most U.S. states already have living-will laws that protect the advance directives regarding life-sustaining treatment. Although such advance directives are becoming more common, provinces in Canada such as B.C. do not legally bind a doctor to refuse medical care even if a patient wishes not to be treated. For example, every patient has a right to effective management of pain, even if such medication shortens life.

In British Columbia about one-third of the $5.4 billion health care budget goes to care for people near the end of their lives. The need to use these resources effectively may involve a certain amount of rationing in the future; proximity of death is not currently a factor in determination of rationing. However, Canada frequently discriminates on the basis of age, usually in favor of the elderly. For example, persons over 65 receive free drugs, or drugs with lower co-insurance fees than those paid by other persons. The ethics of using public money to discriminate in favor of elderly persons, including those with incomes adequate to pay for reasonable quantities of drugs, will be a subject for discussion in Canada's health care reform.

New Legislation

Legislative changes regarding new autonomy for health professions other than physicians are occurring in several provinces including Ontario and Alberta. The hierarchy of health care professionals with the physician at the top, a hierarchy which is the heart of the medical model, is now beginning to wobble, and there is reason to believe the collapse will accelerate. The new health professions legislation in Ontario (consisting of 26 separate statutes), which impacts the province in 1993, embodies principles and mechanisms which permanently change the relationships of the health care professions.

First, the Act describes the area of practice which is thought to be appropriate for each profession. Some areas of practice will be the reserved domain of a single profession. Others will be open to more than one professional group. The approved activities (the "designated acts") were identified by a provincial commission (the Swartz Commission) which made recommendations to the Ministry of Health. These recommendations were only modestly amended through a process of public consultation.

Second, the Act establishes a mechanism through which professions can seek revisions to their powers and roles. This Commission is an agent of the Ministry of Health, not of the medical profession, and therefore, from now on, physicians will not control what can be done by any other profession.

Third, the new legislation replaces many former statutes, including the Act which established the supremacy of physicians and gave them a monopoly on the "practice of medicine."

The new Act increases the number of health care professions who can see patients without referral from a physician. This group includes chiropodists and podiatrists, osteopathic physicians (who are, in the new Act, grouped with allopathic physicians), and midwives. Physiotherapists, nurse practitioners, and others are in the line-up awaiting review by the Commission. They are seeking independent status, including one or more of

    ☐ the right to see private patients (without referral by a physician),
    ☐ the right to order diagnostic tests and prescribe prescription medications,

☐ the right to refer patients to other health care professionals and to health care agencies, and

☐ the right to provide an expanded array of services within their realm of practice.

The new procedures for defining the appropriate range of practice of health care professionals (a process not under the control of physicians) will be much more likely to expand the legal area of practice of non-physicians than was the old process, which was under the control of physicians. Ambulance attendants, for example, will surely seek the right to perform defibrillation and use life-saving drugs without physician approval. Although physician advice will play an important role in determining what changes will take place, the changes themselves will be the product of a public policy process rather than the former physician-controlled process. Non-acceptance by physicians was a serious obstacle to emerging groups like midwives when the right to "practice medicine" was limited to physicians.

As professions become independent, their powers will almost surely be routinely linked to described areas of competence, a principle already routinely applied to physicians with hospital privileges. A psychologist, for example, would be assigned hospital privileges only in psychology.

Physicians have routinely used the argument that expanding the roles of other professionals would be a threat to the public, but the quality of physician decisions has now been sufficiently examined to suggest that many other professionals will do at least as well.

These changes are not part of some Machiavellian anti-doctor plot, but are rather the logical and rational evolution of Canada's health care system. Many health care professionals have special skills quite different from those of most physicians, and these skills are being recognized. The argument that physician control is necessary to protect the patient is no longer saleable or reasonable.

Physicians will remain more powerful than any other health care profession, but they will, in the future to a far greater extent than now, share their former leadership position. As professionals become independent, each will make mistakes, just as physicians do, but there is no evidence to suggest that other health care professionals make, or will make in the future, fewer or more mistakes than physicians.

All independent health care professionals (not just physicians) will be subject to evaluation by outsiders, all will be obliged to routinely seek and accept patient choices, and all will carry malpractice insurance. The ethical dilemmas of resource allocation between the social good, the professions, and the patient will grow even more complex.

Health care professionals with new levels of independence, each with the ability to diagnose and treat in their areas of expertise, will bring new kinds of competition including competition for patients, hospital space, health care dollars, and, most important of all, public support. These new providers will bring new kinds of competition to health care in Canada.

Social Change and Health Care

Throughout health services, there is an unease which began in the 1980s but has become more marked in the 1990s. The theory of social change suggests that unease is normal at this time. Students of the process of social change would say that the evolution of health care is following a predictable pattern.

Social change theory states that as social systems evolve, and as the world in which they operate also changes, it is inevitable that at some point in time the status quo becomes unsatisfactory. The first event in the process of social change is the appearance of unhappiness with, and opposition to, the status quo.

In health care this first stage is largely completed. The status quo as it existed in the 1960s has been discredited. Health services have been shown to be overvalued, and professional domination is incompatible with the consumer era. Former preoccupations with physical health are incompatible with the current emphasis on quality of life. The broadening of the spectrum of competent and responsible health care professions, in combination with new patient rights, has identified the medical model as anachronistic. The almost religious faith of patients in physicians as the "priests of medicine" is being challenged by evidence of the inappropriateness of many professional decisions.

The second stage in the process of social change is the appearance of alternatives to the status quo. Usually many alternatives are proposed. In Canada there are, or are proponents of,

- new professional alignments,
- new organizational options,
- new payment options,
- new social objectives,
- a new distribution of power,
- new roles for government,
- new levels of personal responsibility for health, and
- new approaches to evaluation and monitoring of health care.

This second stage of social change is one of great confusion, and it is the stage in which the health care system currently finds itself. Vestiges of the old are mixed with ideas competing for the future. Institutions, workers, users, and policy writers are at varying levels of agreement with and understanding of what is happening. Simple solutions are being sought for poorly understood complex problems.

The cultural and structural upheaval which began in earlier decades is accelerating. The uncertainty, anxiety, and confusion which are present in our health services network are all inevitable during a process of such massive change, but they cannot be ignored. They will wax and wane until a new status quo is in place, and that will not be for some time.

Some examples of the current confusion follow.

- A wish by users for both perfect health care and a control of spending.
- A wish by politicians for controlled spending on health care, but unlimited access by patients to publicly financed health care.
- Knowledge that perhaps one-third of all health dollars spent contribute little if anything to health status, but minimal attention to the professional decisions that produce the low value care.
- A death due to a failure in the health care system receives major media attention and probably evokes a policy response, whereas a death on the highway or at work hardly merits a story and certainly there will be no policy response.

☐ Ministers and Deputy Ministers of Health regularly make speeches and publish brochures speaking of how spending must be curtailed and how we need to spend our health dollars better, but the ministries of health and the system seldom pay much attention to an examination of the cost-effectiveness of alternatives. The ideas at the top are inconsistent with the skills and culture of the bureaucracy.

☐ The federal government is withdrawing from health care financing (Bill C-69, 1991) but states that the penalties within the *Canada Health Act* (1984) will stay in place. Provincial options are unreasonably limited in an area of provincial jurisdiction by a federal law which is seen as reflecting earlier financing arrangements and in a time in which provincial autonomy is being strengthened.

The Evolution of a New Status Quo

The third stage in the process of social change is the selection of a new status quo. This is still in the future.

Spending changes which bring more "bang for the buck" will not come primarily from new organizations. These may improve equity and promote local control (both desirable trends) but are unlikely in themselves to improve the economic skill with which we buy health care. The spending changes will also not primarily come from better evaluation of technology, including new drugs, although these will contribute because they will eliminate use of selected devices and drugs which have no value or are not competitive with other products available. The spending improvements will also not come primarily from greater efficiency since the system has improved immensely since the first major squeeze at the time of the oil crisis in the early 1970s. Savings will also hopefully not come to any large extent from reductions in worker incomes (although physicians are at risk). Changes will not come from endlessly refining our knowledge of regional variations in utilization. Refining this knowledge now serves no purpose unless there is a plan for the use of this information to alter practices. The big spending changes will come from improvements in professional decision making. Most drugs and health care devices should not come off of the market they should just be used more appropriately. Most surgical and diagnostic procedures should be treated similarly.

Professional decision patterns are highly individual and cultural, and changes will therefore often be much more behavioral than scientific. The process will seldom occur as quickly or as easily as the passing of a regulation, although regulations will, at times, be one of the tools through which the behavioral changes will be stimulated.

Many of the changes listed in Figure 12.1 are substantial and some completely reverse a former position. Managing the system, for example, is very different from merely financing it. To question professional practice patterns and be prepared to change them is a complete rejection of the historical sanctity of professional freedom. New partnerships between ministries of health and providers in the field will, if they develop, require a new kind of public servant with new kinds of skills and attitudes.

The Ethics of Resource Allocation

Ethical questions of resource allocation are the result of

    ☐ shifts in the values of Canadians,
    ☐ the current environment of fiscal constraint,
    ☐ a focus on the outcomes of the health care system, and
    ☐ advances in technology that create more options.

Decision making, whether by consumers, practitioners, administrators, or governments, has cost implications. Canada now has good case-mix data that links costs to units of service and lengths of stay in hospitals. There is as yet, no good information on patient outcomes that result from the services consumed. Many of the best studies in this area are from the U.S.

Figure 12.1

The Evolution of Resource Allocation in Health Care in Canada

Determinants of Resource Allocation in 1950
    -The allocation patterns the year before
    -The preferences of politicians
    -The advice of physicians
    -The date of the next election

Determinants of Resource Allocation in 1970
    -The allocation pattern of the year before
    -The preferences of politicians and bureaucrats
    -The extraparliamentary process — the pressure of advocacy and community groups
    -The date of the next election
    -The coroners' reports
    -The media
    -The advice of health care professionals

Determinants of Resource Allocation in 1990
    -The preferences of politicians and bureaucrats (and these preferences were changing)
    -The allocation pattern of the year before
    -The extraparliamentary process
    -Opinion polls
    -Financial realities
    -A new understanding of the determinants of health
    -A better understanding of the usefulness of specific services

The Possible Determinants in 2001
    -The preferences of an informed public
    -Cost-outcomes relationships (the relative value of options)
    -The allocation pattern of the year before
    -The preferences of politicians and technocrats
    -The pressures of advocacy and self-interest groups

Figure 12.2

The Changing Role of Provincial Governments: Planners and Decision Makers

From	To
Insurance company	Planner, manager, and funder*
Financial protection of patients	Quality protection as well as financial protection*
Open-ended spending (1960s)	Global caps everywhere (1990s)*
Concern regarding total spending (1980s)	Concern regarding amount and quality of spending (1990s)*
Professional decisions unquestioned	Professional discretion limited by public policy*
Health care as the top priority	Health status as the top priority
Health status protected by the "Health Department"	Health status protected by all departments
Emphasis on hospitals and doctors	Emphasis on outcomes/impact*
Sickness policy	Health policy
Centralization	Decentralization
A bureaucratic, authoritarian Ministry	Partnerships with consumers and providers
Everything for everybody	What can be afforded*

*Shows points where ethical issues will be prominent.

Canadian provinces see ethical conflicts emerging with increased resource constraint. The federal government is reducing support for health care as a result of the 1991 *Federal Government Restraint Law* (Bill C-69). As a result, there will be changes in access to traditional programs, setting priorities for services, acquisition of technology, and comparisons of health care spending and other social programs that will focus on health. Canada is also experiencing a growth in business-oriented attitudes in health care and a simultaneous questioning of the charitable role of hospitals. Overall, the question being asked by provincial ministries is "Are we doing the right things right?"

Social values and visible ethical principles are now as prominent in program funding choices as they are in the physician's role in deciding which procedures to perform on which patients.

Canada has three major organizations that deal with health services research and nine ethics research centers mainly affiliated with universities or foundations. These groups have already produced useful findings in program evaluation (cost-benefit, cost minimization, and cost effectiveness) for targeted medical and surgical procedures. Many medical treatments and procedures were introduced in Canada without evaluation of either costs or outcomes, and it is now difficult to use evaluation findings to terminate or reduce funding to these commonly available procedures. Health professionals have been trained to provide them and consumers have come to expect them.

Resource allocation is, perhaps, the area of greatest weakness in quality control in Canada, and our resource allocation will remain weak until we know a great deal more about the benefits of various health services. The annual physical check up was actively promoted until an extensive 1975-76 study by the Canadian Medical Association led to the proposition that, for many years of one's life, the annual physical is not a good use of resources. Nurses took the temperature of all patients in hospital 2 to 4 times a day until someone examined the practice in the early 1960s and found that it was a waste of time. Similar comments have been made about fetal monitoring and the use of ultrasound in normal pregnancy. In terms of quality improvement, there is nothing so beneficial as stopping something that either produces no benefits or is actually a hazard.

The allocation or reallocation of money is one of the important tools for improvement of the quality of health care outcomes. Inability to control the costs in any major expenditure area is, consequently, a threat to quality improvement everywhere.

Many programs are aimed at better use of resources, and better resource use should mean better quality of care. For example, patient categorization in hospitals allows nursing staff to be better distributed to wards. Placement coordination services and regional patient assessment processes improve the matching of patients with programs or facilities. Operating room scheduling can minimize disruption of physician office time. The delivery of care through multidisciplinary teams can allocate work more efficiently and conserve patient resources. The amalgamation of obstetrical units or the designation of only a small number of hospitals as appropriate for highly specialized services also improves quality.

Provincial and federal statutes are fundamental to many quality control activities. The mandatory reporting and follow-up of selected diseases reduces their likelihood of being a hazard to the community. Provincially required certification, licensing, and discipline improve the quality of workers. The restriction of certain duties to certain professionals such as dentists and physicians is thought to protect quality, but negative impacts of these rules may be as great as the positive ones. Drug licensing and the use of federal legislation to ban unsafe equipment are other examples, as are regulations governing the granting of hospital privileges to physicians and dentists.

The Canadian Approach to Rationing: An Example of Resource Allocation

Every public policy choice brings with it some trade-offs, problems or tough choices. Canada has chosen public policy in health care that matches public funding of the insurance side of the industry and essentially private and entrepreneurial delivery of care. Canada offers first-dollar coverage, often described as "health care is free." With no visible disincentives for either consumer or providers, Canadians face rationing for some popular services from time to time, as supply adjusts to meet demand. Just as the early availability of Moosehead beer fluctuated at levels below demand — beer stores ran out and drinkers lined up for more, so the early availability of new technology such as coronary artery bypass surgery caused queuing and efforts to adjust supply.

Health care stories in Canada are also easy media. Physicians with a vested interest in increasing funding to particular services have been known to use the media as an intermediate target to government. Stories of patients dying while waiting for surgery are a media event in Canada, mainly because they are rare. The American media also target these as major events. Data from Canadian studies show that fewer than 1 percent of Canadians on waiting lists for bypass surgery die while waiting. Even after bypass, about 5 percent of those with advanced coronary artery disease face a risk of death each year. This is simply the risk affiliated with coronary artery disease itself. It is also true that watchful waiting is advantageous for some patients, who may be better off *not* receiving a medical or surgical intervention.

The primary decision-maker for a patient's position in a queue in Canada is the physician. Usually an urgent case is placed immediately at the front. Challenges to the government that it is the fault of an elected official that a patient has died are not always completely justified. For some physicians, a long waiting list is a reflection of their personal popularity and a source of self-esteem. Redistribution of these patients to other equally competent doctors is difficult to achieve, except in more progressive group practices.

The linguistic challenge in Canada is in health care no less intense that in many other areas of Canadian culture. In health care the debate revolves around when a managed queue becomes rationing. Most dictionaries define rationing as sharing or dividing equitably among those in need. Equity also implies that those in greater need may receive more. This is precisely what Canada's approach has been in both the funding and delivery of health care.

Rationing Coronary Artery Bypass Surgery in Ontario: An example of the Canadian Approach

A 1991 study of bypass surgery in Ontario found that increases in demand for bypass surgery resulted from increased aggressiveness in testing by cardiologists and increased safety of the procedure, allowing many more patients to become eligible.

Table 12.3

Growth in Bypass Rates in Ontario 1979-88

	Rate Per 100,000 Population
1979	28.6
1981	34.3
1983	41.5
1985	41.0
1988	43.0

Source: C.D. Naylor, A Different View of Queues in Ontario, Health Affairs, 1991, vol. 10, no. 3, p. 110-128.

These two factors caused an increase in the waiting list in Ontario in 1990 to about 1,800 cases. By 1991 this list had dropped to about 1,000 due to an integrated strategy introduced by the Ministry of Health. Phase one included an increase in the capacity of bypass programs by about 800 cases per year, followed by an increase in ICU beds and specialist nurses. Additional dedicated nurses were funded to manage waiting lists, and surgeons adjusted booking procedures to ensure more availability of emergency operating time and to reduce bumping of booked cases. Three hundred cases were done in the United States in 1991, and there was also an increase in angioplasty rates, reducing bypass queues. By the end of 1992, the waiting list will likely approach 500 cases or less. For many of these patients the wait will be only a few weeks.

When the issue of coronary artery bypass queuing is broadened to examine all procedures for which Canadians may wait, it becomes more difficult to set priorities. Measures of quality of life and anxiety over waiting must be paired with measures of cost-effectiveness of care and the value Canadians place on equity. It is outliers who create the media impression of crisis, not the norm.

Ethical issues emerge in the waiting list discussion at all three levels of distributive justice: macro, mezzo and micro. At the macro level is the debate over whether to direct additional capital and operating money to health care and to heart surgery. In both Canada and in the United States, an increasing number of the elderly, including those over 75 years of age, are receiving bypass surgery. This reinforces the notion that rationing in Canada is in favor of the elderly, and the same may hold true in America.

Table 12.4

Bypass Rates for Elderly Persons, Canada and the United States

United States	Per 100,000 Persons	
	1981	1985
Age 65-74	146	296
Age 75 and over	32	100

Canada	Per 100,000 Persons	
	1981	1985
Age 65-74	76	141
Age 75 and over	9	25

Source: G.M. Anderson, J.P. Newhouse, and L.L. Roos, "Hospital Care for Elderly Patients with Diseases of the Circulatory System: A Comparison of Hospital Use in the United States and Canada," The New England Journal of Medicine, 321 (1989): 1443-48

Note: C.D. Naylor notes (ibid) that this represents a 215 percent increase over 1981 for the United States and a 188 percent increase for Canada.

At the mezzo level of justice, decisions are made that alter distribution of resources within an institution. In Ontario, more resources in ICUs were allocated for bypass surgery and fewer were available for other procedures because not all the allocation was done with new money.

At the micro level then is the issue of which patient is determined to be next in line for bypass. This ethical decision has been left primarily in the hands of physicians, who, argues C.D. Naylor, may not distribute cases efficiently across equally skilled providers. This argument is based on the stringent requirements for post-graduate training in surgical specialties in Canada.

The issue of waiting in Canada is not that there are queues, but rather the appropriate management of information so that those in urgent need receive care immediately, while those targeted for an elective procedure are distributed to appropriate providers with shorter queues. In Canada, this queuing is far more acceptable than the notion of rationing American-style which leaves consumers with the decision of whether treatment is needed and worth the price of the user-fee or other deterrent. "Catastrophic coverage" is not in the Canadian vocabulary, as it is in America.

The Evolution of Rights

Patients' rights in Canada have emerged along two pathways: legal rights and moral rights. **Legal rights** are based on case law while **moral rights** are based to a considerable extent on an implicit promise from the professionals in the health care setting. Parallel to this evolution has been the philosophical move away from the medical model of health care delivery and toward the social model, with increased patient participation and partnership becoming the norm.

Two new paradigms are emerging in this environment. The first is the healthy public policy model which has, as a fundamental premise, the idea that health is not solely derived from health services. This implies that resources for health should be allocated to the things that do support health such as education and housing. The second paradigm is called, for want of a better name, the cost-benefit model. This framework states that only health care with a positive outcome will be funded by the public purse, while services with an unknown or undetermined outcome must be purchased with discretionary income. These models will change the fundamental assumptions surrounding patients' rights. The healthy public policy model will demand social responsibility from consumers and providers of health services. Patients will need good information on where best to "spend" the public's resources to best achieve health. Health services will not be provided when they offer less net benefit than some other public service whose programs produce health. The patient advocate will also be society's advocate.

The cost-benefit model will demand health service provision by the least expensive provider or the least intensive form of therapy. The main administrative function will be the denial of health care to those who will not benefit from it. Patients' rights under this model will be limited to access to proven therapy from the least skilled, and therefore least costly worker able to deliver that service. Eligibility and options will likely be outlined by a data processor or management information system. The role of the patient advocate will be to push the system to provide care.

Currently, Canada is probably somewhere between the medical model and the social model, hence the need for "rules" that govern the amount of paternalism and authority in the patient-provider relationship.

Concepts of Advocacy

Patient advocates, as employees of a hospital, walk a fine line between doing a good job and being fired for doing too good a job. Their responsibilities to patients transcend the usual employee relationship with the employer. Advocates have, in the past, focused their attention on patient education to achieve informed consent, patient representation for death with dignity or termination of aggressive therapy, and support of a patient for whom intervention will be of no benefit and is therefore discontinued. Just now emerging is the role of the advocate as an agent of social responsibility.

An advocate is not an ombudsman. This position is not one of redress but one in which patients in need of assistance are actively sought out. The advocate negotiates the complex hospital bureaucracy and tries to assure, wherever possible that the patient is satisfied with the services of the hospital. The **advocate** is a source of information. He or she opens lines of communication and uses patient complaints to improve policies and procedures. The advocate is an integral part of innovation and change in a hospital. Advocates should also have a role in quality assurance, risk management, accreditation, research approval, and liability issues.

The Hospital's Contract With the Patient

One of Canada's most widely read authorities on health law is Lorne Rozovsky. In his 1974 volume *Canadian Hospital Law*, Rozovsky states: "A hospital's responsibility to the patient is largely based on an implied contract with the patient....within the realm of legitimate expectation by the public. (The hospital) is also responsible for the acts of its servants, employees and agents." Of course, as Rozovsky points out, physicians who are not employed by the hospital can be negligent without the hospital being negligent. Nurses, except private duty nurses paid by the patient, are the responsibility of the hospital.

Health law in Canada's provinces, human rights legislation, and the Constitution provide a number of well-defined legal rights for patients, in addition to those mentioned earlier in the chapter. These include

- ☐ the right to be free from bodily harm and interference, from which is derived informed consent to treatment;
- ☐ the right to emergency care;
- ☐ the right to choose a doctor;
- ☐ the right to an acceptable standard of care, from which accreditation is derived;
- ☐ the right to choose or refuse a treatment, from which palliative and hospice care are developing;
- ☐ the right to a confidential medical record including the emerging issues surrounding access to one's own record and the emerging issues surrounding access to one's own record and the ability to destroy one's own record;
- ☐ the right to be treated without discrimination;
- ☐ the right to safekeeping of personal property while in hospital.

Moral rights include

- ☐ the right to be treated with respect;
- ☐ the right to personal privacy;
- ☐ the right not to be subjected to unnecessary diagnostic procedures;
- ☐ the right to have reasonable continuity of care.

The Ethics of Informed Consent

One of the measures of the quality of health care is the extent to which it respects patients' rights.

Perhaps the most important right, and one which is honored most of the time, is the right to refuse to do what a health professional recommends. This concept of informed consent is longstanding but is still evolving. At one time, a general consent form, usually signed at the time of admission to hospital, gave the physicians and institutions permission to proceed virtually as they pleased. Later, it became necessary for the consent to specifically authorize designated procedures. More recently, informed consent required that the patient not only understand what was being proposed, but that he or she also be fully informed about the risks associated with the intended services.

A new requirement has recently been added. An Appeal Court judgment in 1986 confirmed that merely describing the risks of what the caregiver wanted to do was not enough. Caregivers now must explain the available alternative courses of action to a patient so that an informed choice can be made. In this case, an award was made to a patient who became disabled following surgery. The surgery was found to have been adequately performed, but the option of nonsurgical therapy was not presented or explained to the patient. The fact that the possibility of major disability was not clearly spelled out was also criticized. Informed consent cannot now be considered to have been given until all clinical options have been described by the practitioner and understood by the patient.

The necessity for patient agreement when the patient is mentally competent is absolute, but the question of what procedure to follow when the patient may be mentally incompetent is more difficult. Mental health legislation attempts to protect the rights of the individual while also allowing physicians to institute therapy in selected circumstances without patient consent.

Patients probably believe and expect their medical information to be confidential, but they should be aware of the situations in which the confidentiality will not be preserved. Hospital and office medical records, or portions of them, can become partially or fully public through

- □ subpoena by a court,
- □ a request from the Canadian Security Intelligence Service,
- □ the compulsory reporting of a variety of reportable diseases,
- □ the compulsory reporting of vital statistics, or
- □ information provided to medical care insurance agencies so that payment will be received by the person providing service.

Patients in different provinces have quite different degrees of access to their medical records. In Quebec, access at all times is assured by law, but in most provinces patients have access to their records and related documents only at the discretion of an institution or physician or on the order of a court.

In the last few years a number of provinces have passed legislation preventing personal or legal access of patients or the public to peer review documents, which are the product of one professional examining the work of another. When the confidentiality of these records is not assured, it is difficult to find physicians who will adequately perform the peer appraisal process.

When patients consider any aspect of care to be inadequate, they have the right to initiate a civil lawsuit. The incidence of successful suits is likely to increase with an increasing acceptance of American precedents, with the use of juries instead of judges in some provinces, with more generous time limits for commencement of an action, and with increasing general use of contingency fees.

In theory, patients have the right not to be coerced by process or professionals. In practice, however, patients are routinely placed in a take-it-or-leave-it situation or are in other ways convinced they should do what the system recommends. This coercion is particularly the case with the physically disabled, most of whom are elderly, and it is also common with minority groups.

Health care providers and administrators are more often adapting their decisions and services to the religious and cultural preferences of clients.

Religious beliefs may alter diet, days of work, or dress at work. Autopsies, organ donation, circumcision, and the disposal of amputated limbs may have restrictions or protocols. Rituals vary at birth and at death. Blood transfusions and use of blood products may be prohibited.

Workers' Rights

Workers in health care, as with workers everywhere, should have the right to reasonable working conditions, including safety and absence of discrimination. The most contentious current safety issue is the risk involved in contact with patients with AIDS or HIV antibodies. Some American hospitals are now routinely testing a majority of admitted patients for AIDS so that staff may know when to be particularly careful regarding contact with body fluids.

Health and Welfare Canada has, for several years, sought individuals exposed to HIV by needle puncture wound or exposure to body fluids. The first 30 instances followed did not lead to infection. By 1992, however, at least 40 cases of AIDS in health workers in North America had been traced to work-related contact. The risk of hepatitis B, which is also contracted through contact with body fluids, is potentially much greater, but immunization is available. The incidence of hepatitis B in health workers is about five times that of the population at large. Over 1 percent of all hospital admissions are hepatitis B carriers. A Toronto surgeon died of the disease in 1985, an event which sharply increased the use of hepatitis B vaccine by health workers.

Other features of worker safety are no different from those in other industries. Hazards include noise, radiation, back injuries, burnout (especially in intensive care and palliative care units), toxic fumes, and injury from clients. Workers should also be assured of the confidentiality of employee health records, although this protection may not be required by law.

Summary

Ethical issues in Canadian health care are now debated regularly by ethics committees, hospital boards and public enquiries. Common law also influences how patient rights are interpreted and what constitutes informed consent. The emerging health professions in Canada will also be part of the evolving ethics of care, rationing, and public expectations for health care.

When it was generally believed that every health problem would be resolved as soon as enough resources were available, so there was little or no evaluation. All energies went into gathering more resources. Now we know health care cannot be given endless resources, but we also know evaluation costs money, so now we do not evaluate because we want to spend every dollar delivering care, whether or not that care needs delivery or whether or not other services would be a better value.

Planners and administrators who control resource allocation must allocate some of their scarce resources to research, including nonclinical studies, if they are to improve the usefulness of health care. Those who allocate resources must know the relationship between specific health care activities and the health status of individuals and communities. Otherwise, allocation will continue to follow either historical patterns or the winds of medical politics.

The cost of various services or episodes of care in hospital is now well known or can be known. Costs outside of hospital are not so constantly examined but are also measured. There is, occasionally, reasonably good data about selected groups of patients — for example, high-risk pregnancies — and sometimes adequate data describing changes in the health of the group over time. There is virtually never a clear understanding of the extent to which health care is responsible for whatever changes have occurred in the population, and there is even less likelihood that we know what would have happened if health care resources had been cut back or increased. Actions based on the known efficacy or/and cost-effectiveness of various health activities will only become possible when we

- document the health of a population at one point in time,
- measure it again at a later point in time,
- know the health resources and activities that were applied in between the two points in time, and
- are reasonably certain of the part played by the health activities in whatever health changes occurred.

References

Angoff, N.R. (1991). Do physicians have an ethical obligation to care for patients with AIDS? *Yale Journal of Biology and Medicine*, 64:207-246.

Ashby, M., Stoffell, B. (1991). Therapeutic ratio and defined phases: Proposal of ethical framework for palliative care. *British Medical Journal*, 1:1322-1324.

Ashwal, S., Caplan, A.L., Cheatham, W.A. et al., (1991). Session IV: Social and ethical controversies in pediatric heart transplantation. *Journal of Heart Lung Transplant*, 10:860-876.

Astrom, S., Nilsson, M., Norberg, A. et al., (1991). Staff burnout in dementia care — Relations to empathy and attitudes. *International Journal of Nursing Studies*, 28:65-75.

Baylis, F., Downie, J. (1992) *Codes of Ethics: Codes, Standards and Guidelines for Professionals Working in a Health Care Setting in Canada, Bioethics Department*. Toronto: The Hospital for Sick Children.

Benrubi, G.I. (1991). Euthanasia — The need for procedural safeguards. *New England Journal of Medicine*, 16:197-199.

Bergen, A. (1991). Nurses caring for the terminally ill in the community: A review of the literature. *International Journal of Nursing Studies*, 28:89-101.

Bunkle, P. (1991). Women and power: How can we change the system? *Health Care Women International*, 12:379-391.

Car-Hill, R.A. (1991). Allocating resources to health care: Is the QALY (Quality Adjusted Life Year) a technical solution to a political problem? *International Journal of Health Services*, 21:351-363.

Cartwright, A. (1991). Changes in life and care in the year before death 1969-1987. *Journal of Public Health and Medicine*, 13:81-87.

Corley, M.C. (1992. The ethical case analysis: Heroic measures for patients with chronic problems. Part II: Ethical analysis. *Dimensional Critical Care Nursing*, 11:36-40.

Crawshaw, R. (1991). A Piece of my mind. The quality of mercy. *Journal of the American Medical Association*, 266:614-615.

Davidhizar, R. (1992). Honesty: The best policy in nursing practice. *Today's OR Nurse*, 14:30-34.

Davis-Barron, S. (1992). Cold hard death, cold hard doctors. *Canadian Medical Association Journal*, 146:560-563.

Delbanco, T.L. (1992). Enriching the doctor-patient relationship by inviting the patient's perspective. *Annals of Internal Medicine*, 116:414-418.

Dickens, B.M. (1991). Issues in preparing ethical guidelines for epidemiological studies. *Law and Medicine in Health Care*, 23:35-70.

Dimenas, E.S., Dahlof, C.G., Jern, S.C. et al. (1990). Defining quality of life in medicine. *Scandinavian Journal of Primary Health Care*, suppl. 1:7-10.

Downie, J. (1992). Where there is a will, there may be a better way: Legislating advance directives. *Health Law in Canada*, 12:73-89.

Einsenberg, J.M. (1986). *Doctor's Decisions and the Cost of Medical Care, The Reasons for Doctor's Practice Patterns and Ways to Change Them*. Ann Arbor, Michigan: Health Administration Press.

Glassman, A.B. (1991). Ethics: A context for the clinical scientist (editorial). *Annals of Clinical Laboratory Science*, 21:225-256.

Hammes, B.J., Dahlberg, P., Colvin, E. (1991). Advance directives by dialysis patients: A practical approach to tough ethical decisions. *Nephrology News Issues*, 5:18-22.

Harris, M.D. (1991). Angels of the hospice. *Home Healthcare Nurse*, 9:11-12.

Hotter, A.N., McCommon, T.L. (1992). The ethical case analysis: Heroic measures for patients with chronic problems. Part I: The ethical case. *Dimensions in Critical Care Nursing*, 11:35-36.

Hull, R.T. (1992). Withholding and withdrawing life-sustaining therapy. Ethical considerations (editorial). *American Review of Respiratory Diseases*, 145:249-250.

Iserson, K.V. (1992). Emergency medicine and bioethics: A plan for an expanded view. *Journal of Emergency Medicine*, 9:65-66.

Jecker, N.S. (1991). Knowing when to stop: The limits of medicine. *Hastings Center Report*, 21:5-8.

Kluge, E.-H. (1992). Codes of ethics and other illusions. *Canadian Medical Association Journal*, 146:1234-1235.

Kurtz, R.J., Wang, J. (1991). The caring ethic: More than kindness, the core of nursing science. *Nursing Forum*, 26:4-8.

Langford, M.J. (1992). Who should get the kidney machine? *Journal of Medical Ethics*, 18:12-17.

Last, J.M. (1991). Epidemiology and ethics. *Law and Medicine in Health Care*, 19:166-174.

Latimer, E. (1992). Ethical challenges in cancer care. *Journal of Palliative Care*, 8 (Spring):65-70.

Lund, M. (1990). Conflict in ethics. Is DNR the right choice? *Geriatric Nursing* (New York), 11:291-292.

MacDonald, D. (1991). Unlimited claims on limited resources: Entropy, health care, and a hospice world view. Third in a series. *American Journal of Hospital Palliative Care*, 8:27-34.

Magder, S., Burgess, M., McGregor, M. et al. (1992). Resource allocation in the intensive care unit. *Annals of the Royal College of Physicians and Surgeons in Canada*, 25:55-58.

Miedema, F. (1991). A practical approach to ethical decisions. *American Journal of Nursing*, 91:20, 22, 25.

Miller, F.G. (1992). Is active killing of patients always wrong? *Journal of Clinical Ethics*, 2:130-132.

Misbin, R.I. (1991). Physicians' aid in dying. *New England Journal of Medicine*, 325:1307-1311.

Mizetic, B.Z., H.G. Pauli and P.-G. Svennson (eds) (1986). *Scientific Approaches to Health and Health Care*, Copenhagen: World Health Organization.

Moffic, H.S., Coverdale, J., Bayer, T. (1990). The Hippocratic Oath and clinical ethics. *Journal of Clinical Ethics*, 1:287-289; discussion 289-293.

Monsen, E.R., Vanderpool, H.Y., Halsted, C.H. (1991). Ethics: responsible scientific conduct. *American Journal of Clinical Nursing*, 54:1-6.

Moran, R.E. (1991). Working with doctors. Different priorities. *Nursing Times*, 87:35-37.

Overall, C. (1991). Access to in vitro fertilization: Costs, care and consent. *Dialogue*, 30:383-397.

Parsons, A.H., Parson, P.H. (1992). *Health Care Ethics*. Toronto: Wall & Emerson Inc.

Plamping, D., Delamothe, T. (1991). The citizen's charter and the NHS (editorial). *British Medical Journal*, 303:203-204.

Povar, G. (1990). Withdrawing and withholding therapy: Putting ethics into practice. *Journal of Clinical Ethics*, 1:50-56.

Scott, J.F. (1992). Lamentation and euthanasia. *Humane Medicine*, 8:116-121.

Singer, P.A., Lowy, F.H. (1992). Rationing, patient preferences, and cost of care at the end of life. *Archives of Internal Medicine*, 152:478-480.

Singer, P.A., Siegler, M. (1992). Advancing the cause of advance directives. *Archives of Internal Medicine*, 152:22-24.

Singer, P.A., Siegler, M. (1991). Decisions to forgo life-sustaining treatment. In: *Current Therapy in Internal Medicine*, 3rd ed. Kassirer, JP (editor) Philadelphia: Dekker.

Singer, P.A., Choudry, S. (1992). Ontario's proposed consent laws: 1. Consent and capacity, substitute decisions, advance directives and emergency treatment. *Canadian Medical Association Journal*, 146:829-832.

Singer, P.A., Tasch, E.S., Stocking, C. et al. (1991). Sex or survival: Trade-offs between quality and quantity of life. *Journal of Clinical Oncology*, 9:328-334.

Sneiderman, B. (1992). Euthanasia in the netherlands: A model for Canada? *Humane Medicine*, 8:104-115.

Stoddart, G. et al. (1987). *The Economic Evaluation of Health Care*, Oxford Press.

CHAPTER 13

What Can the United States and Canada Learn From Each Other?

The Economic Imperative for Cost Control in Health Care

C ompetition in the global marketplace is one significant factor causing trading nations to evaluate the efficiency and size of their health care systems. Spending more on health care means spending less on other sectors of the economy. Nations with universal insurance as the primary funding service for health care generally draw their resources from consumers through taxation. Employers do not carry the burden of health care premiums at the workplace. One of the reasons why America's products are not as competitive as they could be lies in the fact that an automobile, for example, has included in its price about $900 for health insurance for the workers who made the car. In Japan, Germany, and Canada, the car costs $900 less than its American counterpart.

It is true that America has the highest standard of living on earth. It is also true that Japan and Germany, and to some extent the number two country, Canada, are catching up fast. If growth trends continue, as shown in Table 13.1, America may not be number one for long.

Table 13.1

**Economic Growth Forecast
Annual Percent Change**

Country	1991	Forecast 1992	1993
Britain	-2.2	0.8	3.1
Canada	**-1.5**	**2.3**	**4.9**
Germany	1.2	2.0	3.0
France	1.2	1.8	2.6
Italy	1.0	1.8	2.4
Japan	4.5	2.2	3.9
United States	**-0.7**	**1.5**	**3.5**

Source: International Monetary Fund, 1992.

On April 13, 1992, *Newsweek* reported the tax burden on U.S. earners. It is modest by world standards, but it does *not* include health insurance, as is true for the other nations listed.

Table 13.2

Tax Revenue as a Percent of GDP 1992

Japan	26 percent
U.S.	28 percent
Canada	34 percent
U.K.	37 percent
Germany	39 percent
France	42 percent
Netherlands	48 percent
Sweden	49 percent

Source: International Monetary Fund, Japan's Ministry of Finance, 1992.

If the average U.S. family's private or employer-based health insurance bill was added to this tax level, Americans would likely pay more overall than Canadians. If private or employer-based insurance was replaced by government-based universal insurance like Canada's, Americans would put money in their pockets. The central organization of universal insurance has the capacity to keep the administrative cost down and to eliminate profit from the insurance market.

Table 13.3

Administration Cost Comparison, 1991

Nation	Cost
Canada	5%
Germany	5%
U.K.	6%
U.S.A.	22%

Source: Iglehart, 1991, Health Care Report GAO, U.S.A., 1991 data for Canada.

Note. Canadian sources usually list administration cost as about 2 percent, but the point is made.

There are several reasons why countries like Canada and Germany have significantly lower administrative costs. Canada keeps paperwork down and administration costs down by

☐ collecting the money for health care through income and excise tax, and
☐ having the provinces distribute the money directly to providers of care.

The provinces try to control growth in health care costs by

☐ slowing the introduction of new (and usually costly) technology by requiring the user of the technology to meet planning standards and priorities,
☐ making hospitals accountable for their global budgets,
☐ supporting training for primary care physicians at a higher rate than specialists, and
☐ provincial bargaining on fee schedules for physicians and, in some provinces, salaries for other health workers.

America hears many myths about health care in Canada. Of all the misinformation in the American debates about health care reform, the myth about universal insurance is the most damaging, not to Canada, but to progress in America.

Arguments against universal insurance include the following.

☐ We can't have universal insurance for health care in America because we don't trust our governments to collect taxes and spend them wisely.
☐ There are too many social problems in America for universal insurance: violence, ghettos, traffic, racial strife and AIDS are just a few worth noting.
☐ America's infant mortality is twice as high as Canada's. Although 600,000 women in America will get no pre-natal care this year, pre-natal care is said to be too expensive to be made available to all.
☐ Americans would not tolerate a delay in the delivery of elective surgery or a diagnostic test, even though access to services such as MRI have not been shown to enhance survival or improve quality of life.

What Can Canada Learn From America?

Canada's provinces, as the major funding agencies for health care, are actively involved in health care reform. Canada has the most expensive publicly-funded health care system on earth and this has become a burden in recessionary times. Looking to the United States for leadership in clinical and health services research has been common for decades. Canada also compares its health goals and health programs to those of European countries with better health indices such as lower infant mortality and longer life expectancy. Reducing poverty appears to be one of the most effective sources of health.

The federal funding infusion into capital projects after 1957 left Canada with the largest number of hospital beds per 1000 population by 1987. Most of these beds are currently full and length of stay is longer than in other countries. Health services research has indicated that shorter hospital stays do not usually harm the patient, and may actually improve outcome. Canada will likely move to close about half its existing beds by the year 2000 and not create new ones. Efforts in Canada to reduce length-of-stay to American levels have been successful in some jurisdictions, but not all.

Table 13.4

Canadian and American Hospital Use, 1987

Nation	Population Admitted to Hospital	Average Length of Stay in Days
Canada	14.5%	8.1 (excluding LTC days)
U.S.	14.7%	7.1

Source: Population figures from OECD, 1989; average length of stay from Rakich, J., "The Canadian and U.S. Health Care Systems: Profiles and Policies," Hospital and Health Services Administration, Spring, 1991.

Table 13.5

Hospital Beds Per 1,000 Population, By Country, 1987

Nation	Beds
Canada	16.1
Japan	11.0
Germany	15.2
U.K.	6.8
U.S.	5.3

Source: OECD, 1989.

The Great Technology Debate

Technology is still viewed as a major source of cost in health care by Canadian bureaucrats. Canada is well below America and Germany on the rate of introduction of new technology with the exception of transplants. For example, Canada ranks high in kidney transplants, primarily because it has been shown to be cost-effective and it provides a significantly improved quality of life over renal dialysis. Second, most jurisdictions in Canada allow drivers to identify themselves as organ donors directly on their drivers license. Efforts to constrain the introduction of new and expensive technology will likely continue in Canada.

Table 13.6

High-Tech Units/Million Persons, 1989

Procedure	Canada	Germany	U.S.
Open heart surgery	1.23	0.74	3.26
Cardiac catherization	1.50	2.64	5.06
Organ transplant	1.08	0.46	1.31
Radiation therapy	0.54	3.13	3.97
Lithotripsy	0.16	0.34	0.94
MRI	0.46	0.94	3.69

Source: Rublee, 1989.

Total Expenditure

Canada spends about 75 percent as much per capita for health care as America does. This expenditure creates fairly complete coverage for 100 percent of Canadians, while the larger U.S. expenditure represents about 85 percent coverage.

Table 13.7

Comparison of Health Expenditures Per Capita in 1987

United States	$ 2,051
Canada	1,483
Sweden	1,233
Switzerland	1,225
Norway	1,149
France	1,105
Germany	1,093
Netherlands	1,041
Australia	939
Japan	915
Italy	841
United Kingdom	758

Source: Ministry of Health of Ontario, 1991.

When population health indicators are added to the equation, Canada is spending more and achieving less than European countries while the reverse is true when Canada is compared to the United States. Most analysts in Canada believe that enough resources are allocated to health care in its traditional forms; some analysts say that too much is spent this way. However, the higher the expenditure, the greater the satisfaction consumers express with their country's health services. U.S. consumers are the exception to this finding as recent opinion polls have shown.

Table 13.8

Public Opinion of Health Care, 1990

Nation	Minor Changes Needed	Fundamental Change	Rebuild Completely
Canada	47 %	38 %	5 %
Germany	41 %	35 %	5 %
Japan	29 %	47 %	6 %
U.S.	10 %	60 %	29 %

Source: Blendon, R.J. and others, "Satisfaction with Health Systems in Ten Nations," Health Affairs, 1990, vol 9 no 2: 185-192.

For the remainder of this century, both Canada and the United States are expected to try to constrain health care expenditures. In Canada, the decisions will be political, in America most efforts now are administrative in nature.

Privatization of Health Care in Canada

The United States media has sold the story of Canada as a place where public financing of health care is the cause of delays, limits on technology and, therefore, risk to health. The issue of privatization of health care is one receiving more attention in Canada now than ever before, even though private sector involvement has always been strong in Canada.

- ☐ Private laboratories, private nursing homes, private home care, and private ambulances are part of the system. (Here, private means also "for-profit" even if the fees are paid by the province to a provider.)
- ☐ Alberta and British Columbia charge premiums for health insurance, although everyone pays the same premium regardless of risk.
- ☐ Many hospitals charge extra for private rooms.
- ☐ Doctors extra-billed until 1984; chiropractors still extra-bill in Ontario.
- ☐ Overall about 20 percent of Canada's health care consumption including dental care and prescription drugs is paid for with personal resources or private insurance.

Canadian hospitals are able to sell services to patients from other countries. For example, the University Hospital in London, Ontario, sells transplants; Manitoba has provided world-wide service for RH-negative pregnancies, and the Ottawa Heart Institute repairs hearts for children from eastern European countries.

Volunteers have played an important role in Canada's hospitals and health care institutions. Trustees on hospital boards are usually volunteers, although some may be appointed by provincial or municipal governments. Auxiliaries raise millions of dollars each year for capital projects and equipment. Many institutions also raise money by charging consumers for services not directly related to health care, and some of those are managed by volunteers.

User Fees in Canada

There is now a debate over user fees as a method of controlling excess demand. Canada is also examining whether co-payments in America and in European countries are a way of increasing the public support for health care or a way of lowering demand. About 50 percent of Canadians support the concept of user fees (*Globe* and *Mail*, November, 10, 1991). There is no evidence that user fees prevent access to the system, but there is a belief that for some services the poor may be deterred more than the rich.

Should Canada Have a "Two Tier" System?

If one does not like the public school system one can, as a major personal add-on cost, use a private school. Some argue that the same opportunities should exist in Canada for health care. The opportunities already exist if one chooses to go south to the Mayo Clinic or elsewhere; public subsidy will, in fact, be available to those who wish quicker or more luxurious care. The Ministry of Health in Ontario, until 1992, covered the total cost of health care for an Ontario resident who chose to receive care in the U.S. In 1992, this coverage was limited to the Ontario fee schedule. The consumer therefore pays the difference or purchases private insurance through providers such as Blue Cross. The exception to this rule occurs when a special service is not available in Canada. Under these circumstances the province covers all charges. Usually the Ministry will negotiate the charges ahead of time for an approved treatement. The opportunity is also available for non-Canadians. They can enter a Canadian hospital and be direct-pay patients, a choice which, in Ontario, brings benefits only to the hospital (not to the Ontario taxpayer and certainly not to the Ontario resident who is waiting in the queue).

The private purchase of hospital care and other health services should, analysts argue, be at least as legally possible in Canada by Canadians as by non-Canadians. Whether for-profit private hospitals and other institutions and programs would be built would depend on whether the private sector thought there was sufficient demand. It does seem preferable that these private services be available from hospitals or other facilities or programs that are separate from the public system, as is the case of education.

The major argument against this two tier system is that Canadians view health care as a right and that there should be equality of access for everyone. Other arguments favor the two tiered system. Education at public expense is available to everyone but Canadians and Americans accept the right of individuals to buy their education elsewhere if they wish, and education services are probably as important as health services. In many fields that are fundamental to health such as housing, recreation, occupational choice, and transportation, there is no expectation of equality. In addition, there is already a two tiered or multi-tiered system inherent in one's ability to purchase home support services such as nursing at personal cost or through private insurance, in the benefits associated with access to preferred accommodation, and in the ability of Canadians to seek health care in the United States if they can afford it. The two-tiered system also exists in a Canadian's varying ability to buy uninsured health care services such as dentistry or outpatient pharmaceuticals. As a final argument, the opportunity to spend one's disposable income on things that can be legally bought is a more fundamental and generic right than that of equal, but limited, access to health care services.

Managing Physician Resources in Canada

Canada has one of the highest ratios of doctors to population in the world, exceeded only by Germany and the United States. A 1991 federal study of physician manpower in Canada recommended a reduction in medical school enrollment of 10 percent. The ministers of health of all 10 provinces have endorsed this recommendation, which will be implemented in 1993. It will take about 10 years for this cut to take effect.

Table 13.9

Practicing Physicians Per 100,000 — 1987

Germany	280.8
U.S.	233.7
Canada	215.5
Japan	156.7
U.K.	137.2

Source: OECD, Health Data File, 1989.

Canada can take a lesson from America on better incentives for physicians. America has more doctors on salary than Canada, and America has more visible and enforced practice standards put in place by HMOs, third party payers, Medicare, Medicaid, and preferred provider arrangements. Problems with cost control, like the rapid rise in payments to doctors in Ontario would be better managed by reducing Canada's dependence on fee-for-service.

Canada's provincial governments have commenced a move towards management of physician numbers and have, in several provinces, placed a cap on the total earnings of doctors as a group. For example, the province of British Columbia introduced legislation in mid-1992 to cap the billings of 6,500 doctors at $1.3 billion for the 1992-93 fiscal year (a 2 percent increase over the previous year). This is an average of $200,000 per doctor. Although organized medicine in Canada is lobbying against such moves, this strategy will likely continue, due primarily to its success in managing cost in countries such as Germany. The German reimbursement model works well as a management strategy because the total medical services budget is set in advance and it is mainly physicians who determine how that budget is allocated. The policing of excess consumption is done by doctors. To some degree, this approach is beginning to be used at a micro-level in Canadian hospitals when physician privileges are renewed — not carte blanche, but for specific procedures and for limited numbers of those procedures. Rationing of these services is then clearly a medical decision since the physician determines which patients have first access. For example, if an orthopedic surgeon has privileges for 60 hip replacements within the budget of the department of surgery, the triage of who is most urgent need will rely on the surgeon's assessment of each patient's pain, mobility, occupation, age, probability of successful outcome, and so on. Clearly, it is not simply the existence of universal insurance that causes queuing, but the clinical judgment of providers of care.

When compared to the trends in management of physician resources in Europe and Japan, the United States is closer to the global village approach than is Canada due to its greater number of salaried and group-practicing physicians. Higher overall physician cost in the U.S. appears due to the distribution of 2/3 specialist and 1/3 primary care physicians as well as other factors. In Canada, the majority of physicians are family or primary care providers.

Setting Priorities in Canada

In recent years, most Canadian provinces have completed either a Royal Commission on health care or some form of advisory commission. Most provinces also have developed health goals and objectives. These should become the normative outline for setting priorities for funding. The following list is typical of provincial goals articulated by these commissions:

- ☐ maintain universality,
- ☐ no new money,
- ☐ predictable costs,
- ☐ greater value for money spent,
- ☐ better health,
- ☐ greater consumer participation, and
- ☐ greater provider accountability.

The Emerging Professions

In Canada, and in the U.S. to a lesser degree, nurses are employees of health care institutions. In the past, nurses have responded to, rather than led, changes in technology, evolution of hospital policy, and new patterns of care. Health care professionals such as physiotherapists, dieticians, and others have been under the direction of physicians. Dentists have monitored hygienists and dental technicians. More independent practice and more direct access by consumers to these providers is the trend of the future. This change will increase competition for health care resources and change the concept of who delivers primary care.

Both Canada and the U.S. will be interested in the expanded skills of these emerging professions, primarily as substitutes for more expensive physicians. Total cost savings will occur only if physician unemployment becomes an acceptable health policy in Canada as it is in Germany and other European Economic Community (EEC) countries.

The American Issues: State Reform of Health Care

Health care reform in Canada began in the provinces, with Saskatchewan taking the lead on such issues as non-profit universal insurance. The Canadian federal government saw an opportunity to step in front of this parade for the purpose of re-election. To some degree, much of the innovation in U.S. health insurance reform is being generated by individual states, just as in Canada. For example, Oregon has proposed that employers provide health insurance or pay a tax into a state insurance pool. Oregon's plans for Medicaid reform were blocked by President Bush, although much national and international attention has focused on the "Oregon Experiment." In Hawaii, the state already requires employers to provide health insurance coverage for workers to receive minimum benefits. Florida has a similar law, due to be in effect in December, 1994. Employers can choose the insurance carrier. California asked voters, in late 1992, to determine whether employers should be required to cover full-time workers. Minnesota has taken a different approach, a "Health Right" plan designed to cover low and moderate income families, paid for by a tax on doctors and hospitals.

Canada can learn from the Oregon Health Services Commission and the efforts made to develop a list of health services ranked in order of the greatest comparative benefit to the least. The state ranked 709 medical services in 17 categories. Categories 1 through 9 were essential to basic care; 10 through 13 were very important; while 14 through 17 were valuable to individuals but were either of high cost or of low benefit. The 1991 Medicaid budget in Oregon funded 98 percent of the first group (1-9), 82 percent of the second group (10-13) and 7 percent of the last group.

Efforts to fairly distribute Oregon's resources began in 1983, when the state legislature assembled community leaders to initiate the discussion. Computer models helped to rank medical treatments by cost-effectiveness. Town meetings were held and a telephone survey was conducted. The plan would have provided universal, basic services to Oregonians. Of special interest were 120,000 people, primarily women and children, who lived below the poverty line in Oregon, but did not qualify for Medicaid.

Conflict with Washington seems to have developed over Oregon's willingness to ration care to serious conditions that respond to treatment. The lack of comfort care for exceptionally small premature infants and end-stage AIDS patients was seen by the federal administration as discriminatory.

Public Health Issues

Last year Canada had 125 cases of tuberculosis. About half were found in immigrants from Southeast Asia and about half were among native Canadians. Last year, the U.S. had in excess of 15,000 cases, at an estimated cost of $1 billion. Part of the difference in incidence may be due to the higher number of HIV-positive persons in the U.S. but part is due to the greater importance placed on public health services in Canada. The Atlanta-based Centers for Disease Control (CDC) estimates that half of America's two-year-olds are not adequately immunized. In Canada, more than 90 percent of two-year-olds are fully immunized, either through a public health department or a physician's office, at no cost to the family.

The National Association of Community Health Centers in the U.S. reported that, in 1992, 8 percent of rural children and 18 percent of urban children must wait at least 3 weeks to visit a public health clinic. Two percent of all centers must turn away all new children.

Table 13.10

Oregon's Priority List

Rank	Category	Example
1	Treatment prevents death, full recovery expected	appendectomy
2	Maternity and newborn care	
3	Treatment prevents death, with residual problems	serious head injury
4	Preventive care for children	immunizations
5	Treatment extends life and improves quality of life	Type 1 diabetes, asthma
6	Reproductive services	contraceptives, sterilization procedures
7	Treatment gives comfort care	painkillers for terminally ill
8	Preventive dental care	
9	Adult preventive services	mammograms, blood pressure tests
10	Acute condition: treatment provides full cure	vaginitis, tooth cavities
11	Chronic condition: single treatment improves quality of life	hip replacement
12	Acute condition: treatment achieves partial recovery	arthroscopic knee surgery, cornea repair
13	Chronic condition: repeated treatments improve quality of life	sinusitis, migraines, psoriasis
14	Acute, self-limiting condition: treatment speeds recovery	diaper rash, conjunctivitis
15	Infertility treatments	
16	Adult preventive services	sigmoidoscopy for colon problems under age 40
17	Treatments provide minimal or no improvement in quality of life	treatment of viral warts

Source: "Rationing America's Medical Care," Brookings Institution, adapted from Oregon Health Services Commission report on "Prioritization of Health Services."

Conclusions

By example, Canada can show the United States how an efficient health insurance system can work. Estimated savings of this move are currently in the range of $50 billion annually. The United States, on the other hand, can show Canada how to apply incentives for efficient delivery of health care. Problems that will continue to plague both nations include rationing technology, fair pricing of health care professionals and supplies, reasonable access by consumers, and ethical issues.

Health care costs in Canada are rising about in line with national income, notwithstanding universal access to care on relatively equal terms and conditions. In the United States, health care is eating up an increasing share of national income.

Before 1971, health care costs consumed an almost identical share of the national income — roughly 7.5 percent — in both the U.S. and Canada. This share rose steadily, stabilizing at 8.6 percent in Canada for 1987, compared with an estimate of 11 percent and climbing in the U.S. for that same year. By 1992, Canadian consumption of GNP had risen to 9 percent for health care, while U.S. estimates exceeded 12 percent. This American consumption still left about 35 million people uninsured or underinsured, without good access to appropriate care.

As Dr. Evans and his co-authors stated in a 1989 article in *The New England Journal of Medicine*: "The large and growing gap between the United States and Canada drives home the point that, for good or ill, the form of funding adopted by Canada does permit a society to control its overall outlays on health care. Furthermore, it is unnecessary to impose financial barriers to access in the process."

The authors recognize, on the other hand, that the Canadian process and system, although successful in general, can be a "bruising political process, producing much sound and fury."

Health care in Canada is a complex process, with less than full agreement about causes of illness, treatment choices, and expected outcomes. The organization of systems to support health through health care is also plagued by lack of consensus.

The greatest attributes of universal insurance are: first, the opportunity to provide care quickly to those who need it, regardless of wealth or employer; and second, the almost complete absence of fear of the cost burden of illness, aging, or childbirth that is prevalent in America. Catastrophic illness in America can easily bankrupt a family. An uninsured couple faces hospital bills of $10,000 for childbirth. An elderly person must be without assets to qualify for nursing home care. In Canada, the very idea of these burdens seems outrageous to the public. The press often says Americans would not wait for elective care as Canadians do, conveniently omitting the direct costs to U.S. consumers of many aspects of their care, including long waits in public emergency departments, cash in hand before a doctor will treat an uninsured child who is injured or ill, and sudden de-insurance of a family if one member becomes chronically ill. Health insurance in America is for the employed and the well — far from the universal approach in Canada.

Notwithstanding the larger share of GNP devoted to health care in America, Canadians live longer, have half the infant mortality, and enjoy comprehensive services for acute care, long-term care, and public health.

The common problems of the Canadian system are those found throughout the publicly funded systems in the industrialized world. Current thinking about solutions to those problems involves a refocusing on quality of life rather than length of life, an emphasis on providing services that improve health outcomes, an understanding that there are many factors contributing to health other than medical and hospital care, and a belief that the public should choose how to spend its tax dollars.

The reason for clearly identifying these issues is to assist in an informed debate in America. Every public policy choice brings with it benefits and burdens. Canada has chosen universal insurance, federal principles and legislation, provincial planning, reasonable implementation of technology, and modest public support of medical research. The product of these choices is a system that looks somewhat American in its hospital sector but more like European nations in its community health and social support.

The provinces are now moving towards regional planning, hospitals are using population data to make decisions about programs, and physicians are advising patients about the probabilities of treatment outcomes to achieve fully informed consent. Many of these management strategies were developed in the United States and they have been adapted to Canadian needs. Perhaps Canada's health care system and its positive impact on health and security may show America that it is bordering on the possible.

References

Barer, M.L. and Evans, R.G. (1992). Interpreting Canada: Models, mind-sets, and myths. *Health Affairs*, 11(1): 44-61.

Blendon, R.J. and Edwards, J.N. (1991). Conclusions and forecast for the future in *System in Crisis: The Case for Health Care Reform*, Blendon and Edwards, ed. New York: Faulkner & Gray.

Culyer, A.J. (1989). Cost containment in Europe. *Health Care Financing Review*. Annual supplement.

Enthoven, A.C. (1989). What Can Europeans Learn from Americans Symposium: International comparisons of health care systems. *Health Care Financing Review*, Annual Supplement.

Evans, R.G., et al. (1989). Controlling Canadian health expenditures—The Canadian reality. *New England Journal of Medicine*, 320(9):571-577.

Fuchs, V.R. and Hahn, J.S. (1990). How does Canada do it? A comparison of expenditures for physician's services in the United States and Canada. *The New England Journal of Medicine*, 323: 884-890.

Harvard Community Health Plan (1990). *An International Comparison of Health Care Systems, Annual Report*. Boston: Harvard Community Health Plan.

Hughes, J.S. (1991). How well has Canada contained the costs of doctoring? *Journal of the American Medical Association*, 265:2347-2351.

Iglehart, J.K. (1991). Health policy report: Germany's health care system. *New England Journal of Medicine*, 324(7):503-508.

Jonsson, B. (1989). What Can Europeans Learn from Americans Symposium: International comparisons of health care systems. *Health Care Financing Review*, Annual Supplement.

Klevit, H.D., et al. (1991). A prioritization of health care services: A progress report of the Oregon health services commission. *Archives of Internal Medicine*, 151(5): 912-916.

Luft, H.S. (1991). Translating U.S. HMO experience to other systems. *Health Affairs*, 10(3): 172-186.

OECD Secretariat (1989). Health care expenditure and other data: An international compendium form the Organization for Economic Cooperation and Development. *Health Care Financing Review*, Annual supplement.

Roos, L.L., et al. (1992). Health and surgical outcomes in Canada and the United States. *Health Affairs*, 11(2): 56-72.

Rublee, D.A. (1989). Medical technology in Canada, Germany, and the United States. *Health Affairs*, 8(3).

Sandier, S. (1989). Health services utilization and physician income trends. *Health Care Financing Review*, Annual supplement.

Schieber, G.J. (1990). Health care financing trends: Health expenditures in major industrialized countries, 1960-87. *Health Care Financing Review*, 11(4).

Schieber, G.J., Poullier, J.P., Greenwald, L.M. (1991). Health care systems in twenty-four countries. *Health Affairs*, 10(3): 22-38.

Sutherland, R.W. and Fulton, M.J. (1990). *Health Care in Canada: A Description and Analysis of Canadian Health Services*. Ottawa: The Health Group.

U.S. General Accounting Office (1991). *Canadian Health Insurance: Lessons for the United States*. Washington, D.C.: Government Printing Office.

Woolhandler, S. and D.U. Himmelstein (1991). The deteriorating administrative efficiency of the U.S. health care system. *The New England Journal of Medicine*, 324(18): 1253-1258.

Young, D.W. (1990). Privatizing Health Care: Caveat Emptor. *International Journal of Health Planning and Management*, 5(4): 237-270.

GLOSSARY

A&D Committee—Admission and Discharge Committee

AEC—Atomic Energy of Canada

Alberta Dependent Adults Act—This act was passed in 1978, and provides for flexible arrangements for incomplete as well as complete transfers of powers in the case of incompetence.

Allopathic medicine—A medical practice based on a theory in which all diseases or body disorders have an external neutralizer.

ALS—advanced life support

ALoS—average length of stay

Ambulance Act—All Ontario ambulance services operate under the *Ambulance Act*, and all are fully or primarily financed provincially. Nine area ambulance services are administered directly under the Ministry of Health, five (including that of Metro Toronto) are municipally managed.

Atomic Energy of Canada—Federal organization that controls the use of all radioactive equipment and supplies.

Average Length of Stay—ALoS is the statistic that describes the most common (average) time spent by the patient in hospital. In calculating ALoS, the day of admission is not counted and the day of discharge is counted.

Beveridge Report—This report from Britain had recommended the establishment of national health systems by studying the levels of fitness and health.

Bill 65—This Quebec bill reorganized and regionalized health and social services, establishing a province-wide network of 12 regional councils (later to become 11) each with 21 members. It described the composition of the boards of the four categories of institutions.

Bill 120—Passed in Quebec in August, 1991, this bill enlarges the responsibilities of the existing Regional Health and Social Services Councils, restructuring health and social service delivery into regions.

Bill C-60—*Hospital Insurance and Diagnostics Services Act, 1957*

Bill C-69—*Federal Government Restraint Law, 1991*

Bill C-91—If passed, Bill C-91 will extend the patent protection to drug manufacturers for 20 years, making it more difficult for generic manufacturers to sell new drugs for less. It also contains a proposal to ban compulsory licensing which will conform with GATT rules.

BNA Act—*British North American Act, 1867*

BOND—Business Oriented New Development program

British Columbia Health Surveillance Registry—a group of separate registries covering congenital anomalies, genetic defects, and several chronic disabilities.

British North American Act—The *BNA Act* of 1867, and subsequent interpretations of it, gave the provinces jurisdiction over most health services. The federal government was given jurisdiction over health services only for those specific populations mentioned in the *BNA Act*. These include native peoples, the armed forces, the RCMP, immigrants or refugees at certain stages in the immigration process, those living in the Northwest Territories and the Yukon, and a few other small groups..

Business Oriented New Development program—BOND is a program in Ontario that was introduced in response to the idea that hospitals should be more business-like. Hospitals were encouraged to raise money through business ventures, and money raised is kept by the hospital.

Canada Health Act—Passed in 1984, this federal legislation affirmed the principles of health care in Canada: portability of insurance, non-profit administration, equity, access, and no unnecessary extra-billing.

Canadian Assistance Plan—CAP provides a resource base of up to 50 percent federal funding available for a broad range of rehabilitative, social support, and community based programs so long as the other half is provided by a source other than a federal institution. Fewer resources are available since the recession impact of the 1990s.

Canadian College of Health Service Executives—CCHSE represents health executives but does not offer certification or licensure.

Canadian Council on Health Facilities Accreditation — An accrediting organization similar to the Joint Commission in the U.S.

Canadian Fitness Survey—Conducted in 1981, this survey was carried out to provide basic information on the fitness levels and lifestyles of Canadians.

Canadian Health and Disability Survey—This survey was conducted as a supplement to the Canadian Labour Force Surveys of October 1983 and June 1984. Nineteen screening questions determined mobility, agility, seeing, hearing, speaking, and mental handicap. All persons reporting disability were followed up with a personal interview that examined the effect of the disability on the person's life.

Canadian Health Promotion Survey—Conducted in 1985, this study surveyed health knowledge, attitudes, beliefs, and behavior. The objective was to find out what Canadians think, feel or know about their health.

Canadian Hospital Association—CHA is a national organization representing the hospital industry. It is located in Ottawa.

Canadian International Development Agency—This agency provides a variety of health services and programs as part of their assistance to less developed countries.

Canadian Medical Association—CMA is a national organization for physicians.

Canadian Medical Protective Association—The CMPA is a physician-operated, non-profit insurance company through which all physicians in Canada buy their medical malpractice insurance. In 1986, physician enrollment increased rapidly due primarily to a withdrawal of private insurance from this market.

Canadian National Cancer Incidence Reporting System—This national registry keeps track of incidents of cancer among Canadians.

Canadian National Institute for the Blind—A group that maintains a registry of the blind population in Canada.

Canadian Nurses Association—The CNA is the national policy advisory body for nurses in Canada. Provincial nursing associations are the union or bargaining agent for nurses while the College in each province sets standards.

Canadian Renal Failure Registry—This registry records the pattern, treatment and outcomes of end stage renal disease. It is maintained by HWC and the Kidney Foundation of Canada.

Capitation payments—This form of payment for health care services (a fixed fee per person, per year) is not common in Canada but is in use at the Sault Ste. Marie Health Centre.

CAP—Canadian Assistance Plan

Caries—The decay of a bone or tooth which leads to cavities.

Case conference—At the point of delivery of care, the case conference brings together a number of providers with different skills related to the provision of care to a patient. It improves the coordination of the many disciplines involved in the care of the patient.

Castonguay-Nepveu Report—Published 1970, this report recommended a high degree of local participation and of regional control. The regional network was designed to measure local needs, set local priorities, and deliver a broad range of services to the extent possible given the resources available.

CCHFA—Canadian Council on Health Facilities Accreditation

CDC—Centre for Disease Control

CD—Community development

Centre Locale des Services de Santé—The CLSS is the only Canadian model that operates within a provincially planned regional network and under a comprehensive provincial statute that determines services, board membership, and relationships with other regional services. It is also the only CHC model that performs most of the functions performed in other provinces by public health units, and it is more closely related to a specific geographic area than most other examples.

CFS—Canadian Fitness Survey

Charities Accounting Act—This administers provincial charities and trust legislation in Ontario through a Public Trustee.

Charities Act—This federal legislation primarily allows organizations to become registered with Revenue Canada so as to be able to issue tax receipts for donations.

Charter of Rights—This is an important component of the Canadian Constitution.

CHA—Canadian Hospital Association

CHC—Community Health Center

CHDS—Canadian Health and Disability Survey

CHO—Comprehensive Health Organization

CHS—Canadian Health Survey

CHS—Community Health Services

CIDA—Canadian International Development Agency

CLSS—Quebec local community health center (Centre Locale des Services de Santé)

CMHA—Canadian Mental Health Association

CMPA—Canadian Medical Protective Association

CNA—Canadian Nurses Association

CNIB—Canadian National Institute for the Blind

College of Physicians and Surgeons—Created by provincial statute to protect the public, the colleges carry out licensing and disciplinary functions in accordance with appropriate provincial legislation. They investigate complaints, conduct peer evaluation programs, and identify and work with physicians addicted to drugs or alcohol.

Community development—This process describes physicians working with communities to help them make decisions and to be heard. The CD process is inherent in all activities which promote community involvement in policy selection, planning or administration.

Community Health Organization—The CHO is a type of community health center that approaches care with a view to coordinate and manage a broad range of traditional health and social services (like U.S. health maintenance organizations). CHOs are funded by capitation.

Community Health Center—For the consumer, a CHC provides one-stop shopping without fear of special charges. Community and consumer control increases the likelihood of accountability to those who use the CHC. The average physician consultation is longer, meaning that there is more discussion and patient involvement. To the government, CHCs bring financial predictability. There are fewer units to deal with, more opportunities for regional planning and no incentive to overutilization. For the doctors on the staff of a CHC, there are the pleasures of holidays with pay, regular working hours, sick leave, opportunities for continuing education without loss of income, and few administrative responsibilities. To other health professionals, CHCs offer the chance to make decisions and perform activities beyond the range of opportunities available in fee-for-service settings. To the advantage of all concerned there may, in the long term, be more desirable patterns of health service consumption.

For a small country, Canada has produced an impressive variety of community health center's names and organizational arrangements. British Columbia has Health and Human Resource Centres (HHRC). Saskatchewan has Community Clinics (CC). Ontario has two models, Community Health Centres (CHC) and Health Service Organizations (HSO). Most HSOs have two features which are unique in Canada; they are controlled by physicians rather than consumers and they are funded through capitation. In Quebec the CHC is called a Centre Locale des Services de la Santé (CLSS) or Local Community Health Centre (LCHC).

Community health services—CHSs offer a method of primary, secondary, tertiary and preventive medical care delivery that responds to every kind of medical problem, most social problems, and use most types of technology. CHS programs are located in homes, offices, clinics, the street, shopping centers, schools, work places, jails and recreational sites.

Conseil Régional de la Santé et des Services Sociaux—These regional councils were a key element in the restructuring of health and social services that began in Quebec in 1972 with the passage of Bill 65. The councils develop regional objectives, measure need, establish priorities, are responsible for coordination of the sources of health and social services, evaluate outcomes, to a variable (but usually quite limited) extent approve capital and operating expenditures, and provide advice to the Minister as required.

Coordinated units—These units work within a decentralized arrangement in which they are functionally related, but organizationally separate, and must work together.

Correctional Service Canada—CSC spends about $50 million a year providing health care for the inmates of federal custodial institutions.

CPI—Consumer Price Index

Crown Corporations—These organizations are sometimes referred to as quasi-public agencies.

CRSSS—Conseil Régional de la Santé et des Services Sociaux

CSC—Correctional Services Canada

CSS—Canadian Sickness Survey (1951)

Day hospital—The day hospitals offer an extensive range of professional services (physicians, nurses, physiotherapist, occupational therapist, social worker, and perhaps others), to give greater emphasis to rehabilitation. All usually provide a noon meal; they may or may not provide transportation.

Day surgery—Day surgery occurs when patients are brought in/admitted to hospital only for the duration of the procedure and recovery time which does not require an overnight stay. Day surgery patients may or may not be counted as admissions, depending mostly on which is most financially advantageous to the hospital or what rules have been laid down by the Ministry.

DCH—Department of Community Health (Quebec)

Denture therapist—In Saskatchewan, this person is able to legally fit, produce, and sell a denture or partial denture with little or no contact with a dentist.

Denturists—A person who is legally able to fit, produce, and sell a denture or partial denture with little or no contact with a dentist.

Denturologists—In Quebec, this person is able to legally fit, produce, and sell a denture or partial denture with little or no contact with a dentist.

Department of Indian and Northern Affairs—This federal department manages programs for native Canadians and residents of the Yukon and Northeast Territories.

Department of National Health and Welfare—This department is also called Health and Welfare Canada (HWC) and is the federal bureau for health policy.

Department of Veterans Affairs—This department had at one time a network of veterans hospitals but these have now largely been converted to civilian hospitals. DVA is now more of a paymaster than a deliverer of service.

Deputy Minister—The Deputy Minister is the senior bureaucrat or manager of the department while the Minister is the elected official held accountable for the policy and operations of the department.

Detoxification centers—These centers provide short term care during recovery from bouts of intoxication. Most are nonmedical, with no medical staff and minimal nursing and counseling capability. The medical models are much more expensive and offer few if any proven advantages over the nonmedical model.

DHC—District Health Councils

Distress center—These centers help people with mental or psychosocial health problems to remain stable and out of care (a primary prevention role). At the same time, they advise some people to go elsewhere for help (a diagnostic/secondary prevention role) and also actually being curative for some others (a therapeutic or tertiary prevention role).

District Health Councils—In Ontario, these councils are established by Order in Council, that is, at the request of the Minister of Health, with the support of the cabinet, and with the approval of the Lieutenant Governor. They report directly to the Minister. The mandate of DHCs is to advise the Minister of Health on the planning and coordination of health services. They are expected to identify needs, set priorities, plan a comprehensive health care program, coordinate health services, evaluate and promote cooperation within the regional network, and make recommendations regarding all of these. The councils may initiate studies themselves or may respond to proposals made by agencies or institutions.

DND—Department of National Defense

DNHW—Department of National Health and Welfare

DSC—Départments de Sánte Communautaire (French term for DCH).

DVA—Department of Veterans Affairs

ECC—Economic Council of Canada

Emergency rooms and routine ambulatory care—Seventy-five to ninety percent of patients who come to emergency departments have problems that are not life threatening or that can be dealt with in a relatively ordinary office. ERs are a major source of routine medical care, receiving 0.5 to 1 visit per person per year. There is considerable disagreement over whether or not most of these users are receiving care in the right place.

English Public Health Act—Created in 1875, it is this act on which most Canadian provinces have modeled their public health legislation.

Entrepreneurial model—This is a model of health care delivery in which the government does not play a role as a major provider or a funder of health services.

Envelope funding—A method of funding that includes different services and resources, and that can be used for different things based on decisions of a regional body.

EPF—*Federal Provincial Fiscal Arrangements and Established Program Financing Act* .

Established Program Financing Act—Legislated in 1977, *EPF* stabilized the federal contribution to health costs. After introduction of *EPF*, federal transfer payments to the provinces have been declining in the 1980s and in the 1990s, to date.

Extra billing—This method of billing includes charging resident fees in long term care institutions, requiring client payments towards drug costs, or extra costs charged by chiropractors. Extra billing also occurs when physicians provide services to patients from outside their province. Extra billing under any other circumstances is prohibited by the *Canada Health Act.*

Federal direct expenditures—This term refer to outlays by the federal government in relation to health care services for special groups such as natives, armed forces personnel, and veterans, in addition to expenditures on research, health promotion, and protection services.

Federal Government Restraint Law—Passed in 1991, Bill C-69 reduces the obligation of the federal government to maintain financial contributions to the provinces for health care.

Federal transfer payments—These payments are the amounts of cash (or tax points) that the federal Department of Revenue agrees to return to those provinces whose people actually paid federal income tax. In Canada, only the federal government has the power to coerce or tax individuals. Notwithstanding this power, provincial governments can also generate revenue through excise tax on such commodities as alcohol, tobacco, and gasoline.

Federal transfers to provinces—These include both cash and tax transfers for insured health services under EPF and the health portion of CAP transfers.

Fellow of the Royal College of Surgeons (or Physicians) of Canada—This designation, FRCS (C) or FRCP(C), is an indication of successful completion of a period (usually five years) of organized, practical training (internship and residencies), plus exams. The setting of exams and the awarding of the specialist designation are functions of professional colleges and not of a university. The U.S. equivalents are FACP or FACS.

Flexner Report—Written in early 1920s, this U.S. report found that most physicians were poorly trained and that most medical care badly documented.

FMG—Foreign medical graduate

Food and Drug Directorate—As part of HWC, this group covers drug and equipment testing through its Bureau on Medical Devices.

Foreign medical graduates—FMGs were once an important component of medical manpower in Canada. This group now has limited access to immigration because Canada has an over supply of physicians.

Foster homes—When referring to geriatric care, foster homes generally offer room and board and minimal personal care or supervision. Payment varies with the amount of care provided.

GATT—General Agreement on Tariffs and Trade

GDP—Gross Domestic Product

Geographic full time professor—University acceptance is a prerequisite to the hospital appointment of physicians with this status.

GFT—Geographic full time (professor)

GNP—Gross National Product

Goldberg Report—This 1987 reported on drug utilization reviewed a study showing that pharmacists prescribe more appropriately than physicians in a geriatric facility.

Granny flat—This term refers to small residences located on the grounds of family caregivers.

Granting/continuance of hospital privileges—The Medical Advisory Committee (MAC) through the Credentials Committee provides recommendations to the board regarding new additions to the medical staff. When the MAC feels that the hospital has enough psychiatrists, orthopedic surgeons, etc., it sends negative recommendations regardless of the qualifications of the applicants.

Gross Domestic Product—GDP reflects of the total production of the economy.

Gross National Product—GNP reflects the portion of economic production available for national consumption.

Group practice—This term has a meaning in the United States that is different from its meaning in Canada. In Canada, it means merely a group of physicians (or other professionals) who cooperate or merge for mutual benefit. In the United States, it means prepaid, consumer-sponsored, non-fee-for-service ambulatory care outlets and hospitals. The Kaiser-Permanente organizations were group practices before they became HMOs.

Hall Commission—This Royal Commission, chaired by Chief Justice Emmett Hall, chose to recommend the model of insurance in which essentially the entire population was covered regardless of age, income, or state of health. It is known as medicare.

HCA—Hospital Corporation of America

HCMT—Hospital Council of Metropolitan Toronto

Health agencies—Health agencies are non-governmental boards and agencies organized at the federal or provincial level are likely to have separately incorporated regional or local chapters. These local or regional chapters usually have some degree of management autonomy but also have close structural ties with the central body (Victorian Order of Nurses, Canadian Red Cross, Planned Parenthood).

Health association—This type of association is a single umbrella organization that, in some provinces, perform licensing/certification and regulatory duties as assigned by statute, as well as trade union functions.

Health Disciplines Act—This act defines the status, self-governing powers, and responsibilities of the various health care professions in Ontario. It is soon to be replaced by the broader umbrella legislation, the *Health Professions Regulation Act.*

Health Maintenance Organization—This rapidly growing model includes many famous early names that proved the worth of the CHC concept, such as the Kaiser networks, the Puget Sound Cooperative and the Health Insurance Plan of Greater New York (HIP). HMOs are all capitation based. They are owned and operated by a broad range of profit and nonprofit groups including labor unions, community groups, religious orders, universities, hospitals, physicians, and insurance companies. A number of HMOs have enrollments of half a million people or more and HMOs provide care to close to 10 percent of Americans. More than one quarter of all American physicians now have some relationship with an HMO.

Health Science Centers—HSCs are an early example of a multi-institutional organization.

Health Service Organizations—An HSO is a type of community health center that is most often controlled by physicians, rather than consumers, and are funded through capitation.

HIDSA—*Hospital Insurance and Diagnostics Services Act, 1957*

HIP—Health Insurance Plan of Greater New York

HMO—Health Maintenance Organization

HMRI—Hospital Medical Records Institute

Home care—Care at home lost favor because the best care came to mean care in hospital. This trend toward institutional care was augmented when health insurance tended to cover the costs of institutional care or office care but not the costs of care at home, and when changes in the nature of and dispersion of the family unit made home care more difficult. Care at home is now regaining favor, first, because it is becoming increasingly recognized that care at home is best for some patients and, second, because institutional costs have risen sharply.

Home sharing—This program matches the homeless with persons who have extra space.

Homeopathic medicine—A medical practice based on the theory that minute doses of whatever makes you sick will either make you better or keep you from getting sick in the first place.

Homes for Special Care—see "Residential care."

Hospital autonomy—The Board of Directors of each hospital writes the rules that govern the hospital. This is done within the limits of provincial legislation and regulations. For example, in Ontario, the board operates within the constraints of the *Public Hospitals Act* and its regulations although dozens of other statutes also affect hospitals. The board is responsible for providing the policy while the hospital administration implements the policy.

Hospital bylaws—The hospital's charter sets forth general institutional goals and characteristics. Hospital rules include such things as the responsibilities and functions of the board and the senior staff, the composition of board committees and the schedule of board meetings, financial control procedures such as the use of closed tenders, conflict of interest guidelines, appointments to and review of medical staff membership, duties and constraints associated with medical staff membership, the major organizational divisions of the hospital and the medical staff, the major health care services of the hospital, the process of patient admission, and other similar matters. This detailed set of rules is known as the hospital bylaws.

Hospital Council of Metropolitan Toronto—This is a regional health association that operates, or has initiated, a consulting service, group purchasing, a drug information service, laundry service, instructional media service, nursing registry, specialty food shop, high technology maintenance program, and research support service as well as its other functions.

Hospital foundations—Many hospitals have recently created foundations as legally separate but organizationally affiliated fund-raising branches.

Hospital Insurance and Diagnostics Services Act—Bill C-60, passed in 1957, required that a minimum but broad range of hospital inpatient services be insured, with outpatient coverage being optional. It also required that there be standardized national reporting, that services be available on equal terms and conditions, and that basic standards are met. In return, provinces received a per capita payment for each insured person. The law specifically excluded cost sharing for psychiatric services because those services were already provided, to some extent, at provincial expense.

Hospital Medical Records Institute—The HMRI is a data center for the hospital industry, located in Toronto.

Hospital Without Beds—These facilities offer diagnostic services, usually integrate health and social services, and may offer day care or other quasi-institutional services. They may offer general medical care, outpatient surgical services, usually offer 15-18 hours a day of minor emergency care, and may have a 1-2 bed holding unit for emergency stabilization before transfer.

HSO—Health Services Organization (Ontario)

HWC—Health and Welfare Canada

ICDA—International Classification of Diseases and Injuries

IDRC—International Development Research Corporation

Interlocking board memberships—In Quebec, board member exchange is mandatory for hospitals, regional planning councils, CLSCs and other components of the regional health and social services network.

International Classification of Diseases and Injuries—This refers to the International Classification of Health Problems in Primary Care (ICHPPC). The Emerl Diagnostic Book (E-Book) is a summary of ICHPPC that is sometimes used to describe the profile of an ambulatory care practice.

International Development Research Centre—An organization that provides a variety of health services and programs as part of their assistance to less developed countries.

JCC—Joint Conference Committee

Joint Conference Committee—The JCC is one of the devices commonly used to help resolve administrative conflict regarding such issues as costs and the use of staff. The JCC is composed of equal numbers of representatives from the administrative staff and the medical staff, and reports to the board of directors.

Le Régie—Quebec Health Insurance Board

Licentiate of the Medical Council of Canada—The LMCC provides standard examinations for all medical schools. Having an LMCC confirms the graduate as academically acceptable in all provinces.

LMCC—Licentiate of the Medical Council of Canada

Long term care—LTC in Canada is integrated with other levels of care and is insured except for a limited consumer contribution for the hotel or residence portion. This generally does not exceed the old age pension.

LTC—long term care

MAC—Medical Advisory Committee

Management Information Systems—MIS for the non-clinical side of health services includes schedules for patient rooms, patient visits, operating rooms or public health nurses, inventory distribution and control, routine reports regarding patient census, patient transfers or surgical activity, personnel files, financial records, and other operational data which are now routinely computer handled. MIS also includes imaging processes such as computerized axial tomography (CAT), positron emission tomography (PET), and nuclear magnetic resonance (NMR). MIS covers patient care locations and all laboratories and pharmacies, forming a network that allows instant access in many location to the latest information about a patient. Computer programs are increasingly being used in pharmacies and elsewhere to identify potential drug incompatibilities or interactive effects, and other pharmacy-based programs are identifying patients who are double doctoring for the purpose of drug abuse or trafficking.

Manitoba Infant Deafness Risk Register—This register documents infants at risk of hearing damage. The infants are then followed by regional hearing centers and the Provincial Office of Hearing Conservation.

Marsh Report—This report, developed in Canada, had recommended the establishment of national health systems by studying the levels of fitness and health in Canadians.

Meals on Wheels—A service, usually voluntary, that picks up meals from a hospital or LTC facility and sells them at cost to persons unable to prepare meals.

Medical Advisory Committee—According to the present *Ontario Public Hospitals Act*, the MAC "...shall advise and collaborate with the administration in all decisions affecting patient care including the allocation of space,...of beds by department and the development of facilities,...approve plans and priorities for the use of funds in all departments and divisions." The MAC is composed of all chiefs of clinical departments and major sub-departments or divisions.

Medical associations—The provincial medical associations, syndicates, or societies are fee setting/collective bargaining/political organizations. They are the labor unions or quasi-labor unions of the medical profession. They exist to serve and protect their members, not society. They negotiate fees, lobby for legislative changes and may represent their members when in dispute with the licensing/disciplining professional society. In a number of provinces there has been open conflict between the medical association and the college. Conflict usually centers around the vigor with which the college pursues its quality review functions.

Medical Audit Committee—This committee assesses the appropriateness of medical care.

Medical Care Act—Passed in 1966.

Medical practitioners—Features that most strongly epitomize private MPs are their control of executive functions such as choice of location, hours of operation, hiring of support staff, choice of office procedures, selection of clients, keeping of records, and distribution of revenue. These practitioners provide services to the populations of their choice and limit services in whatever way they choose.

Medical Research Council of Canada—This is a federal agency that manages resources for clinical and biomedical research.

Medical Services Branch—MSB is the branch of the HWC which maintains nursing stations, health stations, health centers, clinics, and small hospitals in the north and on reservations. MSB also trains and employs indigenous health workers and pays directly for care provided by health workers and institutions within the MSB network.

Medicare—This term refers to a system of publicly funded health care insurance based on freedom of choice and directed toward the effective use of the Canada's health resources to attain the highest possible levels of physical and mental well-being.

Members—In terms of CHC management, members tend to be those persons who wish to have a say in the management decisions, at least to the extent of voting at an annual meeting.

Minister of Health—The Minister is an elected member of a provincial or federal legislature appointed by either a Premier or the Prime Minister to the post. The Minister is the most senior person in the health system both provincially and federally.

MIS—Management Information Systems

MORE—Multiple Organ Retrieval and Exchange Program

MP—Medical practitioner

MRC—Medical Research Council (of Canada)

MSB—Medical Services Branch (of Department of National Health and Welfare)

Multiagency committees or boards—These include, for example, federal-provincial committees of ministers of health or of deputy ministers of health, and special federal-provincial technical advisory committees dealing with subjects such as manpower, laboratory services or health insurance. These committees may be standing or ad hoc and may be formal or informal. They exist at all levels of bureaucracy or community.

Multiple Organ Retrieval and Exchange Program—MORE is both a provincial and national program. For example, it is called MORE in Ontario, or the national Organ Waiting List (OWL) based in Winnipeg. Both have increased the likelihood that organs that are available will be used.

National Breast Screening Survey—This study involves 90,000 women aged 40-59 in 15 Canadian centers. Early results of the study released in December, 1992, have suggested that repeated examinations, including mammography, have clarified the role of early screening in breast cancer detection, and determined that early detection changes the course of the disease for women over 50.

National Defence Medical Centre—This is an Ottawa-based organization that has provided health care services to the armed forces.

National Health Research Development Program—An organization that has provided funding for research into clinical aspects of health care.

National Health System—This refers to a centralized model of health care delivery in which a government, usually through a ministry of health, organizes and delivers health services. (Example, U.K.)

NHRDP—National Health Research Development Program

NHS—National Health System

NNAAP—National Native Alcohol and Addictions Program

NP—Nurse practitioner

Nurse practitioner—The NP provides a range of primary care services. In Canada, most nurse practitioners work independently in remote and rural areas.

OCATH—Ontario Council of Administrators of Teaching Hospitals

OECD—Organization for Economic Cooperation and Development

OHIP—Ontario Health Insurance Plan

Ontario Blue Cross—In Ontario, Blue Cross is a non-profit $200 million a year supplementary insurance program covering 60 percent of Ontarians. Insurance may cover travel to the U.S., private hospital rooms, and other non-acute care expenses.

Ontario College of Physicians and Surgeons—A provincial organization responsible for the licensing and discipline of physicians who practice in Ontario.

Ontario Hospital Association—This is a health association in Ontario that offers a provincial hospital computer service and a hospital purchasing program in addition to its other functions.

Ontario Nursing Homes Act—This act controlls the health care funding and standards for nursing homes, most of which are private, for-profit.

Order in Council—This refers to an order made at the request of a minister, with the support of the cabinet, and with the approval of the Lieutenant Governor.

Osteopathic medicine—A medical practice based on the theory that the body, if it is operating well, has the capacity to respond to may diseases and threats of disease through emphasis on nutrition, exercise, manipulation, and lifestyle. There are no osteopathic schools of medicine in Canada and a U.S. Doctor of Osteopathy living in Canada could only be licensed as a drugless practitioner.

OWL—Organ Waiting List (Winnipeg)

Palliative care—PC is a philosophy of care in which care is delivered by teams who follow a patient out into the community as well as continue involvement in the institutional care. PC programs arose because of the inability, or unwillingness, of caregivers and health care institutions to respond appropriately to the needs of the terminally ill.

PAS—Professional Activities Study

PC—palliative care

Policy proposal—This originates within government or from outside. It tends to be examined in one department and reviewed by one minister. If supported at this level, it may then go to a cabinet committee (or several committees) and to various departments for financial, social, political, or organizational evaluation.

POMR—Problem Oriented Medical Record

Postal Alert—This is a program for high-risk patients at home in which the postman alerts authorities when mail has not been picked up.

Potential years of life lost—This statistic measures the negative impact of early injury or death.

Preferred accommodation—If a patient (or his or her insurer) is willing to pay extra, he or she will get a more private room and, in some hospitals, earlier admittance to the hospital. In Ontario, this was made more profitable for the hospital through BOND.

Private expense—This includes various uninsured and privately insured services provided by physicians, dentists, and other specialists, was well as non-funded institutional care costs, drugs, and appliances.

Private practitioners—A term for health care professionals that include physicians, dentists, optometrists, chiropractors, denturists, herbalists, osteopaths, podiatrists, chiropodists, acupuncturists, and clinical psychologists.

Problem Oriented Medical Record—This medical record is created when the case notes are separated on the basis of the problem that is being studied. The POMR is easier to digest, easier to summarize, and easier to use in research or quality review but is probably still less widely used than the traditional format.

Proclamation—Before an act becomes a law in the Canadian legislature, it must be "proclaimed."

Provincial Colleges of Physicians and Surgeons—Colleges are professional organizations that are also quasi-governmental agencies. They were created by statute to perform licensing, regulation, and disciplinary functions for their members. They are funded by fees paid by members.

Public insurance model—A model of health care delivery in which most health services are publicly financed but are administered and delivered by someone other than the government.

PYLL—Potential years of life lost

QA Committee—Quality Assurance Committee

QOL—Quality of Life

Quality assurance—QA is composed of two related but distinctly separate activities. The first of these is quality measurement (or evaluation), the second is quality control. Quality control through prospective medical audits may also be computer based, and a variety of students sharpen their diagnostic and treatment skills through computer assisted education.

Quasi-public agencies—These agencies were created by statute by governments of all levels to perform some specific regulatory, educational, policy-making, evaluative, or managerial function outside of the government bureaucracy, although not fully beyond government influence.

Quebec Health Insurance Board—Also called "La Régie," it is a quasi-governmental agency.

Rand Formula—The term for the change of a medical association to a "closed shop" where all physicians must belong to the association, as in Ontario.

Rationing—The order in which patients are admitted has, until now, been almost entirely the product of physician created priorities. If a patient waits, it is because other physicians have won the power struggles in the MAC. Rationing the number of urgent cases, especially those with proven cancer or a high degree of risk, is limited, and earlier admission of these patients would not seriously disturb the admission patterns of other patients.

RCMP—Royal Canadian Mounted Police

Reception centers—These include halfway houses, day care centers, rehabilitation centers and long term care institutions.

Reibel vs Hughes—A legal case in which the patient was not informed of the risks of the procedure, became hemiplegic as a result of the surgery, and successfully sued his physician.

Residential care—When applied to mental health services, this term refers to a live-in arrangement combined with some level of counseling and supervision. It is provided in a general category called Homes for Special Care.

Revenue Canada—This is the department of the federal government that collects tax.

RNA—Registered Nursing Assistant

Roster—This is a financial term applying to Ontario HSOs. It consists of those persons who consider the CHC to be their primary source of care. Monthly capitation payments are then made to the HSO for all rostered patients who, in that month, did not obtain services from an outside source which could have been provided by an HSO.

Royal Commission—Royal Commissions are appointed to conduct a government mandated evaluation of a defined problem. One example of such a commission is the Royal Commission on Health Care and Costs in British Columbia, which tabled their report "Closer to Home" in 1991.

Saskatchewan Dental Nurses Act—Passed in 1973, this act authorized dental nurses (now called dental therapists) to do selected dental work.

Sheltered housing—This term refers to a variety of architectural and service arrangements in which a number of domiciliary units are supported by on-site staff.

The support staff can be limited to only basic assistance, or it can consist of three shifts of full-time workers able to offer levels of care comparable to those available in long-term care facilities. As many as 5 percent of the elderly in the United Kingdom live in sheltered housing. In Canada, this arrangement is routinely available only for the young physically disabled. Quadriplegics in special housing may require up to six hours of personal care a day, including being turned through the night, being helped in and out of bed, being dressed for school or work, and being fed and the equivalent. This need for a large volume of care does not prevent the disabled from being tenants in the fullest sense rather than institutional residents. The care is delivered as home care rather than as institutional care and costs compare favorably. This model merits major consideration as another residential option for the disabled elderly.

Sheltered workshops—These workshops could be considered a form of psychiatric facility. They allow individuals to work in a protective environment where stress is reduced, production standards are different, and work can have a therapeutic component.

"Single point of entry"—This concept commonly refers to an arrangement in which persons in need of continuing care are referred to and assessed by a standardized process based in a single agency. After review, the person is referred to the appropriate community-based or institutional program for on-going care. This arrangement is a great improvement over unintegrated options in which many types of agencies, programs, and institutions use their own (often unique) referral and assessment practices.

Social drop-in center—These centers provide mental and psychosocial services for the homeless, the poor, the lonely, and the rejected. In addition to prevention, diagnostic, and therapeutic roles, they also provide food, socialization, and counseling.

Social Service Centers—They provide social services to institutionalized and noninstitutionalized persons and groups.

Statistics Canada—The major producer of and repository for a broad range of health and health services information.

Statutes—Statutes set out only general principles in Canadian legislation. The details are written into the regulations.

Teaching hospitals/university relationships—These relationships are made complex by legal, educational, quality of care, and financial factors. They are, as a result, clearly set out in formal agreements. In Canada, the agreement was made more simple by the fact that most of the income of both institutions comes from government. Hospitals may still wish to limit the extent to which their global budget supports costs which they think universities ought to pick up.

Ticket orienteur—A controversial $5 user fee in place in Quebec for those who inappropriately use an emergency room in a hospital.

Tissue Committees—Located in hospitals, Tissue Committees looked for evidence of unnecessary surgery.

Vocational rehabilitation of disabled persons—About 50 percent of this is funded through CAP. The second half of the funds are raised locally.

Voluntary agency—These agencies, as well as the informal caregiver serve an important role as creators and shapers of programs that later become universally accepted. Their track record is impressive. Palliative care, programs for persons with

Alzheimer's disease, sheltered housing for the disabled, and home-support services of various kinds exist because someone in the community saw a need and responded to it.

VON—Victorian Order of Nurses

Waxman-Hatch Act—(U.S.) Passed in 1984, this legislation cut the requirements that forced generic drug manufacturers to reproduce the clinical trials of the original drug company. This act demanded only that the active ingredients of the drug meet the same pharmacological standards as the original product.

WCB—Workers Compensation Board

Wheels to Meals—A service in which volunteer (usually) drivers deliver isolated individuals to central dining locations.

WHO—World Health Organization

Workers Compensation Board—Each province has a WCB funded by both employees and employers which provides income replacement and rehabilitation to injured workers. Most WCBs also support occupational health and safety programs.

INDEX

Abortion, 42
  legalization of, effects of, 51
Accountability, 23
Acquired immune deficiency syndrome
    (AIDS), 223
  hospices, 100
  reported cases, January 1991, 223
Activity, and life expectancy, 217—219
Acute (short term) care, 183
Acute treatment hospitals, 90. *See also*
    Hospital(s)
  organization of, 95
  role in long term care, 187
  short term, 89—117
Addiction recovery programs, 161—162
Addictions Research Foundation, 57
Administration, 2—3. *See also* Bureaucracy
  costs, 255
  services, 59
Administrators, power of, 5
Adolescents, health status of, 219—220
Advance medical directives, 234—235
Advice, 59
Advocacy, 245
AEC. *See* Atomic Energy of Canada
Aesthetics, dental, 198
Aging, 178
Agreements, formal, 11
AIDS. *See* Acquired immune deficiency
    syndrome
Alberta, 8
  health costs, 3
  health financing, 3, 193
    sources, 27, 33
  health insurance premiums, 33
  health services, 55
    utilization of, 41
  home care expenditures, 31
    as percentage of total health care
  expenditures, 1975 and 1986, 44
  hospitals
    expenditures per person, per patient-
  day and per separation, 43
      fees, 39
      municipal, 91
      provincial, 92
      regional boards, 106
      user fees, 33
  legislation in, 235
  medicare premiums, couple with two
  children, 1989-90, 34
  mental health services, 163
  native health in, 221
  physician billings, 1990-91, 41
  privatization in, 259
  public health expenditures as percentage
  of total health care expenditures, 1975
  and 1986, 44
  regionalization, evolution of, 13
  reporting in, 99, 224
Alberta Dependent Adults Act, 167, 269
Alberta Health Annual Report, 1991, 41

Alcohol abuse, 226
Alcoholics Anonymous, 57—58, 161
Allergies, seasonal, physician
    approaches to, 42
Allopathy, 68, 269
Ambulance Act, 207, 269
Ambulance services, 38, 206—209
  cost changes, 1975-87, 207
  provincial systems, 47
  use of, 41
Ambulatory care
  planning networks, 122
  routine, 203—204
American College of Surgeons, 71
American Doctor of Osteopathy (DO), 68
Anti-Tuberculosis League, 58
Appliance expenditures per person, annual
    percentages rates of increase, 1960-70
    and 1970-82, 32
Area-wide (regional) health planning
    agencies, 17—19
Armed forces' medical services, 47
Arthritis Society, 58, 127
Assessment services, 187
Atomic Energy of Canada (AEC), 48, 269
Auditors, 112
Australia, health expenditures per capita,
    1987, 258
Authority to deliver services, 8
Average length of stay (ALOS), 109, 269

Balance billing, 38
Barer-Stoddard Report Toward Integrated
    Medical Resource Policies for Canada,
    85—86
Belgium, organs for transplant in, 100
Beveridge Report, 49, 269
Bill 65, 19, 54, 269, 272
Bill 120, 22, 70, 269
Bill C-22, 143
Bill C-60. *See Hospital Insurance and
    Diagnostic Services Act* (HIDSA)
Bill C-69. *See Federal Government Restraint
    Law*
Bill C-91, 143, 146, 269
Billing
  extra, 38, 53, 66, 84, 116, 259, 274
  fee-for-service, 13, 40, 66—67, 75—76, 80,
  120
  of governments, for drugs, 148
  physician, 41, 75—76, 84
Bill of Rights, patients', 185
Biological factors, 89—90
Biology, 226
Birthing changes, 116
Blue Cross, 150
BNA Act. See British North American Act
Board memberships, interlocking, 11, 17,
  278
Boards of Health, 16

BOND. *See* Business Oriented New
  Development program
Brain-damaged, 183
Britain. *See* United Kingdom
British Columbia, 23
  abortions in, 42
  community health centers, 124, 126, 271
  costs, 3
  dental hygienists in, 198
  financing, 3, 193
  health care budget, 235
  health insurance premiums, 33
  HIV positives in, 223
  home care, 131
    expenditures as percentage of total
  health care expenditures, 1975 and 1986, 44
  hospitals
    expenditures per person, per patient-day
  and per separation, 43
    fees, 33, 39
    regional boards, 106
  hospital workers strike, 9
  household caregiver support devices, 191
  labor-management relations, 9
  living will legislation in, 235
  mental health services, 162
  Minister of Finance, budget address, 1992,
  70
  Ministry of Health, 233
  physicians in
    managing resources, 261
    programs which influence practice
  location, 82
  physiotherapists in, 66
  privatization in, 259
  public health expenditures as percentage of
  total health care expenditures, 1975 and
  1986, 44
  reporting in, 99, 224
British Columbia Health Surveillance
  Registry, 270
British North American (BNA) Act, 47, 55, 270
Budgets
  capping of, 233
  global, 41, 120, 234
  health, 142
Bureaucracy, 5, 16, 83—85
  definition of, 83
Burn centers, 202
Business Oriented New Development (BOND)
  program, 94, 270, 281

Cabinet, 1
Caesarian section rates, 41
California, health care reform in, 263
Canada. *See specific province or territory*
Canada Assistance Plan (CAP), 28, 49, 283
Canada Fitness Survey (CFS), 218
Canada Health Act, 4, 6, 33, 50—51, 66, 270,
  274
  support for, 38

Canada Health Attitudes and Behaviors
  Survey, 220
Canada Health Survey (CHS), 214—215, 217,
  222
Canada Sickness Survey (CSS), 222
Canadian Assistance Plan (CAP), 270
Canadian Association of Pathologists, 111
Canadian Cancer Society, 58
Canadian Charter of Rights, 8
Canadian Coast Guard, 208
Canadian College of Health Service Executives
  (CCHSE), 61, 270
Canadian Council on Health Facilities
  Accreditation (CCHFA), 111, 270
Canadian Fitness Survey (CFS), 270
Canadian Health and Disability Survey
  (CHDS), 217, 270
Canadian Health Coalition, 58
Canadian Health Promotion Survey, 218—219,
  270
Canadian Heart Foundation, 58
Canadian Hospital Association (CHA), 270
Canadian Hospital Law, 246
Canadian International Development Agency
  (CIDA), 48, 270
Canadian Labor Congress, 58
Canadian Labour Force Surveys, 217, 270
Canadian Lung Association, 58
Canadian Medical Association (CMA), 69, 100,
  241, 270
  licensure requirements, 83
Canadian Medical Protective Association
  (CMPA), 61, 76, 270—271
  fee schedule, 1992, 79
  litigation costs
    as percent of payments to plaintiffs,
  1980-86, 78
    total, 1980-86, 78
  membership fees, by specialty, 1983-86, 77
Canadian Mental Health Association (CMHA),
  154
Canadian National Cancer Incidence
  Reporting System, 271
Canadian National Institute for the Blind
  (CNIB), 58, 224, 271
Canadian Nurses Association (CNA), 196—
  197, 271
Canadian Physiotherapy Association, 111
Canadian Red Cross, 58, 98, 127, 276
Canadian Renal Failure Registry, 224, 271
Cancer
  clinics, 96
  mortality rates, 222
  treatment of, 42
CAP. *See* Canadian Assistance Plan
Capital expenditures
  annual percentages rates of increase per
  person, 1960-70 and 1970-82, 32
  health budget allocated to, 1980-90, 142
Capitation, 40, 67, 120, 271
Cardiac catheterization

comparative availability of, 140
  per million persons, 1989, 257
Cardiopulmonary resuscitation (CPR), role of
  public in, 209
Cardiovascular surgery, 137
Caries, 271
Case conferences, 11, 164—165, 271
Castonguay Commission, 166—167
Castonguay-Nepveu Report, 54, 271
Catastrophic coverage, 244
CAT scans, with headaches, frequency of, 42
CCHFA. *See* Canadian Council on Health
  Facilities Accreditation
CD. *See* Community development
Centers for Disease Control (CDC), 263
Central bed registry, 203
Central control, 187
Central monitoring, 202—203
Centre for Occupational Health and Safety,
  budget for 1987-88, 31
Centre Locale des Services Communautaires
  (CLSC), 11, 19—21, 54, 127
Centre Locale des Services de Santé (CLSS),
  11, 19—21, 125—126, 271
Centres d'Accueil. *See* Reception centers
CFS. *See* Canadian Fitness Survey
CHA. *See* Canadian Hospital Association
Change, 13
Charitable Gifts Act, 98
Charities, 97—98
Charities Accounting Act, 97—98, 271
Charities Act, 97—98, 271
Charter of Rights, 52, 271
CHCs. *See* Community health centers
CHDS. *See* Canadian Health and Disability
  Survey
Child psychiatry, 155
Children
  dental program for, 47, 195, 199—200
  health status of, 219—220
  mental health services for, 161
  psychiatric disorders in, prevalence of, 220
Childrens Aid societies, 57
Children's Hospital, 219
Chiropractors, 6
CHO. *See* Comprehensive Health Organization
Chronically ill, 204
Chronically mentally ill, community services
  for, 162
Chronic care, 172, 183—184
CHS. *See* Community health services
CIDA. *See* Canadian International
  Development Agency
Clarke Institute, 163
Clinical (patient care) services, 59
Clinical Staff Advisory Committee, 102
CLSC. *See* Centre Locale des Services
  Communautaires
CLSS. *See* Centre Locale des Services de Santé
CMHA. *See* Canadian Mental Health
  Association
CMPA. *See* Canadian Medical Protective

Association
CNA. *See* Canadian Nurses Association
CNIB. *See* Canadian National Institute for the
  Blind
Cognitively impaired, 183
Co-insurance, 38
  fees, 39
College of Family Physicians of Canada, 61,
  103
  certification by, 83
College of Family Practitioners of Canada, 232
College of Physicians and Surgeons, 69, 272
Communication problems, 204
Communities, 62
Community Clinics (CCs), 124, 271
Community development (CD), 272
Community Health Centers (CHCs), 5, 57, 124,
  127, 271—272
Community health centers (CHCs), 120—126
  advantages of, 123
  community/user control of, 121—122
  cost, quality and benefit of, 123
  disadvantages of, 123—124
  examples, 125—126
  financing methods for, 120
  members of, 122
  Ontario guidelines for, 122
Community Health Organization
  (CHO), 125, 272
Community health services
  (CHS), 119—135, 272
Community hospitals, 91
Community services
  for liaison, 128
  for long term care, 186
    categorization of, 185
  for mental health crisis
    intervention, 159—160
  for mentally ill, 161—166
  programs, 90
Competency, 232
Competition, between agencies or
  individuals, 12
Complaints, 232
Comprehensive Health Organizations
  (CHOs), 124
Computerized tomography scanners, per
  million population in Canada, 1990, 139
Computers, 100
Conference on Reconstruction, 49
Confidentiality, 247
Conseil Régional de la Santé et des Services
  Sociaux (CRSSS), 14, 16, 19—20, 166,
  272—273
Consensus seeking, devices for, 17
Consent, 168
Constitution, 246
Constitution Act, 1
Consumer Price Index (CPI), health care
  component of, 1986, 31
Consumer Reports, 21
Consumers, 62

Coordinated units, 273
Coordination and integration, 9—13
Coronary artery bypass surgery
    rates, 243
    rationing, 242—244
Coroners' inquests, 112
Correctional Services Canada (CSC), 48, 273
Cosmetic surgery, coverage for, 37
Cost(s), 3, 25—44, 249, 265. *See also* Health
    expenditures
    controlling, 233
        actions for, 234
        economic imperative for, 253—255
    growth of, 25
    share of national income, VII
    sharing of, 49
Cost-benefit model, 245
Council of Physicians and Dentists Clinical
    Staff Advisory Committee, 102
Council on Community Health
    Accreditation, 132
Counselling, 13
Courts, 5
CPI. *See* Consumer Price Index
Credentials Committee, 116, 275
Crohns disease, 223
Crown Corporations, 56—57, 273
CRSSS. *See* Conseil Régional de la Santé et
    des Services Sociaux
CSC. *See* Correctional Services Canada
CSS. *See* Canada Sickness Survey

Day care, 186
Day hospitals, 186, 273
Day surgery, 273
DCH. *See* Department of Community Health
Death, 215—217
Death certificates, 223
Deductibles, 38
Deinstitutionalization, 167—168
Dementia, 183
Denmark, LTC beds per 1000 people
    over 65, 180
Dental health, 200
Dental hygienists, 198
Dental nurses, 198, 200
Dental services, 197—201
    childrens' program, 47, 195, 199—200
    costs, payment, and financing
    of, 30, 200—201
    manpower in, 197—199
    programs, 47
Dental therapists, 198, 200, 282
Dentists, 7, 198
    earnings of, 200—201
    expenditures on, annual percentages rates
    of increase, per person, 1960-70 and
    1970-82, 32
Denture therapist, 273
Denturists, 273
Denturologists, 197, 273
Department(s) of Community Health (DCH)

(Départements de Santé Communautaire,
    DSC), 54
Department(s) of health and social services,
    merging of, 12
Department of Indian and Northern Affairs,
    273
Department of Manpower and Immigration, 48
Department of National Defense (DND), 48
    hospitals operated by, 92
Department of National Health and Welfare
    (DNHW). *See* Health and Welfare Canada
Department of Revenue, 275
Department of Veterans Affairs (DVA), 48, 273
Dependency ratios, 179
Deputy Minister, 273
Dermatologist billings, 1990-91, 41
Deterrent fees, 38
Detoxification centers, 161, 273
    costs for, 30
DHCs. *See* District Health Councils
Diagnostic procedures, utilization of, 42
Direct patient payments, 37—38
Disability, definition of, 173
Disability rates, 222
Disabled persons, vocational rehabilitation of,
    283
Disaster plans, components of, 205
Disaster response, 204—206
Disease, types of, 212—213
Distress centers, 157, 274
District Health Councils (DHCs), 14, 16, 18—
    19, 56, 274
    mental health services, 166
    regional committees with multiagency
    representation in, 17
    selection of members, 16
DND. *See* Department of National Defense
Doctor strikes, 2, 5
Douglas, Tommy, 2
Drop-in centers, 157, 283
    costs for, 30
Drug benefit plans, 142, 150
    beneficiaries of, 145
    cost to, 145
Drug expenditures, 29—30, 142—143
    client payments, 38
    dispensing fees, 147
    estimated, public hospitals, 144
    health budget allocated to, 1980-90, 142
    methods to control, provincial, 150
    per person, annual percentages rates of
    increase, 1960-70 and 1970-82, 32
    prices, 6
        control of, 143—146
Drug Prices Review Board, 143
Drugs
    billing governments for, 148
    dispensing of, 148
    generics, 146
    industry, 142, 147
    as measure of health status, 218
    post-marketing surveillance of, 149

prescribing and marketing, 146—147
prescriptions, writers of, 148
prescription sales, retail stores, 144
DVA. *See* Department of Veterans Affairs

Easter Seal Society, 224
ECC. *See* Economic Council of Canada
Economic Council of Canada, 7
Economic growth forecast, 253—254
annual percent change, 254
Edmonton, disaster response in, 206
Education, 191. *See also* Training
Elderly, 177—182. *See also* Geriatrics
bypass rates for, 244
entry age of, 179
rights for, 176—177
Elizabethan Poor Laws, 131
Emergency alarm systems, 189
Emergency care
area-wide approach to, 201—202
information services important to, 209
personnel, upgrading of, 208
public rating of, 209
role of public in, 209
Emergency departments, 202
central monitoring of, 202—203
24-hour, reduction of, 116
psychiatric services, 163
staffing of, 208
Emergency physicians, remunerations, 208
Emergency response system
components of, 201
mobilizing, for usual small scale
emergency, 206
Emergency rooms (ERs), 203—204, 274
central monitoring of, 203
Emergency services, 201
network costs, 207
Emergency transportation system. *See also*
Ambulances
characteristics of, 208
Emergency visits, 41
Emerl Diagnostic Book (E-Book), 278
Emotional health, 212
impact of illness on, 218
End-stage renal disease, 222—223
English Public Health Act, 131, 274
Entrepreneurial model, 46—47, 274
Envelope funding, 274
Environment, 89—90
EPF. *See Federal Provincial Fiscal
Arrangements and Established Program
Financing Act*
Ethics, 8, 229, 248
of constraint, 233—234
hospital, 231—232
of informed consent, 246—248
and legislation, 234—235
in native health, new, 233
norms, 232
of resource allocation, 238—241

Ethics research centers, 241
Europe. *See also specific country*
physician resources in, managing, 261
Evaluation
of health care, 232—233
of hospitals, 111—112
processes for, assessment of, 112—114
Evans, John, 68
Evans, Robert, 42
Extendicare, 59
Extra billing, 38, 53, 66, 84, 115, 259, 274
Extracorporeal shock wave lithotripsy,
comparative availability of, 140
Extramural hospital program, 131
Extraparliamentary processes, 17

Facility care liaison services, 128
Family social services, 128
Federal direct expenditures, 28, 274—275
Federal government, 47—52
grants from
conditional, 49
unconditional, 50
services financed and operated by, 49
Federal Government Restraint Law, 240, 275
Federal hospitals, 92
Federal-Provincial Advisory Committee on
Health Manpower, 1983 Report, 75—76
*Federal Provincial Fiscal Arrangements and
Established Program Financing Act* (EPF),
2—3, 27—29, 50, 274
Federal Restraint Law (Bill C-69), 4, 50
Federal transfer payments, 27—28, 31, 50, 275
Fee-for-service payments, 13, 40, 66—67, 75—
76, 80, 120
Fee-for-service professionals, 66—67
Fees
co-insurance, 39
dispensing, 147
licensing, 82
resident, 38
schedules, 74, 79, 84
setting, 74—75
user, 33, 38—39, 70, 259
Fellow of the Royal College of Surgeons (or
Physicians) of Canada [FRCS(C) or
FRCP(C)], 275
Fetal monitoring, during labor, 42
Field health care personnel, training of, 208
Financial aid, 191
Financing, 3, 25—44
approaches to, 114
methods of, 16, 120
public, history of, 1—2
sources of, 27—34, 44
Finland, national health system in, 47
Flexner Report, 71, 275
Florida, health care reform in, 263
FMG. *See* Foreign medical graduate
Food and Drug Administration (FDA), 147
Food and Drug Directorate, 275

Bureau on Medical Devices, 275
Food commissariats, 14
Food services, regional, 16
Foreign medical graduates (FMGs), 275
For-profit facilities and programs, 59—60, 90, 92
Foster homes, 187, 275
France
   economic growth forecast, annual percent change, 254
   health expenditures, per capita, 258
      and life expectancy and infant mortality, 1987, 26
   tax revenue as percent of GDP, 1992, 254
   total R&D expenditures as percentage of GDP, 1989 or latest year, 141

GDP. *See* Gross Domestic Product
General beds, 99
General consent form, 246
General hospitals, psychiatric services, 163
General practitioners, billings by, 1990-91, 41
Geographic dispersion, 12
Geographic full time (GFT) professor, 104, 275
Geriatrics. *See also* Elderly
   day care, 186
   day hospitals, 186
   definition of, 173
Germany
   administration costs, 1991, 255
   AIDS in, reported cases, January 1991, 223
   economic growth forecast, annual percent change, 254
   health care, public opinion of, 1990, 258
   health expenditures, per capita, 258
      and life expectancy and infant mortality, 1987, 26
   high-tech units/million persons, 1989, 257
   hospital beds per 1,000 population, 1987, 256
   infant mortality rates, per 1000 live births, 221
   physicians
      managing resources, 261
      practicing, per 100,000, 1987, 261
   R&D expenditures as percentage of GDP, 1989 or latest year, 141
   tax revenue as percent of GDP, 1992, 254
Gerontology, definition of, 173
GFT professor. *See* Geographic full time professor
Global budgets, 41, 120, 234
GNP. *See* Gross National Product
Goldberg Report, 149, 275
Government
   billing of, for drugs, 148
   boards, power of, 5
   fee schedule, 74
   health insurance bodies, production and use of doctor billing profiles by, 84
   health insurance plans, participation in, 39

power of, 4—5
role of, 1
   in drug industry, 150
Granny flats, 187—188, 275
Grants
   conditional, 49
   unconditional, 50
Greater Vancouver Mental Health Service, 14, 165
Greenshield, 143
Grenfell Mission hospitals, 104
Gross Domestic Product (GDP), 275
   percentage devoted to health care, 29
   percentage devoted to R&D, 141
   percentage devoted to tax revenue, 254
Gross National Product (GNP), 276
   percentage devoted to health care, 25—26
Group homes, 57—58
Group practices, 126, 276

Halfway houses, 57, 161
Halifax, disaster response in, 206
Halifax-Dartmouth, mental health services, 166
Halifax-Dartmouth Mental Health Planning Board, 11
Hall, Emmett, 50, 276
Hall Commission, 2, 36, 276
Hamilton Civic Hospitals, 91
Handicap, definition of, 173
Hawaii, health care reform in, 263
HCA. *See* Hospital Corporation of America
HCMT. *See* Hospital Council of Metropolitan Toronto
Headaches, CAT scans with, frequency of, 42
Health, 211—228
   blurred margin between sickness and, 212—213
   definition of, 211—212
   determinants of, 227—228
   problems, less serious and short-term, 222
   protection, 227
   standards of, selection of, 214
Health agencies, 276
Health and Human Resource Centers (HHRCs), 124
Health and Human Resource Centres (HHRCs), 271
Health and Welfare Canada (HWC), 47—48, 248. *See also* Medical Services Branch
   budget, 1987-88, 31
   Health Hazard Appraisal exercise, 155
   Home Care Report, 1990, 127
   Medical Research Council 1984 submission to, 5
Health association, 276
Health care
   evaluation of, 232—233
   political nature of, 4—6
   public opinion of, 1990, 258
Health care workers, 65—66

education of, 196—197
entry or function of, 7
male-female mix of, 196
rights of, 248
role of, expanding, legislation for, 235—236
safety of, 248
Health Disciplines Act, 53, 276
Health expenditures. *See also* Cost(s)
    annual percentage rates of increase per
    person for various categories of care, 1960-
    70 and 1970-82, 32
    federal direct, 28
    federal transfers to provinces, 28
    growth in, 29—30, 44
        annual percentage rates per person for
        various categories of care, 1960-70 and
        1970-82, 32
    national
        by category, 29
        by source of funds, 28
    per capita, 27, 258
        and life expectancy and infant mortality,
        1987, 26
    percentage of GDP, 29
    percentage of GNP, 25—26
    percentage of national income, VII
    percentage of total government budgets, 25
    private expense, 28
    provincial, 28
    total, 257—258
Health Hazard Appraisal exercise, 155
Health institutions, budget allocated to,
    1980-90, 142
Health insurance. *See also* Co-insurance
    public agencies, mandatory provision of
    specified information to, 84
    public model, 46, 281
        advantages of, 53
    universal, attributes of, VII, 265
Health Insurance Plan of Greater New York
    (HIP), 126, 276
Health insurance plans. *See also specific plan*
    features that Canadians want, 40
    government, participation in, 39
    premiums for, 33
    provincial, 52—53
Health legislation, 246; *See also specific bill or act*
Health maintenance organizations (HMOs),
    40, 125—126, 276
Health planning, 8—9
    area-wide (regional) agencies, 17—19
Health policy
    bodies which write, 6
    oriented to healthy outcomes, 22
Health professions
    emerging, 195—196, 262
    inside medical model, 80
    outside medical model, 81
    physician power over, 80—81
Health Professions Regulation Act, 53, 276
Health Right plan, 263
Health Science Centers (HSCs), 12, 91, 276

Health Service Organizations (HSOs), 122,
    124—125, 271, 276, 282
    types, 125
Health services, 89—90, 128, 201—209. *See
    also specific care*
    costs of, growth in, 25
    maintenance, 128
    philosophy of, 45—46
    research organizations, 241
    social, political, and structural factors
    in, 45—63
    utilization of, 40—41
Health status, 215
    advances in, socioeconomic and public
    health measures that caused, 227
    cause and effect, 225
    of children and adolescents, 219—220
    data, 223—226
        difficulties with, 224—225
    determinants of, 89—90
    indicators of, 213—214
    reports on, 214—215
    threats to it, 222—223
Hemorrhoids, physician approaches to, 41—42
Hepatitis B, 248
Heredity, 226
HIDSA. *See Hospital Insurance and
    Diagnostic Services Act*
HIP. *See* Health Insurance Plan of Greater
    New York
Hippocratic Oath, 71
Historical trends, 23—24
HMO. *See* Health maintenance organization
HMRI. *See Hospital Medical Records Institute*
Holistic approach, 122
Home(s)
    adaptations, 189
    sharing, 187, 277
    for special care, 282. *See also* Residential
    care expenditures, annual percentages
    rates of increase per person, 1960-70 and
    1970-82, 32
    visits, 190
        by nurses, 190
Home care, 127—128, 277
    client or agent willingness to receive, 129
    costs of, relative, 129
    expenditures, as percentage of total health
    care expenditures, 1975 and 1986, 44
    extent of benefit from, 131
    factors limiting, 128—131
    financial implications of, 130
    issues in, 130—131
    need for, relative, 129
    objectives of, 130
    organizational approach to, 131
    programs, 127
    publicly financed, determinants of
    delivery, 129
    sources of, 127—128
    termination of, delayed, 131
    total potential caseload, 130

Home care services, 128
  maintenance, 189
  support, 41
Homemaker services, 189
Homeopathy, 68, 277
Hospital(s), 90, 116—117. *See also* Emergency
  departments
  accreditation process, 113
  autonomy of, 277
  Board of Directors of, 277
  boards, 57
    control of appointments to medical staff
  by, 84
  bylaws, 101, 277
  classification of, by ownership, 91—92
  competency of, 232
  contract with patient, 246
  costs, 34
  day, 186
  as determinants of community health
  status, 89—90
  efficiency improvements, 114
  ethics of, 231—232
  evaluation of, 111—112
    processes for, assessment of, 112—114
  expenditures per person
    per patient-day, and per separation,
  1985-86, 43
    per patient-day and per separation, 43
  extramural programs, 131
  for-profit (proprietary), 92
  foundations, 97—99, 277
  function of, selection of, 110—111
  general, psychiatric services, 163
  health budget allocated to, 1980-90, 142
  industry, issues and questions that face,
  109—116
  joint ventures, 105
  mergers, 106
  and Ministries of Health, 92—94
  multi-institutional agreements, 104—107
    cooperative dispersion, 106
    one master provider and satellite users, 104
    shared services via new corporate entity, 105
  multi-institutional management of, 107
  objectives of, 112—113
  organization of, 94—104
  out-of-province income and patients in, 115
  religious, 91, 104
  reporting, 99—100
    annual, 109
  responsibilities of, to regional planning or
  service bodies, 110
  senior management teams of, 68
  social expectations of, 232
  special, expenditures, annual percentages
  rates of increase per person, 1960-70 and
  1970-82, 32
  use of, 256
  user fees, 33
Hospital centers, 54
Hospital Corporation of America

  (HCA), 59—60
Hospital Council of Metropolitan Toronto
  (HCMT), 61, 277
Hospital for Sick Children, 202, 204
*Hospital Insurance and Diagnostic Services
  Act* (HIDSA), 1, 49—50, 109, 153, 276—277
  requirements of, 49
Hospital Medical Records Institute (HMRI),
  111—112, 277
Hospital privileges, granting/continuance of,
  116, 275
Hospital services
  definition of, 37
  insurance programs for, 34—40
  utilization of, 42
Hospital statistics
  bed days, number per 1000 (total population
  per year), 109
  bed distribution, 115
  bed supply
    and community health status, 108
    number per 1000 population, 107—108,
  256
  percentage occupancy, 109
  and reporting, 107—109
  separations or admissions, per 1000, 41,
  108—109
Hospital Statistics 1 and 2 (HS1 and HS2), 109
Hospital Without Beds, 208—209, 277
Hospital workers strikes, 9
Hotel services, 59
Household caregivers
  assistance to, 129—130
  maintenance services, 128, 189—192
  stress to, causes of, 190—191
  support devices, 191
House of Commons, 6
House staff, 103
Housing, sheltered, 188
HSOs. *See* Health Service Organizations
Human rights matters, 8
HWC. *See* Health and Welfare Canada

ICDA. *See* International Classification of
  Diseases and Injuries
IDRC. *See* International Development
  Research Centre
Illness
  impact on emotional health, 218
  types of, 212—213
Image, 13
Imaging devices, 137
Immunizations, 263
  coverage for, 37
Improving Health and Well-Being in Quebec, 21
Income
  ceilings, 84
  maintenance of, 184
  regulation of, 8
Income Tax Act, 91, 98
Indemnity insurance, 37

Indians. *See also* Native peoples
    health services to, 47, 51
Individual(s), power of, 4
Individual social services, 128
Infant mortality, 221
    and per capita health expenditures and life
    expectancy, 1987, 26
    rates
        for native peoples, 221
        per 1000 live births, 221
Infection Control Committee, 102
Inflation, 31
Information
    exchange of
        devices for, 11
        easy, legal obstruction to, 13
    physician control over, 81
    services important to emergency care, 209
    unwillingness to share, 12
Informed consent, 230—231, 246—248
Institutionalism, 168
Institutions
    budget allocated to, 1980-90, 142
    regulation of, 7—8
Insurance. *See also* Health insurance
    indemnity, 37
    malpractice, 76
    programs for hospital and physician
    services, 34—40
    single carriers, 39—40
    universal, attributes of, VII, 265
Integration, 9—13
Intellectual health, 212
Interlocking board memberships, 11, 17, 278
International Classification of Diseases and
    Injuries (ICDA), 278
International Classification of Health
    Problems in Primary Care (ICHPPC), 278
International Development Research Centre
    (IDRC), 48, 278
International Statistical Classification of
    Disease and Injury (ICDA), 223
Interns, 103
Interprofessional hostility or disdain, 13
Intraregional liaison, devices for, 17
Inuit. *See also* Native peoples
    health of, 221
    health services to, 47, 51
Issues, 3—4
Italy
    economic growth forecast, annual percent
    change, 254
    health expenditures, per capita, 1987, 258
    total R&D expenditures as percentage of
    GDP, 1989 or latest year, 141

James Bay Clinic, 126
Japan
    AIDS in, reported cases, January 1991, 223
    economic growth forecast, annual percent
    change, 254

health care, public opinion of, 1990, 258
health expenditures, per capita, 258
    and life expectancy and infant mortality,
1987, 26
hospital beds per 1,000 population, 1987,
256
infant mortality rates, per 1000 live births,
221
physicians
    per 100,000, 1987, 261
    resources, managing, 261
tax revenue as percent of GDP, 1992, 254
total R&D expenditures as percentage of
GDP, 1989 or latest year, 141
JCC. *See* Joint Conference Committee
Joint Commission on Hospital Accreditation,
    71—72
Joint Conference Committee (JCC), 96, 278
Joint Liaison Committee, 107
Joint Medical Commission(s), 9
Joint ventures, 105
Justice
    macro level, 229, 243
    mezzo level, 230, 244
    micro level, 230, 243—244
    social, 229—230

Kaiser-Permanente organizations, 126, 276
Kenora (Ontario) Children's Aid Society, 8
Kingston, hospital mergers in, 107

Laboratory networks, provincial, 47
Labor-management relations, 9
Lac Du Bonnet Centre, 126
Laissez-faire model, 36
Lalonde, Marc, 48
Laundries, regional, 16
Leaf, Alexander, 230
Legal obstruction, to easy exchange of
    information or delegation of functions, 13
Legal rights, 244, 246
Legislation, 153. *See also specific bill or act*
    ethics and, 234—235
    health, 246
    human rights, 246
    living will, 234—235
    new, 235—236
Lesage, 54
Letters patent, 16
Lexchin, Joel, 147
Licensure, 82—83
Licentiate of the Medical Council of Canada
    (LMCC), 83, 278
Life expectancy, 177—178, 217—219
    at birth, 1931-89, 222
    and per capita health expenditures and
    infant mortality, 1987, 26
Lifestyle, 89—90
    choices, 226
Lithotripsy, per million persons, 1989, 257

Living Society, 191
Living wills, 234—235
Lloydminster, insurance coverage in, 37
LMCC. *See* Licentiate of the Medical Council
    of Canada
Local Community Health Centres (LCHCs),
    125. *See also* Centre Locale des Services de
    Santé
Long term care (LTC), 5, 172—173, 278
    current structure of, 173—174
    evolution of, 171—173
    financing of, 192—193
    goals or objectives of, 173
    institutional
        direct patient payments for, 38
        use of, 41
    organization and delivery of, principles that
    should govern, 174—177
    placement agencies, 57
    placement services, with authority to
    control placement, 12
    role of acute treatment hospitals in, 187
    users of
        mentally incompetent, 182—183
        physically dependent but mentally
    competent, 180—181
Long term care services, 171, 183—193
    community, 186
        categorization of, 185
    factors affecting size, 173—174
    at home, 185
    outside home, 185
    with primary objectives of prolonging life
    and maintaining physical health, 188
    with primary objectives of protection and
    elevation of quality of life, 188—189
    professional, through administrative
    arrangements, 190
    terminology, 172—173
    which deliver personal care, 190
    which make it possible for user to remain at
    home, 189—190
    which make physical environment more
    tolerable or manageable, 189
    which preserve households, 190—192
    which promote user control, 192
    which provide basic householder
    functions, 189
Long term dependency, definition of, 181
LTC. *See* Long term care

MAC. *See* Medical Advisory Committee
MacNeil, Chuck, 75
Macro-justice, 229
Magnetic resonance imaging (MRI)
    comparative availability of, 140
    per million persons, 1989, 257
Malpractice insurance, 76
Malpractice suits, 112
Mammographies, volume of, 42
Management, 59

citizen and provider participation in, 23
Management Information Systems (MISs), 278
Mandatory reporting, 84, 224
Manitoba
    community health centers, 126
    emergency physicians, remuneration for,
    208
    health care expenditures, growth in, 30
    health services, 55
        government in, 53
        per diem operating cost, 1991-92, 179
    home care, 129, 131
    home care expenditures as percentage of
    total health care expenditures, 1975 and
    1986, 44
    home care programs, 127
    hospital expenditures per person, per
    patient-day and per separation, 43
    hysterectomy rates in, 42
    labor-management relations, 9
    medical imaging in, 139—140
    physicians
        percent increase in, relative to
    population, 36
        professional organizations of, 69
    physician services, response to growing
    expenditures, 35
    privatization in, 259
    public health expenditures as percentage of
    total health care expenditures, 1975 and
    1986, 44
    rural health and social service boards, 14
Manitoba Health Report, 139
Manitoba Health Services Commission, 40, 56
Manitoba Imaging Advisory Committee, 139
Manitoba Infant Deafness Risk Register, 224, 278
Marsh Report, 49, 279
Massachusetts General Hospital, 229
Maternal mortality, 222
Meals on Wheels, 58, 189, 279
Medicaid, 146
    reform, 262
Medical Advisory Committee (MAC), 94—96,
    102, 116, 275, 279
Medical associations, 69, 279
    fee schedule, 74—75
Medical Audit Committee, 72, 279
Medical Care Act, 50, 279
Medical Council of Canada, 83
Medical model, 3, 65
    health professions inside, 80
    health professions outside, 81
Medical Post, The, 75
Medical practitioners, 279
Medical records, access to, 247
Medical Research Council (MRC), 48, 141, 155, 279
    1984 submission to Health and Welfare
    Canada, 5
Medical schools, 52
Medical Services Branch (MSB), 47, 233, 279
    budget for 1987-88, 31
    hospitals operated by, 92

services operated or funded by, 51
Medical staff, 96
  bylaws, 101—102
  committees, 102
  privileges of, process of granting, 102
Medicare, 2, 34, 50, 146, 279
  premiums, couple with two children, 1989-90, 34
Medications. *See* Drugs
Members, 122, 279
Mental competence, 167
Mental health, 166—167, 212
  concepts of, 158—159
  crisis intervention, community-based, 159—160
  facilities, 156—159
  inadequate, 154
  legislation, 247
Mental health services, 153—169
  children's, 161
  clients/users of, 154—155
    functional categories of, 154
  community-based, 161—166
  delivery of, 159—160
  diagnostic, 157
  inpatient, 159
  issues and problems, 167—168
  manpower, 162
  organization and administration of, 162—166
  preventive, 156—157
  programs, 127, 156—159
  public support for, 168
  regional, 165
  role of provincial governments in, 164
  specialization, 168
  therapeutic, 158—159
Mental illness
  characteristics and perceptions of, 155—156
  diagnosis of, 157
  policies and practices related to, 155—156
  prevention of, 156—157
    activities for, 156—157
Mentally ill, rights of, 231
Mentally incompetent, 182—183
  classification of, 183
Mergers, 106
Metropolitan Halifax-Dartmouth Mental Health Planning Board, 166
Metropolitan Toronto Hospital Planning Council, 18
Metro Toronto, 207
Midwives, 116
  education of, 197
Minister(s), 273
  decisions of, 16
Minister of Health, 279
Ministry of Environment, 48
Ministry of Health, 52, 269
  administration of ambulance services by, 207
  impact on hospitals, 92—94
  psychiatric services operated by, 163
Ministry of Health and Social Services, 21

Ministry of Labor, 48
Ministry of Transport, 48
Minnesota, health care reform in, 263
MIS. *See* Management Information Systems
Mississauga, disaster response in, 205
Mobile brain-damaged, 183
Moderately or severely demented, 183
Montreal Neurological Institute, 197
Moral rights, 244, 246
MORE Program. *See* Multiple Organ Retrieval and Exchange Program
Mortality
  infant, 221
  maternal, 222
Mortality rates
  age standardized, 222
  cancer, 222
  infant
    for native peoples, 221
    per 1000 live births, 221
Motor vehicle accidents (MVAs), death rates from, 221—222
MP. *See* Medical practitioner
MRC. *See* Medical Research Council
MSB. *See* Medical Services Branch
Multiagency committees or boards, 11, 280
Multidisciplinary teams, 121
Multi-institutional organizations, 12
Multiple Organ Retrieval and Exchange Program (MORE), 100, 280
Municipal governments, 55—56
Municipal hospitals, 91

National Anti-Poverty Association, 58
National Association of Community Health Centers, 263
National Breast Screening Survey, 280
National Cancer Incidence Reporting System, 224
National Committee on Medical Manpower, 1975 Report, 162
National Defence Medical Centre, 48, 280
National Health Research Development Fund (NHRDF), 141
National Health Research Development Program (NHRDP), 280
National Health System (NHS), 46—47, 280
National models, 46—47
National Native Alcohol and Addictions Program (NNAAP), 51
Native health, 221
  ethics of care in, new, 233
Native peoples. *See also* Indians; Inuit
  health services to, 51—52
    impediments to, 51
    programs, 52
Neighborhood health centers, 126
Netherlands
  health expenditures, per capita 1987, 258
    and life expectancy and infant mortality, 1987, 26
  tax revenue as percent of GDP, 1992, 254

Neurosurgical nurses, education of, 197
New Brunswick
   direct patient payments in, 38
   drug benefit plans, 150
   home care, 131
   home care expenditures as percentage of
   total health care expenditures, 1975 and
   1986, 44
   hospital expenditures per person, per
   patient-day and per separation, 43
   hospital reporting in, 99
   hospitals
      extramural program, 131
      provincial, 92
      regional boards, 105
Newfoundland
   Grenfell Mission hospitals in, 104
   licensing fees in, 82
   public health and home care expenditures
   as percentage of total health care
   expenditures, 1975 and 1986, 44
   ratio of hospital expenditures per person,
   per patient-day and per separation, 43
Newfoundland Medical Association, 82
Newfoundland Medical Board, licensure by,
   82—83
Newfoundland Royal Commission, on hospitals
   and nursing home costs, 1984, 99
New orientations, 22—23
New Perspective on the Health of Canadians, 48
New York City, AIDS in, 223
NHRDP. See National Health Research
   Development Program
NHS. See National Health System
Nisga Tribe, health services for, 233
NNAAP. See National Native Alcohol and
   Addictions Program
Norway, health expenditures, per capita, 1987, 258
Nova Scotia
   fee setting in, 75
   labor-management relations in, 9
   living will legislation in, 234
   professional organizations of physicians in, 69
   public health and home care expenditures
   as percentage of total health care
   expenditures, 1975 and 1986, 44
   ratio of hospital expenditures per person,
   per patient-day and per separation, 43
Nova Scotia Minister of Health, 166
NP. See Nurse practitioner
Nurse(s), 6—7
   home visits, 190
      costs for, 30
Nurse practitioner (NP), 280
Nursing homes, 5

Objectives, 13
OCATH (Ontario Council of Administrators of
   Teaching Hospitals), 18
Occupational health services, 90
OHIP. See Ontario Health Insurance Plan

One-stop shopping, 12, 121
Ontario, 8. See also District Health Councils
   AIDS hospice, 99—100
   ambulance services, 207—208, 269
   cancer clinics, 96
   children, prevalence of psychiatric disorders
   in, 220
   community health centers, 124, 271
      guidelines for, 122
   coronary artery bypass surgery in
      rates, 1979-88, 243
      rationing of, 242—244
   dental health in, 200
   disaster response, 205—206
   doctors strike, 1986, 5
   emergency services, 202
      network costs, 207
   extra billing in, 66, 115
   federal transfer payments to, 50
   financing and costs, 3
   health care expenditures, 25
   health funding, sources of, 27
   health insurance premiums, 33
   health service organizations in, 125
   health services
      government in, 53
      governments in, 56
   home care in, 131
      expenditures as percentage of total
   health care expenditures, 1975 and 1986, 44
   Hospital Boards of Directors in, 277
   hospitals
      acute treatment LTC, 187
      beds, number per 1000 population in,
   107—108
      expenditures per person, per patient-day
   and per separation, 43
      foundations, 98
      July 1990 report of Fundraising
   Programs, 99
      mergers, 106—107
      and Ministries or Minister of Health, 93
   labor-management relations, 9
   legislation in, 235
   long term care
      financing of, 193
      institutional beds, 99
   long term care services, 191
   mental health services, 162, 166
   midwives in, 116
   Minister of Health, 166
   Ministry of Health, 98, 163, 260
   physicians
      payments, 66—67
      professional organizations of, 69
      programs which influence practice
   location, 81
   policy examples, 8
   privatization in, 259
   psychiatric beds, 160
   psychiatric hospitals, 161
   public health expenditures as percentage of

total health care expenditures, 1975 and 1986, 44
public health services, 132—133
public health units, small, merging of, 12
quality of life indicators, 214
regionalization, evolution of, 14
registries, 224
reporting in, 224
Ontario Auditor General, 98
Ontario Blue Cross, 280
Ontario Child Health Survey, 1983, 220
Ontario College of Pharmacy, 147
Ontario College of Physicians and Surgeons, 61, 280
    Peer Evaluation Program, 84, 232
Ontario Council of Administrators of Teaching Hospitals (OCATH), 18
Ontario Crippled Children's Central Care Registry, 224
Ontario Health Insurance Plan (OHIP), 75
    payments
        to professionals, 31
        by type of service and by in and out of province, 1984-85, 33
Ontario Health Service Organizations, 122
Ontario Hospital Association, 61, 280
Ontario Hospital Services Commission, 56
Ontario Nursing Homes Act, 185, 280
Ontario Public Hospitals Act, 95, 279
Ontario Royal Commission into Confidentiality of Health Information, 1980, 7
Ontario Supreme Court, 98
Open heart surgery
    comparative availability of, 140
    per million persons, 1989, 257
Order(s) in Council, 16, 281
Oregon
    health care reform in, 262
    priority list, 264
Oregon Experiment, 263
Oregon Health Services Commission, 263
Organization, 2—3, 23—24
Organ transplantation, 137
    comparative availability of, 140
    organs for, 100
    per million persons, 1989, 257
Organ Waiting List (OWL), 100, 280
Orthodontists, 198—199
Osteopaths, training of, 68
Osteopathy, 68, 281
Ottawa
    birthing in, 116
    emergency units, 202
    federal drug regulatory agency in, 147
    food commissariat, 14
    privatization in, 259
    psychogeriatric clinics, costs for, 30
Ottawa-Carleton
    addiction recovery programs, 161
    detoxification centers, 161
    long term care institutions, utilization of, 41
    mental health services, 162—163

regional food services and laundry, selection of members, 16
Ottawa-Carleton Placement Coordination Service, selection of members, 16
Ottawa Civic Hospital, 6, 91
Ottawa Heart Institute, 259
Ottawa-Hull, insurance coverage in, 37
Ottawa Riverside Hospital, 91
OWL. *See* Organ Waiting List

Palliative care (PC), 186—187, 281
Palliative Care Foundation of Canada, 186
Pap smears, volume of, 42
Paramedics, training of, 208
PAS. *See* Professional Activities Study
Paternalism, definition of, 181
Patient records, integrated, 13
Patient registries, 209
Patient satisfaction surveys, 112
Patients' Bill of Rights, 161, 185
Patients' rights, 231, 246
    evolution of, 244—245
    principles that support, 174—176
Payments, 53
    capitation, 40, 67, 120, 271
    fee-for-service, 13, 40, 66—67, 75—76, 80, 120
    methods of, effects of, 80
    salary, 67
    sessional, 67
PC. *See* Palliative care
Peer review, 247
Peer review documents, access to, 247
Personal care services, 128, 190
Pharmaceutical Advertising Advisory Board, 147
Pharmaceuticals, 137—138, 142. *See also* Drugs
    earnings, growth in, 143
Pharmacists, 147—149
    historical perspective on, 147—148
    role of, 149—150
    rural and urban, 148—149
Philanthropy, definition of, 98
Philosophy, 2
Physical emergencies, response to, 201
Physical fitness, benefits of, 218
Physically dependent but mentally competent, 180—181
Physician(s), 5—7
    associations, 68
    autonomy of, 70—74
    billing, 41
        pattern changes, 75—76
    billing profiles, 84
    control over information, 81
    in decision-making, 114—115
    expenditures, 30
        per person, annual percentages rates of increase, 1960-70 and 1970-82, 32
    fee schedule, 74

health budget allocated to, 1980-90, 142
income, 69—70
    sources of, 31
licensing of, 82—83
in management, 96—97
payments, 53
    capitation, 40, 67, 120, 271
    methods of, effects of, 80
    salary, 67
    sessional, 67
in policy roles, 67—68
power over other professions, 80—81
practice location, programs which influence, 81—82
practicing, per 100,000, 1987, 261
professional functions of, 82—83
professional organizations of, 69
representatives, 68
resources
    managing, 260—261
    planning, future directions in, 85—86
role of, 65—87, 236
training of, 68
Physician services
    approaches to common ailments, 41—42
    insurance programs for, 34—40
Physiotherapists, 7, 66
Placement, central control over, 187
Placement agencies, 57
Placement services, 187
Planned Parenthood, 58, 276
Planning, 3, 6—9
    area-wide (regional) agencies for, 17—19
    citizen and provider participation in, 23
Poison information centers, 209
Policy, 3, 6—7
    examples of, 8
    oriented to healthy outcomes, 22
    proposals, 281
Polyclinics, 126
POMR. *See* Problem Oriented Medical Record
Population
    aging, 178—180
    percentage by age, 216
Postal Alert, 188, 206, 281
Potential years of life lost (PYLL), 281
Power
    and quality of life, 181—182
    restoration of, strategies for, 182
Preferred accommodation, 281
    use and cost of, 115
Price regulation, 8
Prince Edward Island
    hospital expenditures per person, per patient-day and per separation, 43
    public health and home care expenditures as percentage of total health care expenditures, 1975 and 1986, 44
    regionalization in, evolution of, 14
Priorities, 2, 13
    setting, 262
Private expense, 28, 281

Private Hospitals Act, 92
Private practice, 66—67
Private practitioners, 66, 90, 281
Private sector
    for-profit, 59—60
    nonprofit agencies or facilities, 57—58
    role of, 1
Privatization, 259
Problem Oriented Medical Record (POMR), 281
Problems, 3—4
Procedures, rates of, 41
Proclamation, 281
Professional Activities Study (PAS), 111—112
Providers
    organizations, 60—62
    regulation of, 7—8
Provinces. *See also specific province*
    Colleges of Physicians and Surgeons, 57, 281
    federal transfers to, 275
    goals of, 262
    governments, 52—55
        role of
            changing, 240
            in mental health services, 164
    health expenditures, 28
    hospitals, 92
    ministries, 53
    ministries of health, 111
    Office of Hearing Conservation, 224, 278
Psychiatric disorders, prevalence in children, 220
Psychiatric facilities, 47
    admissions, 160—161
    beds, 160
    hospitals, 104, 161
Psychiatrists, salaried, 167
Psychogeriatrics, 155
    clinic costs, 30
Psychosocial problems, and health services utilization, 42
Public financing, history of, 1—2
Public health
    clinics, 263
    expenditures, as percentage of total health care expenditures, 1975 and 1986, 44
    hospital drug expenditures, estimated, 144
    inspectors, responsibilities of, 132
    issues, 263
    measures, 227
    programs, 127
    units
        chief executive officers of, 68
        small, merging of, 12
Public health services, 47, 131—134
    costs of, 133
    issues in, 133
    problems of, 265
Public Hospitals Act, 92—93, 98, 101, 277
Public Hospitals Act Review, 116
    Report of the Steering Committee, 114

Public insurance agencies, mandatory provision of specified information to, 84
Public insurance model, 46, 281
   advantages of, 53
Public opinion, 258
   support for mental health services, 168
Public policy, 89
   adoption of, legislative stages of, 7
   as determinant of health, 227
Public policy model, 245
Public programs, financing of, 3
Puget Sound Cooperative, 126, 276
PYLL. *See* Potential years of life lost

QOL. *See* Quality of Life
Quality, 7
Quality assurance (QA), 282
Quality Assurance Committee, 102
Quality of life
   indicators of, 214
   power and, 181—182
Quarantine stations, 92
Quasi-public agencies, 56—57, 111, 282
Quebec
   abortion clinics, 99
   access to medical records in, 247
   acute treatment hospitals in LTC, 187
   community health centers, 124, 126, 271
   denturologists in, 197, 273
   doctors in, under Bill 120, 70
   health and social services system, 19—22, 54—55
      current reform issues in, 21—22
      government in, 53
      government structure of, 19—20
      organization of, current issues in, 22
      regional network of institutions in, 20—22
   health funding, sources of, 27
   home care, 127, 131
   home care expenditures, 31
      as percentage of total health care expenditures, 1975 and 1986, 44
   hospital expenditures per person, per patient-day and per separation, 43
   hospitals, professional staff organizations in, 102
   information, 81
   interlocking board memberships, 11, 17, 278
   labor-management relations, 9
   life expectancy in, 217
   living will legislation in, 234
   local community health center. *See* Centre Locale des Services de Santé
   local community service centers. *See* Centre Locale des Services Communautaires
   mental health in, 166—167
   Ministry of Health, 54
   Ministry of Social Affairs, 54
   Ministry of Welfare, 54
   physician practice, programs which influence location of, 81—82
   physicians, professional organizations of, 69
   psychiatric beds, 160
   public health expenditures, as percentage of total health care expenditures, 1975 and 1986, 44
   public health services, 132
   quality of life indicators, 214
   regional committees with multiagency representation, 17
   Regional Health and Social Services Council. *See* Conseil Régional de la Santé et des Services Sociaux (CRSSS)
   regionalization, evolution of, 14
Quebec Health Insurance Board (La Régie), 56, 278, 282
Quebec Medical Association, 69
Queen Street Mental Health Centre, 162
Queen's University, 107
Queensway General Hospital, Toronto, 59

Radiation therapy
   comparative availability of, 140
   per million persons, 1989, 257
Rand Formula, 69, 282
Rate or price regulation, 8
Rationing, 115, 241—242, 282
   of coronary artery bypass surgery, 242—244
Reception centers (Centres d'Accueil), 54, 282
Records
   access to, 247
   integrated, 13
Recreation, 185
Referral arrangements, 203
Régie, La. *See* Quebec Health Insurance Board
Regional agencies, characteristics of, variability of, 15—17
Regional authorities, characteristics of, variability of, 15—17
Regional boards
   characteristics of, variability of, 15—17
   methods of selection of members, 16
Regional body
   decision by, 16
   degree of influence or authority of, 16
Regional commissions
   characteristics of, variability of, 15—17
   methods of selection of members, 16
Regional committees
   methods of selection of members, 16
   with multiagency representation, 17
   variability of characteristics, 15—17
Regional councils
   characteristics of, variability of, 15—17
   methods of selection of members, 16
Regional departments, variability of characteristics, 15—17
Regional food services, 16
Regional Health and Social Services Councils, 22, 166, 269

Regional health planning agencies, 17—19
Regional Hospital Planning Councils, 14, 18
Regionalization, 14—15
    authority for, sources of, 16
    evolution of, 13—15
    institutional or program obstruction of,
    techniques for, 17
    objectives and philosophy of, 15—16
    prerequisites or devices for strengthening,
    17
Regional laundries, 16
Regional mental health services, 165
Regional programs, variability of
    characteristics, 15—17
Registered nurses (RNs), 196—197
Registered nursing assistants (RNAs), 196
Registries, 203, 209, 224, 270—271
Regulations, 7—8
Reibel vs Hughes, 231, 282
Religious hospitals, 91, 104
Reporting, 224—225
    errors in, 225
    hospital, 99—100
        annual, 109
    mandatory, 224
Report of the Steering Committee, 114
Research, 137—138, 141
Research and development, 143
    total expenditures as percentage of GDP
        1989 or latest year, 141
        selected countries, 1989 or latest year,
    141
Researchers, 112
Resident fees, 38
Residential care, 159, 282
Residential options, 185—186
Residents, 103
Resources, 3
    allocation of, 248
        ethics of, 238—241
        evolution of, 239
        rationing, 241—242
            example, 242—244
        matching to health needs, 23
Respiratory Technologists, 195
Respite care, 191
Revenue Canada, 98, 282
Rights, 8. *See also* Bill of Rights
    for elderly, 176—177
    legal, 244, 246
    moral, 244, 246
    patients', 231, 246
        evolution of, 244—245
        principles that support, 174—176
    workers', 248
RNA. *See* Registered Nursing Assistant
Rochon, Jean, 68
Roemer's Law, 39
Roster, 122, 282
Royal College of General Practitioners, 65
Royal College of Physicians and Surgeons, 103,
    111

certification by, 83
Royal Commission(s), 47, 50, 74, 282
    on Health Care and Costs in British
    Columbia, 282
Rozovsky, Lorne, 246

Sabbaticals, from work, 191
Safety, 7
Salary payments, 67
Saskatchewan
    1992 budget, 75
    children, dental work in, quality of, by type
    of provider, 1976, 199
    childrens' dental program, 47, 195, 199—
    200
    community health centers, 124, 271
    dental therapists (dental nurses), 198
    denture therapists in, 273
    direct patient payments in, 38
    doctors strike, 1962, 2, 5
    drug benefit plans, 150
        beneficiaries of, 145
        cost to, 145
    drug expenditures, 143
    drugs, prescribing and marketing, 146
    health financing in, methods of, 16
    health services, government in, 53
    hospital expenditures per person, per
    patient-day and per separation, 43
    hospital insurance in, 34, 36
    mental health services, 165
    physician ethics in, 80
    psychiatric beds, 160
    public health and home care expenditures
    as percentage of total health care
    expenditures, 1975 and 1986, 44
    reporting in, 224
Saskatchewan Dental Nurses Act, 199, 282
Saskatchewan Medical Care Insurance
    Commission, 56
Saskatoon, mental health services, 165
Saskatoon Community Clinic, 126
Satisfaction surveys, 112
Sault Ste. Marie Health Centre, 125—126, 271
Saunders, Cecily, 186
Scrip writers, 148
Security, 189
Self-image, 13
Self-regulation, 82
Senate, 6
Senior citizen centers, 57
Senior citizens, 173
    client visits to, costs for, 30
Senior's Health Benefits Program, 150
Sessional payments, 67
Severely cognitively impaired, 183
Severely demented, 183
Sheltered housing, 188, 282—283
Sheltered workshops, 162, 283
Short term acute treatment hospitals, 89—
    117. *See also* Hospital(s)

Short term care, 183
Single point of entry, 12, 283
Smith Falls, hospital mergers in, 107
Smoking, 226
Social activities, 185
Social and Health Maintenance Organizations, 126
Social change, 236—244
Social drop-in centers, 157, 283
    costs for, 30
Social expectations, 232
Social expenditures, 25—34
Social factors, 46
Social health, 212
Social justice, 229—230
Social model, 244—245
Social Planning Councils, 57
Social responsibility index, 114
Social Service Centers, 19—20, 54, 283
Society of Obstetricians and Gynecologists of Canada, 41—42
Special hospitals
    beds, 99
    expenditures, annual percentages rates of increase per person, 1960-70 and 1970-82, 32
Specialization, 168
St. John Ambulance, 209
St. Michaels, 202
Staff, secondment of, 11
Standardized assessment practices, 187
Statistics Canada, 48, 143, 283
    reports on health status, 214—215
Status quo, evolution of, 238
Statutes, 7, 16, 283
Stress, 168
Strikes
    doctors, 2, 5
    hospital workers, 9
Structure, 1—24
Studies, 224
Sudbury General, 202
Sudbury Laurentian, 202
Sudbury Memorial, 202
Sunnybrook, 202
Support services, 128
Surgery
    cardiovascular, 137
    coronary artery bypass
        rates, 243
        rationing, 242—244
    cosmetic, coverage for, 37
    day, 273
    open heart
        comparative availability of, 140
        per million persons, 1989, 257
Swartz Commission, 235
Sweden
    health expenditures, per capita
        1987, 258
        and life expectancy and infant mortality, 1987, 26

national health system in, 47
tax revenue as percent of GDP, 1992, 254
total R&D expenditures as percentage of GDP, 1989 or latest year, 141
Switzerland
    health expenditures, per capita, 1987, 258
    research and development in, 143

Taxation strategies, 44
Tax revenue, as percent of GDP, 1992, 254
Teaching hospital/university relationships, 103—104, 283
Technology, 100, 137—138, 257
    assessment of, 138—139
    comparative availability of, 140
    high-tech units/million persons, 1989, 257
    managing, example of, 139—140
Telecommunication networks, 209
Telephone monitoring services, 188
Terminally ill, 204
Terminology, 37
Territories. See also specific territory
    public health and home care expenditures as percentage of total health care expenditures, 1975 and 1986, 44
    ratio of hospital expenditures per person, per patient-day and per separation, 43
Ticket orienteur, 70, 283
Tissue Committees, 72, 283
Toronto
    ambulance services in, 269
    burn centers, 202
    CPR training in, 209
    hospital mergers in, 107
    mental health services, 163, 166
    trauma centers, 202
Toronto City Council, health services budget, 1987, 56
Toronto General Hospital, 60
    referral arrangements, 203
Training, 191
    of health care workers, 196—197
    of nurses, 196—197
    of paramedics, 208
Transplantation, of organs, 137, 140
    per million persons, 1989, 257
Transplant organs, 100
Transportation, 184
    emergency system. See also Ambulances
        characteristics of, 208
Trauma care hospitals, 201
Trauma centers, 202
Travenol Canada, 60
Trends, 221—223
Tuberculosis, 263
Two tier system, 259—260

Ultrasound, during pregnancy, 42
Uninsured services, 37
Union Hospital Districts, 16

Union Hospitals, 91
United Kingdom
    administration costs, 1991, 255
    AIDS in, reported cases, January 1991, 223
    economic growth forecast, annual percent
    change, 254
    health care delivery model of, 280
    health expenditures, per capita, 258
        and life expectancy and infant mortality,
    1987, 26
    hospital beds per 1,000 population, 1987,
    256
    infant mortality rates, per 1000 live births,
    221
    long term care beds per 1000 people over
    65, 180
    midwives in, education of, 197
    national health system in, 46—47
    practicing physicians per 100,000, 1987, 261
    regional hospital boards in, 105
    research and development in, 143
        total expenditures as percentage of GDP,
    1989 or latest year, 141
    sheltered housing in, 188, 283
    tax revenue as percent of GDP, 1992, 254
United States
    addiction recovery programs, 161
    administration costs, 1991, 255
    AIDS in, reported cases, January 1991, 223
    community health centers, 126
    coronary artery bypass surgery rates, for
    elderly, 244
    CPR training in, 209
    economic growth forecast, annual percent
    change, 254
    health care, public opinion of, 1990, 258
    health care reform in, state, 262—263
    health expenditures
        per capita, 258
            and life expectancy and infant
        mortality, 1987, 26
        as percentages of GNP, 1960-92, 26
        total, 257—258
    health services in, 47
    high-tech units/million persons, 1989, 257
    hospital beds per 1,000 population, 1987,
    256
    hospital use, 1987, 256
    infant mortality rates, per 1000 live births,
    221
    learning from, 256, 265
    osteopaths in, 68
    physician ethics in, 80
    physician licensing in, 82
    physician resources in, managing, 261
    practicing physicians per 100,000, 1987, 261

quality of life indicators, 214
    research and development in, 143, 146
        total expenditures as percentage of GDP,
    1989 or latest year, 141
    tax revenue as percent of GDP, 1992, 254
Universal insurance
    arguments against, 255
    attributes of, VII, 265
University Hospital, 59—60, 259
University of Manitoba, 52
User fees, 33, 38—39, 70, 259
Utilization, 3, 40—41
Utilization fees, 38

Valley Health Board, 233
Vancouver
    hospital mergers in, 107
    mental health services, 165
Veterans' hospitals, 92, 104
Victorian Order of Nurses (VON), 58, 127, 276
Vital statistics, 223
Vocational rehabilitation, of disabled persons,
    283
Voluntary agency, 58, 127, 283—284
Volunteers, 259
VON. See Victorian Order of Nurses

Walk-in clinics, 208
Waxman-Hatch Act, 146, 284
WCB. See Workers Compensation Board
Wellesley Hospital, 202
West Germany, research and development in,
    143
    total expenditures as percentage of GDP,
    1989 or latest year, 141
Wheels to Meals, 189, 284
White House Conference on Aging, 176—177
WHO. See World Health Organization (WHO)
Winnipeg, physician growth in, 1980-91, 35
Women's Health Centres, 126
Worker safety, 248
Workers Compensation Boards (WCBs), 53,
    57—58, 94, 284
    fee schedule, 74
Workers' rights, 248
Workshops, sheltered, 162
World Health Organization (WHO), 89
    definition of health, 211—212

Yorkton, mental health services, 165
Yukon
    financing and costs in, 3
    health insurance premiums in, 33